CLINICAL PROBLEMS IN
Gastroenterology

Jonathan M Rhodes

MA, MD, FRCP

Professor of Medicine (Gastroenterology)

Royal Liverpool University Hospital

Liverpool, UK

and

Her Hsin Tsai

MD, MRCP (UK)

Consultant Physician and Gastroenterologist

Castle Hill Hospital

Cottingham

North Humberside, UK

 Mosby-Wolfe

London Baltimore Bogotá Boston Buenos Aires Caracas Carlsbad, CA Chicago Madrid Mexico City Milan Naples, FL New York Philadelphia St. Louis Sydney Tokyo Toronto Wiesbaden

Copyright © 1995 Times Mirror International Publishers Limited

Published in 1995 by Mosby-Wolfe, an imprint of Times Mirror International Publishers Limited

Printed In Italy by G. Canale & C.S.p.a., Turin.

ISBN 0 7234 1943 4

For full details of all Times Mirror International Publishers Limited titles, please write to Times Mirror International Publishers Limited, Lynton House, 7–12 Tavistock Square, London WC1H 9LB, England.

A CIP catalogue record for this book is available from the British Library.

Library of Congress Cataloging-in-Publication Data applied for.

Project Manager:	Louise Cook
Developmental Editor:	Jennifer Prast
Designer/Layout Artist:	Lara Last /Lindy van den Berghe
Cover Design:	Lara Last
Illustration:	Lynda Payne
Production:	Joe Lynch
Index:	Nina Boyd
Publisher:	Richard Furn

CONTENTS

CONTRIBUTORS

Edward Eastham MB BS, FRCP
Consultant Paediatrician, Royal Victoria Infirmary, New-
castle upon Tyne, UK

Brian Eyes MB ChB, DMRD, FRCR
Consultant Radiologist, Aintree Hospital, Liverpool, UK.

Tim Helliwell MD, MRCPath
Senior Lecturer and Consultant Histopathologist, Royal
Liverpool University Hospital, Liverpool, UK.

Barry Taylor MA, MCh, FRCS
Consultant General and Gastrointestinal Surgeon,
Warrington Hospital NHS Trust, UK

Lawrence Weaver MD, FRCP
Consultant in Paediatric Gastroenterology and Reader in
Human Nutrition, Royal Hospital for Sick Children
and University of Glasgow, UK

PREFACE

Most gastroenterology textbooks are arranged according to organ, for example, stomach, liver and colon. While this layout may appear logical and allow easy reference to information on specific diseases, it is often unhelpful to the reader who is seeking help with diagnosis or clinical management. Our aim has been to structure this book according to clinical problems as they are likely to confront the practising clinician. These are sometimes symptoms (pain) or signs (jaundice), but may also arise from the results of 'screening' tests, which are increasingly performed (e.g. unexpected abnormal results of liver function tests). We hope this approach will help the reader improve his or her diagnostic skills; gaining a sort of 'instant clinical experience' as well as factual knowledge.

Each chapter begins with a logical approach to diagnosis and then continues with a description of the natural history and management of specific disease. In order to avoid repetition, arbitrary decisions have sometimes been made when deciding where to discuss aspects of certain conditions. The natural history and management of Crohn's disease, for example, is covered fully in the chapter on diarrhoea, while it is also relevant in the differential diagnosis of pain, bleeding and anaemia. The accounts of the natural history and management of each condition are clearly identified by indexing, cross referencing and headings to allow the reader to locate the relevant section easily. We have also tried to make the figure legends as informative as possible for easy browsing.

Each chapter ends with a bibliography consisting mostly of recent comprehensive review articles plus papers of historical interest. Particularly important aspects of diagnosis or management are emphasised in teaching point tables throughout the text.

JM Rhodes
HH Tsai
1995

ACKNOWLEDGEMENTS

We are extremely grateful to our co-authors Barry Taylor, Edward Eastham and Lawrence Weaver for their excellent chapters on the acute abdomen and gastrointestinal problems in infancy and childhood, without which this book would have been incomplete. We also owe thanks to Brian Eyes and Tim Helliwell who uncomplainingly responded to numerous requests for figures.

Much of the approach to diagnosis and management in this book has inevitably been influenced by our own teachers to whom we owe a great debt, including particularly Robert Allan, Roy Cockel, Elwyn Elias, Derek Jewell, Neil McIntyre, Dame Sheila Sherlock and Sir Thomas Thomsom.

Many thanks also to our colleagues in gastroenterology (particularly Ian Gilmore, Martin Lombard and Tony Morris), and in surgery, radiology and pathology, who have all shown great tolerance for the provocative clinical discussions which help to make clinical medicine so much more fun than writing grant applications, attending committee meetings and following other similar pastimes of the middle-aged physician.

We are very grateful to all our other friends and colleagues who helped provide figures (which we have acknowledged individually in the legends), Martina Sheelan for her secretarial help and Richard Evans for reading the text. Our friends at Mosby-Wolfe, Jennifer Prast and Louise Cook, have been cheerfully tolerant of biro scrawl defacing their proofs as we add 'just one more bit' and we are very grateful to Lynda Payne for her superb artwork. Finally, many thanks to our families (and dog) who have tolerated our mute immobility with enormous patience.

I
CHRONIC OR RECURRENT ABDOMINAL PAIN

REACHING A DIAGNOSIS

Is the pain functional or organic?

About 50% of patients consulting a doctor with chronic abdominal pain have a functional rather than an organic cause for the pain. If such patients are extensively investigated they undergo unnecessary investigation at considerable cost and tend to equate the large number of tests with serious illness. It is therefore essential to have a screening process that identifies these patients positively (rather than negatively by excluding organic disease).

The important first consideration is the patient's age. It is unsafe to label any chronic abdominal pain developing for the first time in a person over 40 years of age as functional without investigation. If the patient is under 40, attempt to make a positive diagnosis of functional pain (i.e. irritable bowel syndrome) from the history and ask the following questions if the answers are not provided spontaneously:

- Is the pain associated with gaseous distension?
- Is the pain associated with constipation or diarrhoea?
- Is the pain relieved by defecation?
- Is the pain intermittent and interspersed by trouble-free days or weeks?

A positive answer to a majority of these questions strongly suggests functional pain. Conversely, the pain is more likely to be organic, and warrants further investigation regardless of age if it:

- Wakes the patient at night.
- Persists for weeks or months.
- Is associated with persistent rather than intermittent alteration of bowel habit.
- Is accompanied by weight loss or rectal bleeding.

A thorough general examination including a rectal examination, a few blood tests, and a smear of faeces tested for occult blood should suffice in a young patient. Blood tests should include a full blood count, erythrocyte sedimentation rate (ESR), and 'liver function tests' (LFTs), or automated serum profile. If these are normal, the only fairly

▶ **Diagnosing functional abdominal pain**

Points in favour	Points against
Intermittent colicky pain	Over 40 years of age at presentation
Associated with distension	Nocturnal pain
Intermittent diarrhoea	Weight loss
Relief with defecation	Rectal bleeding
	Persistent pain
	Persistent diarrhoea
	Anaemia
	Raised CRP

common organic disease that still needs exclusion in developed countries is Crohn's disease. A blood test for the acute phase-reactant C-reactive protein (CRP) is useful because a normal CRP more confidently excludes active Crohn's disease than a normal ESR, but a raised CRP is not specific for the disease. Parasites and tuberculosis need exclusion if the patient is from a tropical or Middle Eastern country.

If the history suggests irritable bowel syndrome, the patient is less than 40 years old, and general examination and blood tests are normal, the patient should be reassured and not investigated further unless the symptoms become unusually persistent.

Is it due to gastric or duodenal disease?

Many patients with a duodenal ulcer give a typical history of epigastric pain that wakes them at night and is periodic (i.e. lasting a few weeks separated by weeks or months without pain). Other patients may have atypical pain or no symptoms at all.

The only way to make a diagnosis is by endoscopy or barium meal examination. Some doctors simply prescribe antacids or anti-ulcer drugs and investigate only if the symptoms persist. This is not unreasonable in a younger

▶ **Points supporting a diagnosis of duodenal ulcer**

Strong points	Weak points
Patient points to site of pain in epigastrium with one finger	Relief of pain with antacids or H_2 antagonists
Nocturnal pain	Poorly localised upper abdominal pain
Family history	Nausea or vomiting
Smoking	
Periodicity of pain (i.e. pain-free weeks or months interspersed with painful weeks or months)	
Similarity to previous episodes of endoscopy-proven ulceration	

▶ **Symptoms of gastritis, benign gastric ulcer and gastric cancer are indistinguishable and include any or none of the following**

- Bloating
- Postprandial fullness
- Upper abdominal pain
- Nausea
- Vomiting

patient, but most patients prefer to have a firm diagnosis, and this usually justifies the initial investigation of all patients with ulcer pain. Further recurrences of the same pain do not require investigation unless the patient is of an age (i.e. over 40 years old) when carcinoma of the stomach needs exclusion. As pain and ulceration associated with gastric cancer may be temporarily relieved by ulcer-healing drugs, all patients over 40 years of age should be investigated as soon as possible after presentation and not given a blind trial of therapy.

A case has been made for the prompt investigation of all patients with dyspepsia regardless of age because curable early (pre-invasive) gastric cancer may be detected. Early gastric cancer is relatively common in the Far East, but in the UK symptomatic gastric cancer is almost always well advanced so it is probable that early gastric cancer can be

detected only by screening asymptomatic patients. This will be impracticable unless high-risk groups can be better defined (**Figs 1.1 and 1.2**).

Duodenal ulcer is associated with *Helicobacter pylori* infection in 98% of patients. A variety of tests are available for identifying IgG antibodies to *H. pylori* in serum or saliva. It seems quite likely that these tests will be used increasingly as part of the initial assessment of abdominal pain, particularly in younger patients (less than 40 years of age), and that a positive result will be followed by *H. pylori* eradication therapy, with subsequent endoscopy only if symptoms persist. This topic still needs further study.

Barium meal versus endoscopy

The choice between barium meal and endoscopy (**Figs 1.3–1.5**) is to some extent arbitrary and depends on local

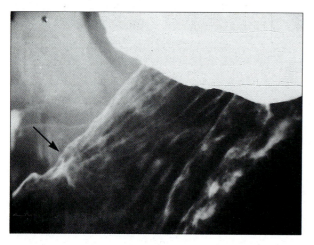

Fig. 1.1 Barium meal showing early gastric cancer (arrowed). Early gastric cancers may be ulcerated, flat or raised, and are often not visible on good quality double-contrast barium studies.

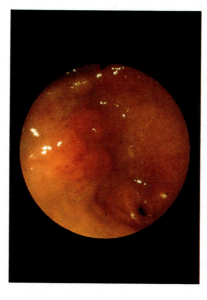

Fig. 1.2 Endoscopic appearance of an early gastric cancer in the gastric antrum.

availability. A well-performed endoscopy in an appropriately sedated patient will provide more information than a barium meal and will be well tolerated. Usually the procedure is not remembered if intravenous sedation is sufficient. A clumsily-performed endoscopy, however, will provide less information than an average barium meal, and be less well tolerated. Patients should not normally have both investigations unless a lesion requiring biopsy is seen on barium meal (e.g. gastric ulcer or carcinoma, **Figs 1.6–1.8**). If a normal double-contrast barium meal is not going to be accepted as proof of normality (although it usually can be), an endoscopy should be performed as the first investigation.

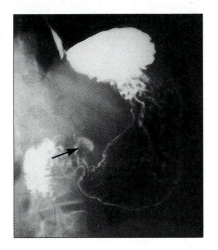

Fig. 1.3 Barium meal showing an ulcer in the duodenal bulb (arrowed). There is also antral gastritis.

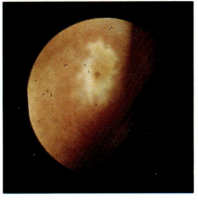

Fig. 1.4 Endoscopic appearance of an acute duodenal ulcer with a dark haematin spot indicating recent bleeding.

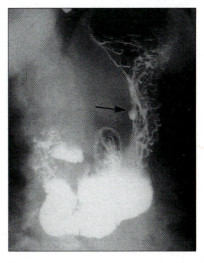

Fig. 1.5 Barium meal showing a benign lesser curve ulcer (arrowed).

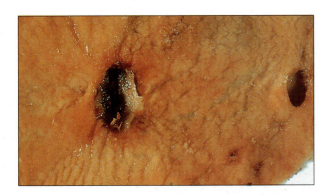

Fig. 1.6 A punched-out benign antral ulcer is seen in this resection specimen. The surrounding mucosa is flat. There is also a superficial erosion. Courtesy of Dr D Day.

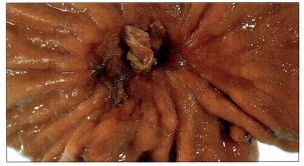

Fig. 1.7 This ulcerated gastric cancer has an irregular margin with slough in its base. Radiating folds are expanded at the edge of the ulcer due to infiltration by tumour. Courtesy of Dr D Day.

Fig. 1.8 There are several small shallow ulcers in the gastric antrum. The surrounding mucosa is reddened and slightly nodular. Histological examination showed the presence of adenocarcinoma, which extended no further than the submucosa (early gastric cancer). Courtesy of Dr D Day

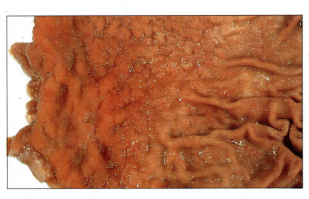

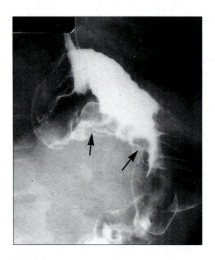

Fig. 1.9 Barium meal showing extensive infiltration of the gastric body by carcinoma (arrowed).

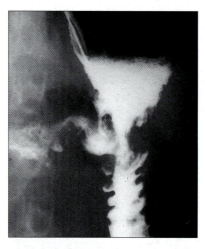

Fig. 1.10 Barium meal showing the appearance following Polya gastrectomy. Stomal ulcers and early premalignant change in the stomach are easily missed, and endoscopy is preferable for investigating the operated stomach.

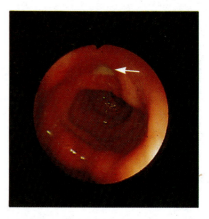

Fig. 1.11 Endoscopic appearance of a stomal ulcer (arrowed).

The only situations when endoscopy is clearly a better investigation than barium meal are for investigating the previously-operated stomach and for the diagnosis of acute bleeding. Following gastric surgery it is usually very difficult to see the stoma clearly with a barium meal and gastric dysplasia or early recurrence of malignancy will require biopsy and histology for diagnosis (Figs 1.9–1.11).

Zollinger–Ellison syndrome

A diagnosis of Zollinger–Ellison syndrome (gastrin-producing tumour) should be considered for:

- Any patient with extensive or multiple duodenal ulcers, particularly if they occur in the distal duodenum.
- Patients with ulcers that are resistant to conventional treatment.
- Patients with ulcers and diarrhoea.
- Patients with ulcers and a family history of other endocrine disorders, particularly hyperparathyroidism.

Diagnosis is suggested if fasting serum gastrin is elevated in a patient with excessive basal acid secretion who has not received H_2 antagonists for at least 48 hours and proton pump inhibitors for at least one week. An elevated serum gastrin alone is not sufficient to make the diagnosis unless it is over 1000 pg/ml because in about 30% of patients the levels overlap the normal range for people with duodenal ulcer. In Zollinger–Ellison syndrome basal acid output is typically higher than 60% of the peak stimulated acid output. A rise of more than 50% in serum gastrin concentration and an acid output higher than 18 mmol/hour after intravenous secretin confirms the diagnosis.

Computerised tomography (CT scanning) offers the best chance of localising the primary tumour, but some tumours are small and multiple and may be sited in the duodenal wall (Fig. 1.12). These are often best visualised by transillumination of the bowel wall at laparotomy. Angiography may also be used (Fig. 1.13).

Approximately 40% of patients with Zollinger–Ellison syndrome have inherited (autosomal dominant) multiple endocrine neoplasia type 1 (MEN 1) syndrome. They are prone to tumours in the three 'Ps': pituitary (e.g. prolactinoma), pancreas (gastrinoma, occasionally insulin, glucagon, or vasoactive intestinal peptide - VIP), and parathyroid. The gastrinomas are usually multiple and resection is rarely, if ever, curative.

▶ **Diagnostic features of Zollinger–Ellison syndrome**

- Persistent or multiple duodenal ulcers
- Diarrhoea
- Jejunal ulceration
- Elevated serum gastrin
- Basal acid output higher than 60% of peak stimulated acid output, but exclude achlorhydria, which is the commonest cause of raised serum gastrin
- Rise of more than 50% in serum gastrin and acid output higher than 18 mmol/hour after intravenous secretin

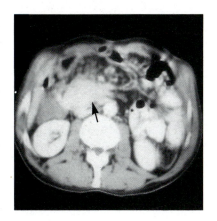

Fig. 1.12 CT scan showing a pancreatic gastrinoma (arrowed) in a patient with Zollinger–Ellison syndrome.

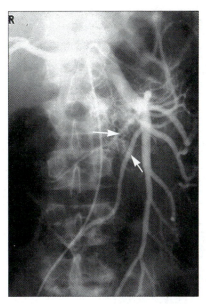

Fig. 1.13 Superior mesenteric angiogram showing abnormal tumour vessels (arrowed) supplying a pancreatic gastrinoma in the same patient as in Fig. 1.12.

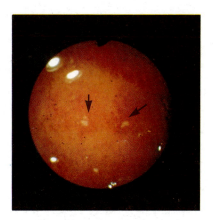

Fig. 1.14 Endoscopic appearances of erosive duodenitis (the erosions are arrowed).

Duodenitis

Duodenitis is usually an endoscopic or histological rather than a clinical diagnosis. Some patients with erosive duodenitis have symptoms indistinguishable from those of duodenal ulceration, but other patients have vague discomfort and nausea. Often there are no symptoms (**Fig. 1.14**).

Is it gallbladder disease?

Gallstones are common, but frequently asymptomatic. The commonest error in diagnosis is to attribute nebulous symptoms of abdominal discomfort and fat intolerance to the presence of gallstones. A firm diagnosis is often difficult in the absence of an acute event such as acute cholecystitis or obstructive jaundice.

Gallstones undoubtedly cause pain if they become impacted in the cystic duct or common bile duct. This pain usually lasts for 30 minutes or more, so is not truly a colic, but is severe and memorable. The patient will typically give a history of several specific attacks of pain and be able to remember the days on which they occurred. Biliary pain is usually felt either in the right upper quadrant or in the epigastrium. It is often associated with nausea or flatulence and may mimic the pain of an irritable bowel syndrome, peptic ulceration, or even cardiac ischaemia. Tenderness in the right upper quadrant is a helpful sign, but some patients without gallstones are tender over a normal liver.

Constant vague pains are unlikely to be relieved by cholecystectomy and fat intolerance has been shown to be common, even in people without gallbladder disease.

Stones in the common bile duct are usually, but not always, associated with some disturbance in liver function tests: often just an elevation of serum alkaline phosphatase with a normal serum bilirubin (**Fig. 1.15**).

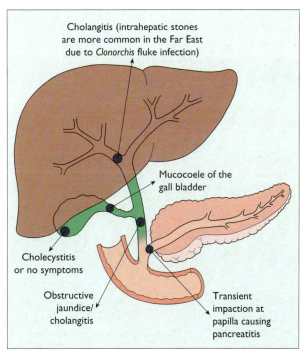

Fig. 1.15 Gallstones and the symptoms they cause.

Radiology

The best initial investigation for gallbladder disease is probably ultrasound (**Fig. 1.16**). It will reliably show whether the gallbladder contains stones, and whether the intrahepatic bile ducts are dilated. It can also fairly reliably exclude malignant disease of the liver or pancreas, but is much less reliable at visualising stones in the common bile duct. If serum alkaline phosphatase is elevated, endoscopic retrograde cholangiography (ERCP) should be performed. If not available, intravenous or percutaneous fine-needle cholangiography are alternatives. Intravenous cholangiography has the disadvantage that some patients have severe reactions to the contrast media and the quality of imaging of the common bile duct is often inadequate. Percutaneous cholangiography is more invasive, though very safe in experienced hands, but will fail in up to 40% of patients with non-dilated bile ducts.

Adenomyomatosis of the gallbladder

If the ultrasound and liver function tests are normal, but the history suggests biliary disease, it may be worth performing an oral cholecystogram because adenomyomatosis of the gallbladder is often missed on ultrasound examination (**Figs 1.17–1.19**). Adenomyomatosis of the gallbladder is often dismissed as irrelevant, but the rather limited clinical studies that have been published suggest that it can cause right upper quadrant pain that is relieved by cholecystectomy.

Gallstones

About 10–15% of British adults have gallstones. It is common to find gallstones in a patient with upper abdominal pain, but in the absence of acute cholecystitis or stones in the common bile duct, it is often difficult to be certain whether the stones are responsible for the pain. If the pain is frequent or constant rather than episodic, endoscopy or a barium meal should be performed to exclude peptic ulceration as an alternative cause of the pain.

About 25% of patients still have symptoms after cholecystectomy. The majority of these patients have a variant of the irritable bowel syndrome and their pain can be reproduced by inflating a balloon in the upper small intestine. It is possible that patients with pain due to gallstones might also get pain from balloon dilatation of the small intestine so this is probably not a useful preoperative diagnostic test. In

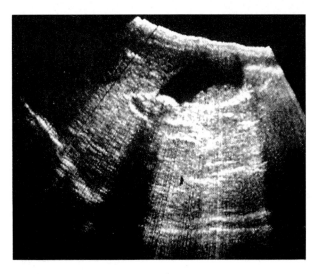

Fig. 1.16 Ultrasound scan of a gallbladder containing a gallstone casting an acoustic shadow.

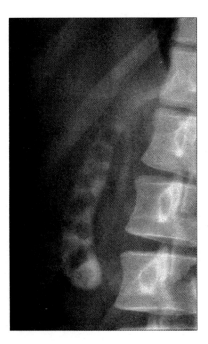

Fig. 1.17 Oral cholecystogram showing multiple radiolucent stones. There is also opacification of the common bile duct on this occasion.

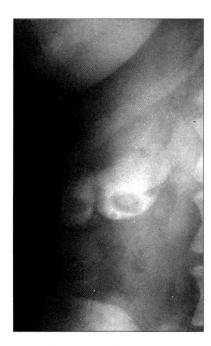

Fig. 1.18 Oral cholecystogram showing a gallbladder with segmental and fundal adenomyomatosis and containing two radiolucent gallstones

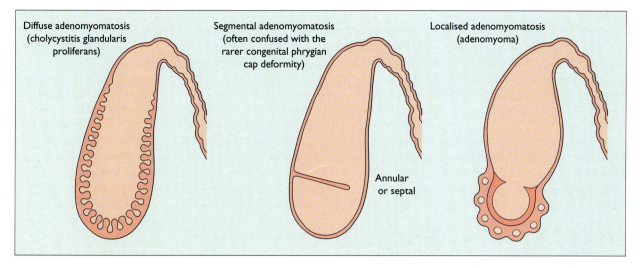

Fig. 1.19 Types of adenomyomatosis of the gallbladder.

practice, the age and fitness of a patient are usually the most important considerations when deciding whether or not to proceed to cholecystectomy.

Is it pancreatic disease?

Investigation of the pancreas is difficult. Patients with chronic upper abdominal pain and normal upper gastro-intestinal endoscopy and gallbladder ultrasound are common. The vast majority of these patients have the irritable bowel syndrome, but there is often a concern that there may be underlying pancreatic disease.

The site of pancreatic pain may vary depending on the site of disease in the pancreas:

- Lesions in the head cause right-sided upper abdominal pain.
- Lesions in the body cause epigastric pain, commonly radiating to the back.
- Lesions in the tail cause left-sided, upper abdominal pain.

At first pain may be precipitated by meals, but later in the course of the disease it may be constant and severe. It may radiate to the back or left shoulder and the patient is often more comfortable sitting forward. None of these features are, however, specific for pancreatic pain.

Biochemical tests for pancreatic disease

Serological tests can be helpful in diagnosing or excluding pancreatic cancer, but only if used appropriately. The most useful detect carbohydrate antigens expressed by mucus glycoproteins, which are shed abnormally into the blood in pancreatic cancer (e.g. CA19-9, CAM17.1/WGA, DUPAN2). As similar glycoproteins are present in normal

▶ **Diagnostic features of gallstones**

Helpful features	Unhelpful features
Ability to remember specific days when pain occurred	Fat intolerance
Right upper quadrant pain with radiation to right shoulder	Vague upper abdominal pain most days
Strong family history of gallstones	Nausea

bile, these tests are not helpful in jaundiced patients. They are also not sufficiently specific to be useful for screening asymptomatic populations. In non-jaundiced patients their sensitivity and specificity is about 85% so they are probably a useful adjunct to ultrasound scanning in the investigation of patients with endoscopy-negative abdominal pain or weight loss. There is no satisfactory blood test for chronic pancreatitis. Serum amylase is usually normal and serum trypsin levels tend to be low in chronic pancreatitis, but overlap with the normal range. Conventional tests of pancreatic function such as the secretin test and PABA (para-aminobenzoic acid) test are too insensitive when pain is the main symptom because pancreatic function is often well preserved until late in the course of both diseases.

Radiology

A normal ultrasound scan performed by an experienced operator will exclude pancreatic disease with 80% confidence and is the best initial test. The results of a CT scan, if available, are probably slightly more reliable. It is less operator dependent and poor visualisation of the pancreas as a result of overlying intestinal gas is less common (**Figs 1.20–1.23**).

If the ultrasound is abnormal, ERCP may be necessary. This is the most reliable test for detecting pancreatic cancer: adequate radiographs will be obtained in approximately 90% of patients and the pancreatogram will be abnormal in 95% of these. It is, however, an expensive and time-consuming test and is not available in all centres. It also induces acute pancreatitis in 3% of patients, who therefore need careful selection (**Fig. 1.24**).

In a patient under 40 years of age with unexplained upper abdominal pain and no weight loss the yield from ERCP is so low that efforts should be made to obtain an adequate pancreatic scan.

A patient with epigastric pain that radiates through to the back and is unrelieved by alkali and who has lost weight clearly merits investigation. A plain abdominal radiograph should be performed first to look for pancreatic calcification (**Fig. 1.25**). If present this is diagnostic of chronic pancreatitis and further tests are usually unnecessary unless surgery is being considered to relieve intractable pain or jaundice. A pancreatic pseudocyst should be considered if there is a recent history of acute pancreatitis; only the largest pseudocysts are palpable, but a pseudocyst should be reliably detected by ultrasound or CT scanning. Serum amylase is elevated in about 50% of patients. An ERCP should not be

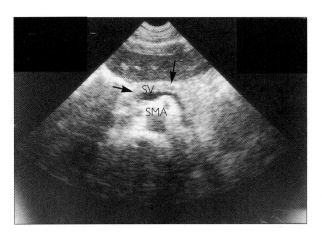

Fig. 1.20 Abdominal ultrasound scan of normal pancreas (arrowed). (SV, splenic vein; SMA, superior mesenteric artery.)

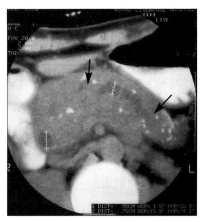

Fig. 1.21 CT scan showing calcific chronic pancreatitis (arrowed).

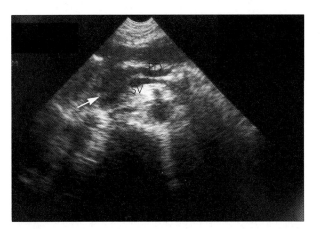

Fig. 1.22 Ultrasound scan showing pancreatic cancer (arrowed) with dilatation of the pancreatic duct (PD). (SV, splenic vein.)

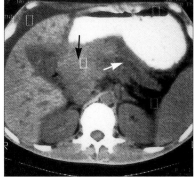

Fig. 1.23 CT scan of a pancreatic cancer (black arrow) with dilatation of the obstructed pancreatic duct (white arrow) Courtesy of Dr C Garvey.

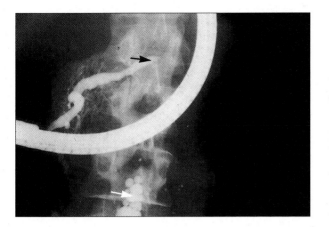

Fig. 1.24 ERCP showing a block in the main pancreatic duct (arrowed) in a patient with carcinoma affecting the tail of the pancreas. The patient had severe back pain in relation to the tumour and myodil can be seen (arrowed) as a result of a previous myelogram.

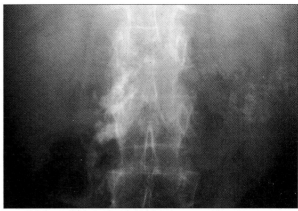

Fig. 1.25 Plain radiograph showing extensive calcification in a patient with alcohol-related chronic pancreatitis.

performed except immediately before surgery (i.e. the same day) because there is a high risk of introducing infection and converting the cyst into a pancreatic abscess with a high morbidity and mortality.

Rupture of the pancreatic duct should be considered if there has been recent trauma to the upper abdomen (e.g. in a road traffic accident). The serum amylase will usually be raised and if ultrasound does not show cyst formation an ERCP should be performed to confirm the diagnosis and identify the site of the rupture.

Is there intestinal disease?

Pain caused by intestinal disease is nearly always due to distension of obstructed bowel. It is colicky and associated with abdominal distension, and may also be associated with altered bowel habit. All these features also apply to the pain associated with the irritable bowel syndrome. Because the irritable bowel syndrome is so common, a screening process must be applied to identify patients who require further investigation. Further investigation is indicated if symptoms develop for the first time in a person over 40 years of age, or if there is anaemia, weight loss, or a marker of underlying disease, such as an elevated erythrocyte sedimentation rate or CRP, or if the test for faecal occult blood is positive.

Radiology

In a younger patient with pain, but no alteration of bowel habit, small bowel disease such as Crohn's disease is more likely than colonic disease; in an older patient, colonic carcinoma would be more likely. A small bowel barium meal is therefore the more useful first radiograph in the younger patient, and a barium enema is more useful first radiograph in the older patient (**Fig. 1.26**). Better detail of the upper

small intestine can be obtained by introducing dilute contrast medium at a rapid rate into the upper jejunum via a naso-enteral tube (small bowel enema or enteroclysis, **Fig. 1.27**). This is not necessary routinely because a conventional small bowel barium meal will give equally good visualisation of the distal small intestine in which Crohn's disease is more common. If there is a likelihood of proximal small bowel disease (e.g. lymphoma) and particularly if malabsorption is suspected, a small bowel enema should be performed.

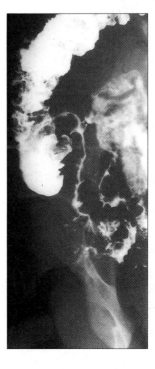

Fig. 1.26 Small bowel barium meal showing extensive stricturing of the terminal ileum in a patient with Crohn's disease.

Volvulus or intussusception

Occasionally patients have intermittent very severe abdominal pain, but normal investigations. An intermittent volvulus of the intestine or stomach or an intermittent intussusception should then be considered (**Fig. 1.28**). The simplest policy is to give the patient a filled-in X-ray form and ask him to report to the casualty department for a plain abdominal radiograph as soon as the pain recurs.

Mesenteric ischaemia

Mesenteric ischaemia should be considered in older patients with abdominal pain after meals and weight loss if no lesion can be found in the stomach, biliary tree, or pancreas. Pain typically starts 15–30 minutes after eating, but may persist several hours. It often causes fear of eating, resulting in weight loss; this may be compounded by fat malabsorption. Diagnosis is by mesenteric angiography, which only supports the diagnosis if it shows more than 50% narrowing of at least two of the three major arteries (i.e. coeliac axis and superior and inferior mesenteric arteries, **Fig. 1.29**).

Is there underlying metabolic disease?

Metabolic causes of chronic abdominal pain such as hypercalcaemia and porphyria are rare and are therefore often diagnosed late. Serum calcium is easy to check and is now commonly included in autoanalyser biochemical profiles. It is sensible to check serum calcium of all patients presenting for the first time with acute or chronic abdominal pain.

In hypercalcaemia:

- Acute pain may be due to acute pancreatitis.
- Chronic pain may be due to dyspepsia or ulceration induced by hyperacidity resulting from the rise in serum gastrin associated with hypercalcaemia.

Porphyria (the forms associated with increased porphobilinogen: acute intermittent porphyria (**Fig. 1.30**) and porphyria variegata, but not porphyria cutanea tarda) causes intermittent episodes of severe abdominal pain rather than chronic pain. Neurological complications of porphyria include behavioural disturbance, epilepsy, coma, and peripheral neuropathy. During an acute attack hyponatraemia, hypertension, and uraemia are common.

Lead poisoning should be considered in a child or an adult with a history of psychiatric illness. Clinical features include colicky pain, constipation, anaemia, and encephalopathy. Other rare causes to consider include complement C1-esterase inhibitor insufficiency, which can be readily excluded by a serum assay, and familial Mediterranean fever in which there is usually a family history. In the absence of a family history a diagnostic therapeutic trial of oral colchicine therapy may be necessary. Familial Mediterranean fever has been reported in Ireland, presumably reflecting introduction of the gene by sailors shipwrecked at the time of the Spanish Armada.

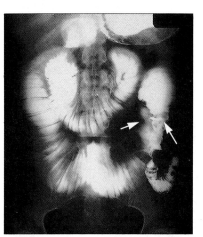

Fig. 1.27 Small bowel enema (enteroclysis) showing jejunal infiltration by lymphoma (arrowed) with proximal dilatation.

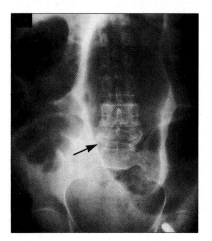

Fig. 1.28 Plain abdominal radiograph showing a sigmoid volvulus (arrowed).

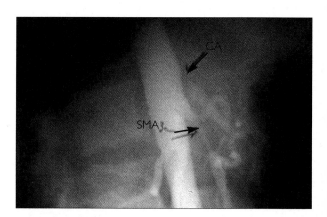

Fig. 1.29 Angiogram showing stenoses at the origins of the coeliac (CA) and superior mesenteric (SMA) arteries (arrowed) in a patient with chronic mesenteric ischaemia.

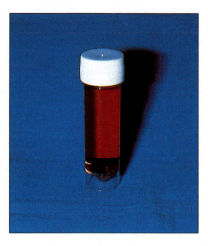

Fig. 1.30 Urine from a patient with acute intermittent porphyria showing the typical red colour that develops when the urine is left to stand.

CONDITIONS CAUSING CHRONIC OR RECURRENT ABDOMINAL PAIN: NATURAL HISTORY AND MANAGEMENT

Irritable bowel syndrome

Natural history

SYMPTOMS

Most patients have abdominal pain, which may be a continuous dull ache, but is frequently colicky. It may involve any quadrant of the abdomen and is often associated with abdominal distension due to wind. Most of the distension is probably due to subconscious air swallowing, exacerbated in some patients by heartburn from oesophageal reflux, which frequently coexists.

Constipation with 'rabbit pellet' faeces is common. The pain is often relieved by defecation, but there is often a remaining sensation of inadequate rectal voiding. Patients may pass mucus either alone or coated on hard faeces. Alternating constipation and diarrhoea is common and patients often pass a formed stool in the morning, but develop diarrhoea later in the day. A few patients have persistent watery diarrhoea and require more thorough investigation to exclude organic disease.

PSYCHOLOGY

Anxious, obsessional patients are more likely to consult their doctor if they develop irritable bowel symptoms, but the psychological aspect of the condition has probably been overemphasised and many psychologically normal people have the syndrome. Patients will however often notice that their symptoms are worse at times of mental stress.

EPIDEMIOLOGY

A recent survey found that 14% of apparently healthy British subjects had irritable bowel syndrome. Furthermore, it has been estimated that about 50% of patients attending British gastroenterology clinics have a variant of the syndrome and that these patients are probably a selected minority of the total population with this syndrome. Approximately 65% of patients are women and although symptoms may persist until old age, most patients develop their first symptoms in early adult life or childhood.

AETIOLOGY AND PATHOGENESIS

The aetiology is unclear. Intraluminal pressure recordings have shown that pain is usually associated with an increased frequency and force of contractions in the colon and small intestine. This probably accounts for the common association of the syndrome with the development of diverticulosis in later life. Pressure studies are usually normal when the patient is unstressed and free from symptoms, and the

Is there occult malignant disease?

If thorough investigations have proved negative, but the patient remains unwell with persistent pain, there will inevitably be concern that underlying malignant disease (carcinoma or lymphoma), has been missed. The next step should be a careful review of all investigations to ensure that all common lesions have been adequately excluded. Abdominal CT scanning should then be performed to exclude retroperitoneal malignancy and to obtain further views of the pancreas and liver. If this also proves negative, the choice will be between a traditional exploratory laparotomy or an expectant 'wait and see' policy. The patient should be carefully re-examined for lymphadenopathy and any suspicious lymph node biopsied. The chances of the patient benefitting from a laparotomy in these circumstances are generally slim and depend on the discovery of a relatively treatable condition, such as a lymphoma; carcinomas presenting in this way have almost invariably metastasised. Laparoscopy may be a useful compromise.

Is it endometriosis?

Lower abdominal pain related to menstruation suggests endometriosis. In up to 25% of patients there is bowel involvement, most commonly affecting the rectosigmoid, and less commonly the appendix, caecum, or ileum. Obstructive symptoms, rectal pain, tenesmus, and constipation may then develop. Rectal bleeding is rare and there is usually no weight loss.

A rectal examination should be performed and induration in the cul-de-sac felt anteriorly through the rectal wall supports the diagnosis. Barium enema examination may show stricturing, but with an intact mucosa. Sometimes a tissue diagnosis (needle biopsy or laparotomy) may be required to exclude carcinoma.

changes observed when the patient is stressed are an exaggeration of normal responses to stress.

The role of diet is controversial. There is a strong association between low fibre intake, high intraluminal pressure, and diverticulosis. Patients with constipation usually benefit from increased fibre intake, but some people develop the syndrome despite apparently adequate fibre intake. Food intolerance may be responsible for symptoms in some patients, but true food allergy is very rare.

Management

REASSURANCE

The most important part of management is reassurance. The mechanisms of pain and alteration of bowel habit in a healthy intestine should be explained simply and clearly. It should be made clear that the doctor understands the severity and genuine nature of the patient's symptoms, but the patient should be reassured that the condition is not harmful and that the frequency and severity of symptoms will diminish with time. Treating the patient dismissively as neurotic will lead the patient to assume that the symptoms have not been taken sufficiently seriously. This will increase any cancer phobia and the patient will almost certainly seek a second opinion!

DIETARY ADVICE

- Constipation usually responds to an increase in cereal fibre. If this fails, the addition of a bulking agent (e.g. ispaghula husk) is the next step. (See also Chapter 4.)
- Diarrhoea is more difficult to manage. If there is a history of milk intolerance, hypolactasia should be sought (see page 87); if confirmed, a low milk intake is recommended.

A recent study suggests that a high proportion of patients benefit from excluding certain foods from the diet, particularly wheat, dairy products, and brassicas. However, this needs confirmation and the mechanism for the food intolerance is obscure. It is unlikely to reflect true food allergy, which is rare in adults. It seems sensible to inform patients about this study so that they can experiment if they wish with stepwise exclusion of foods from the diet.

OTHER ADVICE AND TREATMENT

Pain is often related to abdominal distension, which is usually due to air swallowing. This should be explained because air swallowing is often partly voluntary and can be diminished if the patient is aware of the problem. Oesophageal reflux may worsen air swallowing and should be treated appropriately with antacids.

Painful bowel spasm can be treated pharmacologically. The musculotropic drug mebeverine and sustained-release preparations of concentrated peppermint oil have both proved beneficial in controlled trials, but tend to work too slowly to treat pain that is already present. Maintenance prophylaxis should be prescribed with reluctance for this chronic yet benign condition. A reasonable compromise is to prescribe a short course of either agent for patients with severe pain in an attempt to break the cycle of pain, anxiety, air swallowing, and more pain. Diarrhoea unresponsive to dietary manipulation may need symptomatic treatment with loperamide. This should be taken only as necessary, not as maintenance treatment.

▶ **Management of patients with irritable bowel syndrome**

Do	Don't
Try to make a positive diagnosis in the younger patient	Overinvestigate young patients (i.e. those under 40 years of age)
Make it clear that you understand the severity of the pain	Diagnose a functional problem without further investigation in a patient over 40 presenting with new symptoms
Explain the nature of spasm-related pain	Tell the patient "Its all in the mind"
Examine thoroughly, including sigmoidoscopy if diarrhoea is a feature. The patient will rightly not accept your reassurance if you don't	Prescribe drugs that are addictive (e.g. codeine) or have unpleasant side-effects (e.g. propanthelene)

Duodenal ulcer

Natural history

SYMPTOMS

No symptoms are specific for duodenal ulceration; duodenal ulcers may be completely asymptomatic and it is common for patients admitted to hospital with a bleeding ulcer to give no history of previous dyspepsia (Fig. 1.31). The most commonly associated symptoms are epigastric pain that wakes the patient at night and periodic pain (i.e. relapses of the pain lasting several days or weeks interspersed by pain-free periods of weeks or months). A less reliable association is relief of pain with antacids or food. Death due to duodenal ulceration is rare in young people, but is much more common in the elderly.

EPIDEMIOLOGY

It has been estimated that approximately 9% of women and 12% of men have been told at some time by a doctor that they have had a duodenal ulcer. Duodenal ulcers are typically recurrent and about 85% of patients relapse within one year of healing if no maintenance treatment is prescribed. Duodenal ulcers are three times more common in first degree relatives of people with ulcers than in the general population and blood group O confers a 40% increase in risk, which is increased still further if the individual is a non-secretor (i.e. secretes gastric mucus glycoproteins that do not express the group O-related H antigen, fucose).

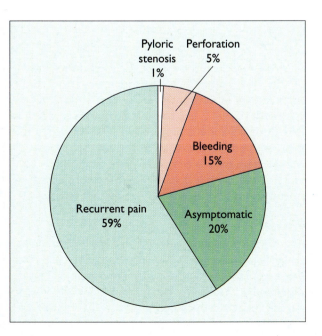

Fig. 1.31 Presentation of duodenal ulceration.

AETIOLOGY AND PATHOGENESIS

The aetiology of duodenal ulceration is unclear; the rate of acid secretion in about 65% of patients falls within the normal range. There is circumstantial evidence that psychological stress may provoke a relapse of duodenal ulceration, but no good evidence that the psyche of ulcer patients is essentially different from control groups.

It seems likely that duodenal ulcers develop as a consequence of a number of factors (Fig. 1.32), which include:

- Exposure to acid and pepsin.
- Defects in the mucus/epithelial barrier.
- Defects in prostaglandin-mediated cytoprotection within the epithelium.
- *H. pylori* infection.

Smoking and stress both increase basal acid output and reduce mucus synthesis, while anti-inflammatory drugs such as indomethacin and aspirin that inhibit prostaglandin synthesis are associated with an increased risk of ulceration (typically prepyloric rather than duodenal) presumably as a result of decreased cytoprotection.

The link between duodenal ulceration and corticosteroid treatment is controversial. People receiving corticosteroids clearly have significant underlying pathology, which may itself carry an increased risk of duodenal ulceration. Although corticosteroid therapy is suspected of causing ulcers the association has not been clearly established.

Many of the elderly ulcer patients are receiving nonsteroidal anti-inflammatory drugs (NSAIDs), which may contribute to the risk of haemorrhage and perforation.

Chronic airways obstruction, alcoholic cirrhosis, and chronic renal failure are all associated with increased risks of duodenal ulceration. In chronic renal failure, gastrin levels are high resulting in increased acid secretion, but the reason for the increased risk in alcoholic cirrhosis and chronic airways obstruction is not clear. Acute alcohol abuse is associated with gastric erosions, but not with any clear increase in risk of duodenal ulcer.

Helicobacter pylori

There is an extremely strong statistical association between duodenal ulcers and the presence of the bacterium, *Helicobacter pylori* in the stomach (*Helicobacter* is a spiral rod). Up to 98% of patients with duodenal ulcer disease have it. It is however common in the stomachs of asymptomatic patients, occurring in about 50% of the adult population in developed countries, with increased frequency in the elderly. Its causative association with duodenal ulcers has been controversial. The bacterium is not found in normal duodenum, but may be present in the duodenum on patches of metaplastic gastric-type mucosa. It has therefore been suggested that duodenal ulcers may occur on or around these

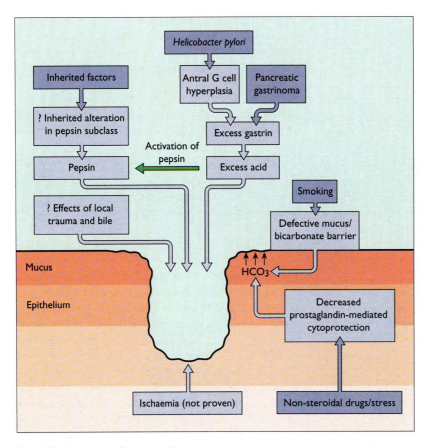

Fig. 1.32 Mechanisms of ulcerogenesis.

metaplastic areas, but the mechanism for this is obscure. It has also been reported that the presence of *H. pylori* in the stomach is associated with increased secretion of gastrin and that this may explain the link with duodenal ulceration. The most striking evidence for a causal association is provided by studies of ulcer relapse after healing with H_2 antagonists. These show that relapse is much more likely in the first year after healing (90% or greater) if the patient is *H. pylori* positive than if the patient is *H. pylori* negative (less than 30%). The source of the organism is unclear, but there seem to be few non-human reservoirs.

Most infection is thought to occur in childhood as a result of close contact with parents or siblings, and its prevalence is higher if there is a history of overcrowding in childhood. The increased frequency of *H. pylori* in the elderly is thought to represent a cohort of people who were exposed to *H. pylori* in childhood and it is hoped that the incidence of *H. pylori* is going to fall steadily as living standards improve.

H. pylori infection is associated statistically, and probably causally, with both atrophic gastritis and gastric cancer, particularly of intestinal type. It has been shown that the secretion of vitamin C into gastric juice that occurs in healthy individuals is naturally suppressed by *H. pylori*, and this might be a possible mechanism for the increased cancer risk. It is therefore speculated that *H. pylori* eradication might result in a substantial reduction in gastric cancer. Efforts are currently being made to develop a satisfactory vaccine.

Management of duodenal ulceration

The management of patients with duodenal ulceration has changed markedly over the last 20 years. Bed rest and bland diets have been shown to be of little or no value, and potent ulcer-healing drugs have become available. High doses of antacids such as aluminium hydroxide (which constipates) or magnesium trisilicate (which causes diarrhoea) or combinations of the two may be used to heal ulcers, but the volumes of antacid required are large and inconvenient for the patient. There is now a wide choice of ulcer-healing agents, which include:

- Histamine H_2 receptor antagonists (H_2 antagonists) such as cimetidine and ranitidine.
- Tripotassium dicitratobismuthate (DeNol).
- Proton pump inhibitors such as omeprazole.
- Sucralfate (a basic aluminium salt of sucrose octasulphate).
- The anticholinergic pirenzepine.
- Synthetic prostaglandin E_2 derivatives.

Of these the H_2 antagonists, the proton pump inhibitors, and the bismuth preparations probably have the best healing rates and differ mainly in terms of convenience, cost, and side-effects. The most convenient are the H_2 antagonists and the proton pump inhibitors.

H_2 ANTAGONISTS

All available H_2 antagonists seem at least as effective when given as a single night-time dose as twice daily and produce healing rates of 80–90% in six weeks. All the rival preparations are remarkably free from side-effects and newer drugs offer no significant advantage over cimetidine and ranitidine. Very rarely, cimetidine causes reversible gynaecomastia. It also potentiates the effects of warfarin, phenytoin, propranolol, theophylline, and diazepam by inhibiting cytochrome P450, and may cause confusion in elderly patients. These side-effects have been reported less frequently with ranitidine, but otherwise there is little to choose between the available H_2 antagonists.

TRIPOTASSIUM DICITRATOBISMUTHATE

Tripotassium dicitratobismuthate used to be available only in an unpalatable liquid form, but it is a very effective drug and is now available in tablets. Its action is unclear, but it has a cytoprotective effect in addition to its anti-Helicobacter effect. Its main disadvantages are that it has to be taken at least twice daily and tends to turn the stools black, causing potential confusion with melaena. It does, however, seem to produce a lower rate of relapse within the first year after cessation of treatment. This has been attributed to its anti-Helicobacter effect. Because of the potential poblems of chronic bismuth neurotoxicity, tripotassium dicitratobismuthate should not be used as maintenance therapy.

PROTON PUMP INHIBITORS

Proton pump inhibitors such as omeprazole block the final pathway of acid secretion and are its most potent inhibitors. As a result they may achieve healing when other agents have failed, particularly in the rare patients with Zollinger–Ellison syndrome. However they produce almost complete anacidity and this might not always be beneficial in a patient with common duodenal ulcer disease. It would presumably increase bacterial colonisation of the stomach and small intestine for example. This group of drugs have however proved very safe and fears about the possible development of gastric carcinoid tumours that were reported in animals given very high doses of the drugs have so far proved unfounded.

ANTI-HELICOBACTER THERAPY

The therapeutic approach to duodenal ulceration is changing rapidly and it is becoming increasingly common for anti-Helicobacter regimens to be used as the initial treatment. Permanent cure is probably achievable in 70–80%, but if the patient is still experiencing ulcer pain at the time of initiating treatment, therapy should include a potent ulcer healing drug such as a proton-pump inhibitor or H_2 antagonist. Futher studies are continually seeking better regimens for H. pylori eradication. but current regimens usually consist of a bismuth preparation or proton-pump inhibitor, each combined with one or two antibiotics (amoxycillin or oxytetracycline or clarithromycin plus metronidazole or tinidazole) taken for one or two weeks.

SUCRALFATE

Sucralfate binds preferentially to ulcerated mucosa and probably has local buffering, pepsin-inhibiting, and bile acid-binding effects without significantly affecting the properties of the gastric or duodenal juice. It has to be taken four times daily, and there is appreciable aluminium absorption, which probably precludes long-term maintenance treatment.

PIRENZEPINE

Pirenzepine is useful as an addition to the H_2 antagonists for resistant ulcers, but is less potent as a single agent.

FAILURE TO HEAL

Check endoscopy is not necessary to check healing if the patient is symptom free, but 10–20% of patients still have an ulcer after six weeks of treatment. Most of these will heal with double dose H_2 antagonist therapy. If the ulcer still fails to heal a change of therapy is indicated, either to a proton pump inhibitor or to a bismuth preparation.

Most patients with slow-healing ulcers are smokers and should be encouraged to stop smoking completely or at least late in the evening when the damage done is probably greatest. Lack of healing despite three months of high-dose H_2 antagonist, standard-dose proton pump inhibitor, or tripotassium dicitratobismuthate, raises the possibility of Zollinger–Ellison syndrome. Such patients should be further investigated (see page 4).

Relapsed duodenal ulceration

Approximately 85% of patients with healed duodenal ulcers relapse within one year without treatment. This is particularly likely if the patient is H. pylori positive. It is at present unclear how to cope best with this problem, but there are four main alternatives:

- Maintenance treatment, usually with half the healing dose of H_2 antagonist given once at night.
- Discontinuation of treatment and treatment of the almost inevitable relapses with further short courses of drugs.
- Attempted eradication of *H. pylori* with two weeks of 'triple therapy' for example bismuth subcitrate one tablet four times daily, oxytetracycline (or amoxycillin), 500 mg four times daily, and metronidazole, 400 mg four times daily; this regimen achieves eradication of *H. pylori* in about 70–80% of patients and when eradication is successful the relapse rate for ulceration is very low (probably less than 10%). An alternative regimen is omeprazole, 20 mg twice daily, and amoxycillin, 500 mg four times daily, for two weeks, but this probably achieves a slightly lower eradication rate.
- Surgery.

MAINTENANCE TREATMENT WITH H_2 ANTAGONISTS

Maintenance treatment with H_2 antagonists is probably the most effective management, but carries the theoretical concern that reducing gastric acidity will increase bacterial colonisation and formation of carcinogenic nitrosamines. No increased risk of gastric cancer has so far been shown and H_2 antagonists have been very extensively used for nearly 20 years. Furthermore gastric acidity reaches normal levels during the day if the H_2 antagonist is taken only at night.

TREATMENT OF EACH RELAPSE WITH NO MAINTENANCE TREATMENT

Treatment of each relapse with no maintenance treatment is reasonable for the patient who has no more than two or three relapses each year.

TRIPLE THERAPY FOR *H. PYLORI* ERADICATION

Triple therapy for *H. pylori* eradication is increasingly used and the inconvenience of the polypharmacy is worthwhile for the patients who achieve eradication of the organism and long-term remission of symptoms.

SURGERY

Surgery is rarely required for uncomplicated ulcer disease, but may occasionally be indicated if triple therapy fails and lifelong maintenance drug therapy is the alternative. It is difficult to decide between maintenance therapy and surgery. There is almost no ulcer-related mortality in either group (**Fig. 1.33**). The theoretical long-term risk of potentiating gastric malignancy by acid suppression probably applies equally to surgery and drug treatment. The main considerations are

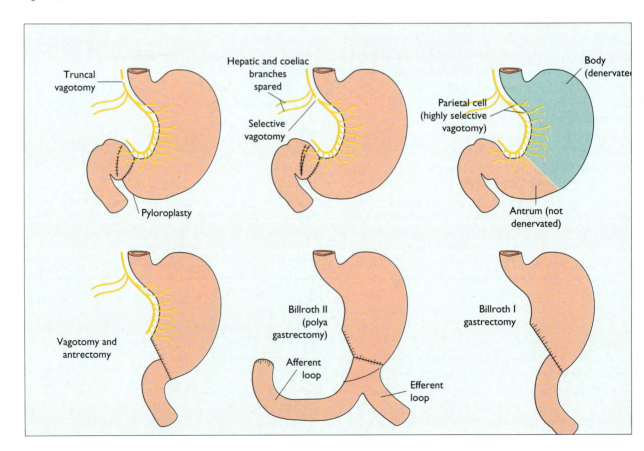

Fig. 1.33 Surgical procedures for ulcers.

therefore the risk of dumping syndrome or diarrhoea after surgery, which probably occurs in 5–10% of patients, and the inconvenience of chronic drug ingestion. With a sensible patient it is probably best to present the alternatives as clearly as possible and allow the patient to decide.

If surgery is chosen, the operation will largely depend on the surgeon:

- **A highly selective parietal cell vagotomy** probably carries the lowest risk of dumping syndrome.
- **Vagotomy and antrectomy** have a lower ulcer recurrence rate than highly selective parietal cell vagotomy (about 3% *vs* 8%, though published series vary considerably).
- **Truncal vagotomy with a drainage procedure** is easiest to perform.

Gastrin assays are widely available and fasting serum gastrin should be checked to exclude Zollinger–Ellison syndrome in any patient referred for surgery. H_2 antagonists should be stopped for 48 hours before blood sampling (**Fig. 1.34**).

Duodenitis

Duodenitis is a nebulous condition that is difficult to define and the correlation between endoscopic and histological appearances is poor. Some patients with duodenal ulcers have an associated erosive duodenitis that heals with treatment of the ulcer and is presumably a form of duodenal ulcer disease. Other patients have erythema of the duodenum, which is sometimes associated with nonspecific inflammation in duodenal biopsies. Possible diagnoses then include duodenal Crohn's disease, coeliac disease, Whipple's disease, and small bowel lymphoma. Usually however the inflammation is confined to the first part of the duodenum, is unassociated with other disease, and seems to be of little consequence to the patient. Endoscopic biopsies from the distal duodenum usually sort this out.

Non-ulcer dyspepsia

Natural history

Non-ulcer dyspepsia is an unsatisfactory term with different meanings for different clinicians, including:

- Abdominal pain.
- Nausea.
- Bloating.
- Belching.
- Fat intolerance.
- Heartburn.

Management

The varying symptoms attributed to this condition have resulted in the publication of many conflicting and confusing clinical trials. It is not surprising that most clinical trials have failed to show any convincing association with any pathology (e.g. *Helicobacter* gastritis) or benefit from any therapy (e.g. H_2 antagonists or triple anti-*Helicobacter* therapy). Further studies are needed in patients with more tightly defined symptom complexes.

The management of symptoms that may be described as non-ulcer dyspepsia includes the following:

- If a patient has **endoscopy-negative upper abdominal pain**, an alternative organic cause should be carefully sought, and if not found a diagnosis of irritable bowel syndrome should be considered.
- **Heartburn** should usually be assumed to be due to acid reflux, even in the absence of endoscopic oesophagitis and treated accordingly. Many patients with heartburn have associated waterbrash, leading to air swallowing and bloating, all of which may resolve with appropriate therapy for the acid reflux.
- Anti-*Helicobacter* therapy may be worth considering for patients with nausea and bloating, but evidence to support its use is inconclusive. If it fails a prokinetic drug such as cisapride may be helpful. This has been shown to be effective in conditions such as diabetic gastroparesis where there is unequivocal evidence of abnormally delayed gastric emptying.

Zollinger–Ellison syndrome

Natural history

In Zollinger–Ellison syndrome there is duodenal ulceration due to increased acidity. The ulcers are often multiple and may be unusually distal or even jejunal. The syndrome is rare, and probably accounts for less than 1/10,000 of all patients with duodenal ulceration, but it is almost certainly under diagnosed.

Normally gastrin is produced mainly by the G cells of the gastric antrum and is under feedback control, but in the Zollinger–Ellison syndrome excessive gastrin is produced by non-beta islet cell tumour(s) of the pancreas or duodenum, which are not under feedback control. This leads to constant over stimulation of the parietal (oxyntic) cells in the body of the stomach resulting in hypertrophy of the gastric body mucosa and very high basal (unstimulated) acid output. This in turn leads to ulceration in the stomach, duodenum, or upper jejunum.

The gastrin-secreting tumour is malignant in about 65% of patients. Up to 25% of tumours are sited in the duodenal wall and may be only 2 mm in diameter, and 90% occur within the 'gastrinoma triangle' bound by the third part of duodenum, the neck of the pancreas, and the porta hepatis. Diarrhoea is common and is the only symptom in about 7% of patients. It is related to hypersecretion of acid and is

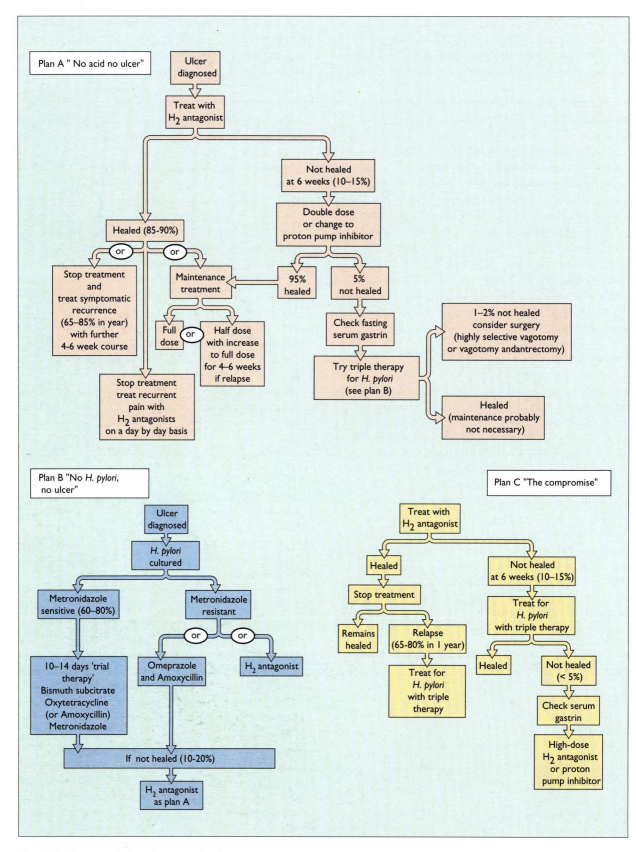

Fig. 1.34 Management policies for duodenal ulcers.

partly due to fat malabsorption, which results from the inactivation of pancreatic lipase at low pH. Vitamin B_{12} malabsorption that is not correctable by intrinsic factor may also occur.

Management of Zollinger–Ellison syndrome

The management of the Zollinger–Ellison syndrome has changed since the advent of H_2 antagonists and proton pump inhibitors. Ulceration and diarrhoea can usually be controlled by proton pump inhibitors so that total gastrectomy is now rarely necessary. This means that an attempt to remove the primary tumour may be reasonable. In the past, combined total gastrectomy and partial pancreatectomy carried an unacceptable morbidity and mortality.

About 65% of patients with Zollinger–Ellison syndrome have malignant tumours, which are often multifocal or have already metastasised. Chemotherapy with streptozotocin can occasionally produce useful tumour regression.

Somatostatin analogues, although often effective suppressors of gastrin release in patients with benign gastrinomas, are commonly ineffective in malignant disease. Leucocyte interferon has been tried with encouraging preliminary results. Survival is surprisingly long however, with a mean survival in the presence of hepatic metastases of 3–5 years. Some patients, particularly those with the MEN 1 syndrome, may have very small duodenal gastrinomas, which may be identifiable only by endoluminal transillumination at laparotomy.

Benign gastric ulcer

Natural history

SYMPTOMS
Symptoms of benign gastric ulceration are variable and often vague. Pain is usually, but not always, present in the upper abdomen. Periodicity is less prominent than with duodenal ulcer. Response to food is variable; more than 50% of patients get some relief from eating, while in about 33% the pain is exacerbated. Other symptoms include discomfort, belching, nausea, and waterbrash (a sudden outpouring of saliva). Bleeding occurs in about 25% of patients at some time. Weight loss is common, making it impossible to distinguish benign from malignant gastric ulceration on the basis of the history.

EPIDEMIOLOGY
The ratio of gastric ulcers to duodenal ulcers is approximately 1 to 4. In recent years they have become as common in women as in men and have a peak incidence in the 50–60-year age group (i.e. 10 years higher than the peak age for duodenal ulcers).

AETIOLOGY AND PATHOGENESIS
In elderly patients, particularly women, gastric ulcers are commonly associated with the use of NSAIDs. They are typically sited on the lesser curve of the stomach in antral mucosa close to the junction between antral- and body-type mucosa. The pathogenesis of gastric ulcers is unknown. Although inhibition of acid secretion usually results in ulcer healing, patients with lesser curve gastric ulcers have normal or low gastric acid outputs. Hypotheses being pursued at present include the following:

- A possible defect in the mucus–bicarbonate barrier, which results from bicarbonate secretion by the gastric epithelium into the overlying mucus.
- A defect in cytoprotection within the mucosa, which is probably prostaglandin-mediated.

Pre-pyloric ulcers are usually associated with higher acid outputs and behave like duodenal ulcers, both symptomatically and in response to treatment. 'Stress' such as burns (Curling's ulcer), trauma, or sepsis is associated with acute erosions, usually of the antrum. They tend to be more superficial and transient than 'peptic' ulcers, but may be prevented by inhibiting acid secretion although they are not usually associated with hypersecretion.

Management

ESTABLISH THAT THE ULCER IS BENIGN
The first priority is to establish that the ulcer is truly benign. This will require endoscopic biopsy and brush cytology. If the diagnosis has been made on barium meal examination, endoscopy should be performed even if the ulcer looks typically benign because there is an appreciable error rate in diagnosis made from the appearance of the ulcer alone (**Figs 1.35** and **1.36**).

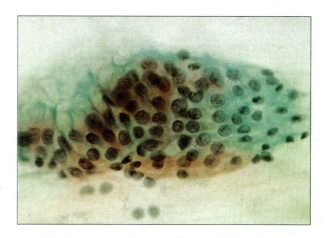

Fig. 1.35 Normal gastric mucosal cytology obtained by endoscopic brushing. Courtesy of Dr D Day.

DRUG TREATMENT

The choice of drugs for healing gastric ulcer is similar to that for duodenal ulcer and includes histamine H_2 antagonists such as cimetidine and ranitidine, proton pump inhibitors such as omeprazole, bismuth subcitrate, sucralfate, pirenzipine, and antacids (see page 15 for further discussion of the mechanisms of action and side-effects of these drugs).

Gastric ulcers take longer to heal than duodenal ulcers, particularly if they are large. Full-dose treatment should be given for 6–8 weeks before an endoscopy is performed to check healing. If the ulcer is still present, further endoscopies should be performed at 6–8 week intervals. Even very large ulcers will heal given time, but large ulcers are more likely to be malignant and should be followed endoscopically and rebiopsied at intervals until complete healing has occurred (**Fig. 1.37**).

FOODS AND MEDICINES TO AVOID

There is no evidence that diet affects healing of gastric ulcers, but it seems sensible to avoid strongly spiced foods. Alcohol certainly damages the mucosa and may stimulate gastric acid secretion and should therefore be avoided. More importantly cigarettes and NSAIDs should be avoided. All prostaglandin synthetase inhibitors carry a risk of ulceration, even if taken by suppository and should be avoided if possible. Simultaneous treatment with H_2 antagonists does not reliably protect against ulceration due to prostaglandin inhibition. There is more evidence to support the use of prophylactic prostaglandin analogues such as misoprostol in patients receiving NSAIDs, but further studies are needed.

RECURRENCE

Approximately 50% of healed gastric ulcers recur within one year. Maintenance prophylaxis with H_2 antagonists has not been properly tested for gastric ulcer and the best management of recurrent gastric ulcer is not clear. Continued H_2 antagonist therapy carries the theoretical risk that chronic lowering of gastric pH predisposes to bacterial overgrowth and increased production of carcinogenic nitrosoamines. Conversely it is well established that partial gastrectomy for gastric ulcer is associated with an increased risk of subsequent gastric cancer.

At present it seems reasonable to recommend maintenance H_2 antagonists for all patients with gastric ulcer. The evidence for any association between gastric ulcer and *H. pylori* is much weaker than for duodenal ulcer. Partial gastrectomy is indicated if gastric ulcers fail to heal after four months of medical treatment and should be considered if recurrence occurs in a patient receiving low-dose maintenance H_2 antagonist therapy.

Gastritis

Natural history

Gastritis may be classified as acute erosive gastritis, chronic atrophic gastritis, reflux gastritis, chronic hypertrophic gastritis (Ménétrier's disease), eosinophilic gastritis, or chronic superficial gastritis (**Figs 1.38–1.45**). Chronic superficial gastritis is probably the commonest.

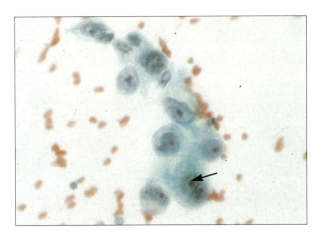

Fig. 1.36 Gastric cytology, at the same magnification as Fig. 1.35, showing a group of malignant cells. Individual cells have an increased nuclear to cytoplasmic ratio and contain prominent nucleoli (arrowed). Courtesy of Dr D Day.

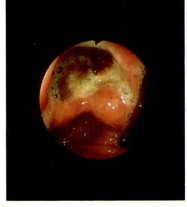

Fig. 1.37 Endoscopic appearance of a large ulcer in the gastric fundus. This ulcer was benign and healed completely after treatment for three months with an H_2 antagonist. Histology and cytology should always be obtained from gastric ulcers because it is impossible to exclude malignancy from endoscopic appearances alone.

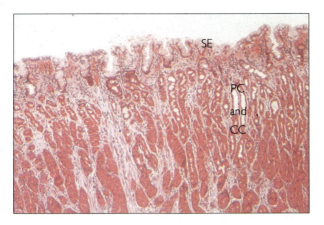

Fig. 1.38 Photomicrograph of normal gastric body mucosa showing surface epithelium (SE), parietal cells (PC) which produce acid and chief cells (CC) which produce pepsin. Courtesy of Dr D Day.

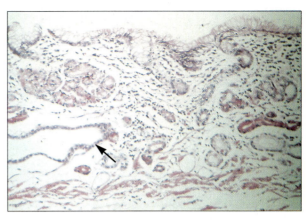

Fig. 1.39 This biopsy from the gastric fundus of a patient with pernicious anaemia shows the features of gastric atrophy. There is thinning of the mucosa and replacement of the specialized gastric glands by simple mucus-secreting glands, one of which is cystically dilated (arrowed). Courtesy of Dr D Day.

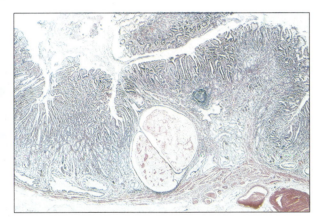

Fig. 1.40 Ménétrier's disease. The body mucosa is markedly thickened and mucus-secreting cells line the gastric glands. There is some glandular dilatation. Courtesy of Dr D Day.

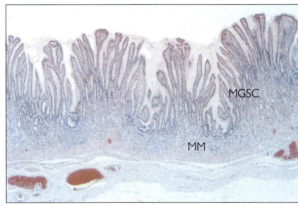

Fig. 1.41 Photomicrograph of normal gastric antral mucosa. MGSC, mucous and gastric secreting cells; MM, muscularis mucosa.

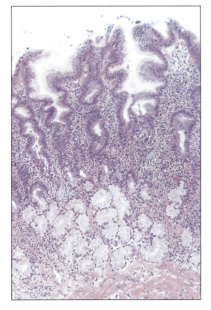

Fig. 1.42 Superficial gastritis in antral-type mucosa. Inflammation affects the supra-glandular layer, and is associated in this example with lengthening of the gastric pits. Courtesy of Dr D Day.

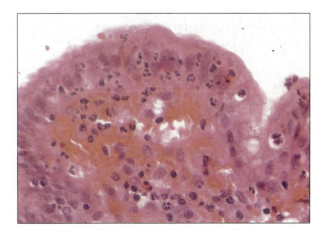

Fig. 1.43 High power magnification of a gastric antral biopsy showing polymorphonuclear leucocytes in the lamina propria and extending into the epithelium in some areas. This is the typical appearance of *H. pylori*-associated gastritis. Courtesy of Dr D Day.

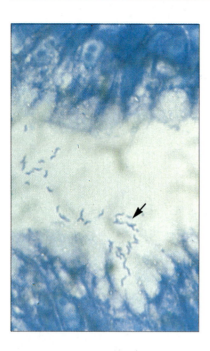

Fig. 1.44 Giemsa stain demonstrates the presence of numerous *H. pylori* organisms (arrowed) in the lumen of a gastric pit. Courtesy of Dr D Day.

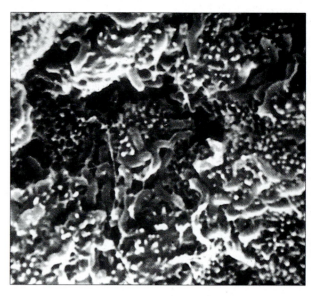

Fig. 1.45 Scanning electron micrograph of a gastric antral biopsy showing *H. pylori* organisms in the lumen of a gastric pit. Courtesy of Professor C A Hart.

ACUTE EROSIVE GASTRITIS

Acute erosive gastritis particularly affects the antrum and occurs after major trauma, burns, sepsis, renal failure, and ingestion of alcohol or aspirin. It is often asymptomatic, but is a common cause of acute upper gastrointestinal bleeding. Its mechanism is unknown, but it has been suggested that it may be due to decreased cytoprotection within the mucosa as a result of altered prostaglandin metabolism.

ATROPHIC GASTRITIS

Atrophic gastritis is a common finding in the elderly patient and arguably occurs normally as part of the ageing process. In younger patients its presence usually implies an immunologically-mediated attack on the gastric mucosa. There are two distinct forms of atrophic gastritis:

- In **type A**, the fundus is primarily affected and patients develop an appropriate hypergastrinaemia in response to reduced acid secretion and there may be pseudopolyposis due to hyperplasia of the gastrin-producing G cells.
- In **type B**, the antrum is primarily affected and patients have a normal serum gastrin.

The immunological attack is probably cell-mediated rather than antibody-mediated because circulating levels of parietal cell antibodies, which are present in only 60% of patients with type A gastritis, correlate poorly with the degree of atrophic gastritis. Both familial (inherited autoimmunity) and acquired (*H. pylori*) factors are involved in the aetiology.

The long-term course of atrophic gastritis is unclear, but it is much more common than pernicious anaemia and it seems likely that only a minority of patients subsequently develop vitamin B_{12} deficiency.

HYPERTROPHIC GASTRITIS (MÉNÉTRIER'S DISEASE)

Hypertrophic gastritis (Ménétrier's disease) is a rare condition in which the normal fundic glands are replaced by hypertrophic epithelium forming massively enlarged mucosal folds. There is a variable degree of inflammation. It may present with pain, vomiting, bleeding, or signs of hypoalbuminaemia, which results from excessive protein loss in mucus shed from the gastric mucosa.

EOSINOPHILIC GASTRITIS

Eosinophilic gastritis is also very rare. It is usually associated with peripheral blood eosinophilia and sometimes with asthma or other allergic disease. Patients may present with abdominal pain, fever, diarrhoea, or ascites. Enlarged antral folds may simulate other infiltrative conditions and cause gastric outlet obstruction.

CHRONIC SUPERFICIAL GASTRITIS

Chronic superficial gastritis is the commonest form of gastritis. Endoscopic appearances of patchy erythema in the antrum correlate poorly with the histological appearances, which consist of an increase in lamina propria mononuclear cells and invasion of the surface epithelium by poly-morphonuclear cells. There is almost 100% correlation between the presence of histologically-proven superficial gastritis with polymorphonuclear cell infiltration and the presence of *H. pylori* on the surface epithelium under the mucus layer. Patients also have detectable serum antibodies to the organism and it is likely that the organisms have a causative role.

Superficial gastritis is a common finding at endoscopy and does not seem to correlate well with any symptom, but there are reports that it causes nausea and flatulence. It is arguably sometimes a cause of non-ulcer dyspepsia.

BILIARY OR ALKALINE REFLUX GASTRITIS
A reddened bile-containing stomach is an almost invariable consequence of partial gastrectomy and is usually termed biliary or alkaline reflux gastritis. It is a specific histological entity, recognisable by foveolar hyperplasia. It is not clear what its significance is because it is common in asymptomatic patients. It may also occur in people with an intact stomach, but further studies are needed to define its natural history.

Management

ACUTE EROSIVE GASTRITIS
Acute erosive gastritis may cause severe bleeding requiring resuscitation or even gastric resection. More usually bleeding stops within 48 hours, particularly if NSAIDs have been stopped. H_2 antagonists should be prescribed, and trials have shown that they also prevent 'stress'-related erosions and should be given prophylactically to patients in septicaemic shock or renal or hepatic failure.

ATROPHIC GASTRITIS
Atrophic gastritis usually requires no treatment unless vitamin B_{12} supplements are required. There is an increased risk of gastric carcinoma, but the size of the risk is probably not sufficient to justify regular endoscopic surveillance if initial biopsies show no evidence of dysplasia or metaplasia (the occurrence of patches of intestinal or colonic type mucosa). However this is still controversial, and it is a sensible policy to follow-up young patients with atrophic gastritis closely.

HYPERTROPHIC GASTRITIS
Hypertrophic gastritis may respond to some extent to treatment with histamine H_2 antagonists or anticholinergics (propanthelene, initially 15 mg four times daily). Partial gastric resection is occasionally necessary to relieve discomfort and reduce protein loss.

EOSINOPHILIC GASTRITIS
Eosinophilic gastritis is sometimes due to a genuine food allergy and exclusion diets are worth trying at first. If there is no improvement, corticosteroid therapy is usually effective.

CHRONIC SUPERFICIAL GASTRITIS
Chronic superficial gastritis due to *H. pylori* can be eradicated by triple therapy in 70–80% of patients. This therapy is given for two weeks and consists of:

- Bismuth subcitrate tablets, one tablet four times daily.
- Oxytetracycline (or amoxycillin), 500 mg three times daily.
- Metronidazole, 400 mg three times daily.

There is considerable controversy as to which, if any, symptoms are relieved by eradicating gastritis. Currently it seems reasonable to attempt eradication of *H. pylori* in patients with unexplained persistent nausea or bloating. Antacids may sometimes produce symptomatic relief, but there seems to be no justification in using H_2 antagonists.

BILIARY REFLUX GASTRITIS
Biliary reflux gastritis sometimes responds to bile acid chelation with cholestyramine, but aluminium hydroxide is worth trying initially because it also has a bile acid-binding effect, albeit weaker than that of cholestyramine.

Carcinoma of the stomach

Natural history

SYMPTOMS
Gastric cancer is usually asymptomatic until invasion occurs into the submucosa or beyond. Common symptoms are then weight loss, abdominal pain, and vomiting. Pain may mimic peptic ulceration, being relieved by H_2 antagonists or antacids, but more commonly it is a vague upper abdominal discomfort, often associated with a feeling of fullness. Frank haematemesis is uncommon, but vomit will often contain some altered blood. Patients may present with lethargy due to anaemia. A tumour mass is palpable in about 50% of patients on presentation.

EPIDEMIOLOGY
The incidence of gastric cancer seems to be declining in developed countries, but its prevalence in the Far East is still very high. The increased risk in lower socio-economic groups may be associated with *H. pylori* infection.

AETIOLOGY AND PATHOGENESIS
Epidemiological links with achlorhydria and a high dietary intake of nitrates have led to the widely proposed hypothesis that an increased content of nitrate-reducing bacteria in the stomach combined with a high dietary nitrate intake will result in increased nitrosation of food, producing carcinogenic nitrosamines. People with pernicious anaemia have been said to have a 10% risk of developing gastric cancer although some surveys suggest this may be an overestimate.

A statistical link has been demonstrated between gastric cancer and the presence of *H. pylori* in the stomach. There is no clear explanation for this association, but the presence of *H. pylori* has recently been shown to result in a marked lowering in the vitamin C content of gastric juice (normally vitamin C is secreted in high concentration in gastric juice). A low dietary intake of vitamin C is also associated with an increased risk for gastric cancer.

Genetic factors are also involved. There are reports of several families with a high occurrence of gastric cancer and there is a 10% increase in risk in association with blood group A. About 65% of patients are male.

Gastric cancer can be subdivided into two types on the basis of pathological appearance:

- Intestinal type resembles colon cancer with glandular formation and mucus synthesis and is probably associated with previous *H. pylori* infection.
- Diffuse type is more disorganised, with malignant cells scattered haphazardly among sheets of fibrous stroma without glandular formation.

Management

Surgery offers the best hope for cure and palliation. A simple screen for metastases should be performed before surgery. A reasonable screen is ultrasound scanning of the liver followed by biopsy if the presence of liver secondaries is going to be a contraindication for surgery. Surgery may still provide the best means of palliating persistent pain or vomiting for some patients with metastases. Surgery varies with the surgeon between:

- Resecting the tumour with a partial gastrectomy.
- Radical total gastrectomy with extensive lymph node clearance and resection of adjacent colon and pancreas.

There is no clear evidence so far to show any advantage for the more radical approach.

Chemotherapy of gastric carcinoma is not curative, but occasionally produces a degree of tumour regression and palliation of symptoms. Controlled trials have established that 5-fluorouracil (5-FU) alone is ineffective, but combinations such as 5-FU with mitomycin C and 5-FU with adriamycin have proved of limited value. They should only be used under supervision by an oncologist and should not be continued if side-effects become troublesome. Irradiation is generally not very effective, but some trials have shown benefit, particularly in the treatment of adenocarcinoma of the gastric cardia.

Treatment with ulcer-healing drugs such as H_2 antagonists or carbenoxolone may reduce pain by promoting healing of ulcerated epithelium, even in malignant ulcers.

PROGNOSIS AND SCREENING

The cure rate of patients with early gastric cancer confined to the mucosa is over 90%, but five-year survival for invasive gastric cancer is only 10%. Recently great efforts have been made to detect gastric cancer earlier. However endoscopic screening of all patients with 'dyspepsia' does not seem to be the solution because symptomatic gastric cancer is almost never 'early' (i.e. confined to the mucosa). In Japan where the incidence of gastric cancer is particularly high, endoscopic screening of asymptomatic patients has had some effect. The proportion of gastric cancers diagnosed at an early stage has risen as a result from 6% to approximately 30%.

The only high-risk groups defined so far are people with pernicious anaemia or previous partial gastrectomy, but they account for a very small proportion of the total number of people with gastric cancer. The risk of gastric cancer in the general population (even in those who are *H. pylori* positive) is not sufficiently high in developed countries for annual endoscopic surveillance to be cost effective, even if it were acceptable to patients. Further work is required to identify aetiological factors in order to define a population at high risk in whom endoscopic surveillance might be feasible (Figs 1.46 and 1.47).

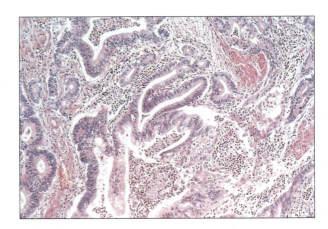

Fig. 1.46 Moderately well-differentiated intestinal-type glandular carcinoma of the stomach. Courtesy of Dr D Day.

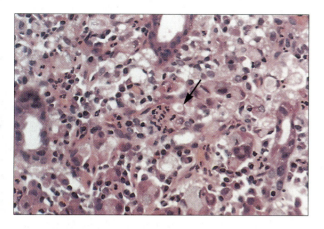

Fig. 1.47 Early gastric cancer showing groups of 'signet ring' cells in which intracellular mucin displaces the nucleus to the periphery (arrowed). Some residual gastric pits and glands can be identified. Courtesy of Dr D Day.

Gastric lymphoma

Natural history

Gastric lymphoma accounts for about 5% of gastric malignancies and for about 60% of gastrointesinal lymphomas. Symptoms and endoscopic features are usually indistinguishable from those of gastric carcinoma and they may be polypoid, ulcerating or infiltrating. Almost all gastric lymphomas are of B cell origin and their histology resembles that of mucosa-associated lymphoid tissue (MALT) rather than primary lymph node lymphoma. Approximately 50% are low grade and these are almost always associated with *H. pylori* infection. High-grade gastric lymphomas often occur in association with low-grade lymphoma elsewhere in the stomach and are probably also due to *H. pylori* infection.

Management

The prognosis is excellent (90–100% five-year survival) if the tumour can be completely excised, whether low-grade or high-grade. There is increasing evidence, however, that early low-grade lymphomas may be curable simply by *H. pylori* eradication therapy. Conventional combination chemotherapy may be required for incompletely resected high-grade lymphoma but further trials are needed to establish optimal therapy.

Gastric polyps

Natural history

Most gastric cancers arise from flat lesions and most gastric polyps are relatively innocuous. They are uncommon, being found at about 2% of endoscopies and are usually asymptomatic unless they ulcerate and bleed (e.g. leiomyomatous polyps, see page 128). Adenomas account for about 5% of gastric polyps but have a similar premalignant potential to colonic adenomata. At least 90% of gastric polyps are hyperplastic. These are almost always harmless, but if very numerous and particularly if present in the gastric fundus, should raise the possibility of familialadenomatous polyposis and lead to investigation of the colon.

Hamartomatous gastric polyps are found in polyposis syndromes such as Peutz-Jeghers (see page 129) and also in familial adenomatous polyposis (see page 134). Fundal polyps found in a patient with pernicious anaemia are likely to be gastric carcinoids, which account for 0.3% of all gastric neoplasms. They arise from enterochromaffin cells, possibly as a result of the trophic effects of gastrin which is elevated in achlorhydria. These tumours have relatively low malignant potential, metastasise rarely, and are therefore a rare cause of carcinoid syndrome.

Management

The polyp should be removed by endoscopic snaring if possible. If this is not possible because of the size or sessile nature of the polpys, multiple biopsies should be taken. If these show an adenoma or carcinoid, then local resection should be performed, whilst hyperplastic polyps can generally be left if asymptomatic.

Gallstones

Natural history

SYMPTOMS

It has been estimated that about 50% of patients with gallstones are asymptomatic. Several series have assessed the risks of leaving stones *in situ*. Overall about 35% need surgery for severe pain or complications during the ten years after diagnosis. The risk of biliary colic or jaundice falls to about 15% over a 10–20 year follow-up of patients who are asymptomatic on diagnosis and whose gallstones are discovered inadvertently during investigation of unrelated problems. Acute cholecystitis occasionally occurs without

▶ **Facts about gallstones**

- 50% of people with gallstones are asymptomatic
- If left untreated, 35% of people with gallstones will need surgery for severe pain or other complications within ten years
- If 'dyspepsia' is the only symptom, 25% of people with gallstones will have the same symptom after cholecystectomy

associated gallstones (see page 33, 44), but chronic cholecystitis is almost invariably associated with stones. The gallbladder is contracted with a thickened and sometimes calcified wall and symptoms are indistinguishable from those associated with gallstones.

EPIDEMIOLOGY

Approximately 4% of Caucasian adults have gallstones, and 80% of these people are female. The prevalence increases with age and is approximately 10% for women aged 40–60 years. There are marked racial variations, with a prevalence of 70% in North American Indians.

AETIOLOGY AND PATHOGENESIS

Approximately 90% of gallstones in Caucasians are cholesterol-based, but the initial nidus for stone formation is probably mucus glycoprotein. An increased risk of cholesterol stones is associated with obesity, diabetes mellitus, multiparity, ileal disease, and hyperlipidaemia. Pigment stones are common in patients with chronic haemolytic anaemias and their prevalence is increased in all forms of cirrhosis. Cholesterol is almost completely insoluble in water and its solubility in bile depends on the detergent effect of bile acids and lecithin. North American Indians have particularly lithogenic bile with a high cholesterol and low bile acid content. It seems that all humans have a tendency to produce lithogenic bile to some extent, and the bile of Caucasians who form gallstones is usually more lithogenic than that of Caucasians without gallstones. Some other factor, possibly accretion of mucin, must be responsible for formation of the initial nidus on which the gallstone crystallises, and gallbladder stasis, which is often marked in diabetes mellitus, probably plays a major role (**Fig. 1.48**).

Management of gallstones

In the absence of acute cholecystitis or obstructive jaundice, it is often difficult to be certain of the relationship of gallstones to a patient's symptoms. If dyspepsia is the only symptom, about 25% of patients with gallstones find that it persists after cholecystectomy. Moreover if cholecystectomy is not performed, one study of 600 patients suggests that only 1.5% develop gallstone complications each year.

As the risk associated with cholecystectomy increases with age, there must be an age above which it is safer to leave asymptomatic gallstones alone, but there are not sufficient data to define this age accurately. It therefore seems reasonable to recommend cholecystectomy to any fit patent under 50 years of age with proven gallstones, and to reserve cholecystectomy for people over 65 years of age to those with acute cholecystitis, non-alcohol-related recurrent acute pancreatitis, or obstructive jaundice. It is often difficult to decide upon the treatment for 50–65-year-olds, and it will depend on the severity and frequency of symptoms and the general health of the patient.

Laparoscopic cholecystectomy has made cholecystectomy a much less invasive procedure for many patients, but it is still associated with a morbidity and mortality, and it is too early to assess whether it will be safer in elderly patients than open cholecystectomy.

Calcification of the gallbladder is uncommon, but is associated with a high risk of subsequent carcinoma of the gallbladder and is an indication for cholecystectomy.

Medical treatment of gallstones

Medical treatment of gallstones has proved rather disappointing. Two bile acids are available for prescription:

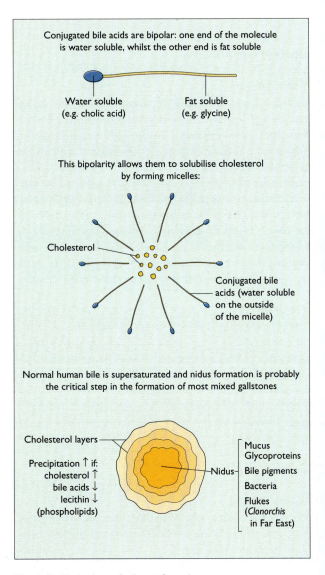

Fig. 1.48 Mechanisms of gallstone formation.

- Chenodeoxycholic acid, 15–20 mg/kg/day.
- Ursodeoxycholic acid, 10 mg/kg/day.

These bile acids expand the bile acid 'pool' and make the bile less lithogenic, but have no effect on pigment stones or on the 10% of cholesterol stones that are calcified. The gallbladder must be functioning on oral cholecystography. If these criteria are met and the gallstones are less than 15 mm in diameter, approximately 75% will dissolve within one year, but the recurrence rate after stopping treatment is extremely high and probably reaches 100% within a few years. Chenodeoxycholic acid is mildly hepatotoxic and causes diarrhoea. It is also expensive for long-term maintenance. Medical treatment is therefore suitable only for elderly patients with symptomatic small non-calcified stones in a functioning gallbladder. There is increasing interest in the use of aspirin as a prophylactic agent, probably acting by inhibiting mucus production by the gallbladder.

Adenomyomatosis of the gallbladder

It is commonly assumed that adenomyomatosis of the gallbladder causes no symptoms, but the relatively few published studies suggest that it causes right upper quadrant pain, which is relieved by cholecystectomy. Adenomyomatosis of the gallbladder predominantly affects the fundus of the gallbladder; the smooth muscle is hyperplastic and packed with epithelial-lined sinuses.

In its mildest form it results in a hypertrophic band or kink across the fundus that mimics a phrygian cap deformity (congenital kinking), and if severe it produces 'cholecystitis glandularis proliferans' or diverticulosis of the gallbladder.

Treatment
Adenomyomatosis of the gallbladder in the absence of gallstones would not be accepted by many as an indication for cholecystectomy, but there is evidence that it may be associated with pain. If symptoms are severe, cholecystectomy is probably indicated.

Chronic mesenteric ischaemia
Natural history
SYMPTOMS AND SIGNS
Clinically significant obstruction to one of the mesenteric vessels (i.e. coeliac axis or the superior or inferior mesenteric arteries) most commonly presents acutely with infarction of the bowel. More rarely, milder intermittent ischaemia results in abdominal angina. Although sudden occlusion of one of the major mesenteric vessels may cause infarction, gradual occlusion allows the development of considerable collateral circulation, so there needs to be more than 50% narrowing of at least two of the three major vessels before symptoms result. Typically, severe central abdominal pain develops 15–30 minutes after meals and may last for several hours. This often leads to a fear of eating which, compounded by malabsorption, causes marked weight loss. Patients are usually elderly with evidence of atheroma elsewhere. There may be an abdominal bruit, but this is not a reliable sign.

Management
Untreated the outlook is poor with rapid deterioration, frequently terminated by infarction of the bowel. Reconstructive vascular surgery produces good short-term results, but there are inadequate data on long term follow-up.

FURTHER READING

Peptic ulcer disease

Aabakken L. Review article: non-steroidal, anti-inflammatory drugs—the extending scope of gastrointestinal side effects. *Aliment Pharmacol Ther* 1992 ; **6**(2): 143–62.

Arens MJ, Dent J. Acid pump blockers: what are their current therapeutic roles? *Baillière's Clin Gastroenterol* 1993; **7**(1): 95–128.

Bardhan KD. Is there any acid peptic disease that is refractory to proton pump inhibitors? *Aliment Pharmacol Ther* 1993; **7** (Suppl. 1): 13–24, discussion 29–31.

Bynum TE. Non-acid mechanisms of gastric and duodenal ulcer formation. *J Clin Gastroenterol* 1991; **13** (Suppl. 2): S56–64.

Curtis WD, Griffin JW. Non-steroidal anti-inflammatory drug-induced gastroduodenal injury: therapeutic recommendations. *Aliment Pharmacol Ther* 1991; 5 (Suppl. 1): 99–109.

Fennerty MB Helicobacter pylori Arch Intern Med 1994; 154, 721–727.

Heatley RV. Review article: the treatment of *Helicobacter pylori* infection. *Aliment Pharmacol Ther* 1992; **6**(3): 291–303.

Holcombe C. *Helicobacter pylori*: the African enigma. *Gut* 1992; **33**(4): 429–31.

Lewis JH Safety profile of long-term H$_2$-antagonist therapy *Aliment Pharmacol Ther* 1991; **5** (Suppl. 1): 49–57.

Moore JG. Stress ulceration in the intensive care unit: use of H$_2$-receptor antagonists. *Aliment Pharmacol Ther* 1991; **5** (Suppl. 1): 111–9.

Peura DA, Graham DY *Helicobacter pylori*; consensus reached: peptic ulcer is on the way to becoming an historic disease *Am J Gastroenterol* 1994; **89**, 1137–1139.

Pounder RE. Degrees of acid suppression and ulcer healing: dosage considerations. *Aliment Pharmacol Ther* 1991; **5** (Suppl. 1): 5–13.

Robert ME, Weinstein WM. *Helicobacter pylori*-associated gastric pathology. *Gastroenterol Clin North Am* 1993; **22**(1): 59–72.

Schiessel R, Feil W, Wenzl E. Mechanisms of stress ulceration and implications for treatment. *Gastroenterol Clin North Am* 1990; **19**(1): 101–20.

Talley NJ. Non ulcer dyspepsia: myths and realities. *Aliment Pharmacol Ther* 1991; **5** (Suppl. 1): 145–62.

Zollinger–Ellison syndrome

Maton PN. Review article: the management of Zollinger–Ellison syndrome. *Aliment Pharmacol Ther* 1993; **7**: 467–475.

Maton PN. Role of acid suppressants in patients with Zollinger–Ellison syndrome. *Aliment Pharmacol Ther* 1991; **5** (Suppl. 1): 25–35.

Mignon M, Ruszniewski P, Podevin P, Sabbagh L, Cadiot G, Rigaud D, Bonfils S. Current approach to the management of gastrinoma and insulinoma in adults with multiple endocrine neoplasia type I. (Review). *World J Surg* 1993; **17**(4): 489–97.

Norton JA Advances in the management of Zollinger–Ellison syndrome Adv Surg 1994; 27, 129–159.

Pasieka JL. Screening and surgical intervention in the multiple endocrine neoplasia patient. (Review). *Sem Surg Oncology* 1993 ; **9**(5): 433–6.

Rhodes JM. The medical management of Zollinger–Ellison syndrome (editorial; comment). *Q J Med* 1991; **78**(287): 191–3.

Thakker RV. The molecular genetics of the multiple endocrine neoplasia syndromes. (Review). *Clin Endocrinol* 1993; **38**(1):1–14.

Gastric carcinoma

Akoh JA, Macintyre IM. Improving survival in gastric cancer: review of 5-year survival rates in English language publications from 1970. *Br J Surg* 1992; **79**(4): 293–9.

Blaser MJ, Parsonnet J. Parasitism by the 'slow' bacterium *Helicobacter pylori* leads to altered gastric homeostasis and neoplasia. *J Clin Invest* 1994; **94**: 4–8.

Bleiberg H, Gerard B, Deguiral P. Adjuvant therapy in resectable gastric cancer. *Br J Cancer* 1992; **66**(6): 987–91.

Colin Jones DG, Rosch T, Dittler HJ. Staging of gastric cancer by endoscopy. *Endoscopy* 1993; **25**(1): 34–8.

De Koster E, Buset M, Nyst JF, Deltenre M. Gastric screening prospects. *Eur J Cancer Prev* 1993; **2**(3): 263–8.

Farley DR, Donohue JH. Early gastric cancer. *Surg Clin North Am* 1992; **72**(2): 401–21.

Lightdale CJ. Endoscopic ultrasonography in the diagnosis, staging and follow-up of esophageal and gastric cancer. *Endoscopy* 1992; **24** (Suppl. 1): 297–303.

Macdonald JS. Gastric cancer: chemotherapy of advanced disease. *Hematol Oncol* 1992; **10**(1): 37–42.

Macintyre IM, Akoh JA. Improving survival in gastric cancer: review of operative mortality in English language publications from 1970. *Br J Surg* 1991; **78**(7): 771–6.

Parsonnet J. *Helicobacter pylori* and gastric cancer. *Gastroenterol Clin North Am* 1993; **22**(1): 89–104.

Smith JW, Brennan MF. Surgical treatment of gastric cancer. Proximal, mid, and distal stomach. *Surg Clin North Am* 1992; **72**(2): 381–99.

Stalnikowicz R, Benbassat J. Risk of gastric cancer after gastric surgery for benign disorders. *Arch Intern Med* 1990; **150**(10): 2022–6.

Weese JL, Nussbaum ML. Gastric cancer—surgical approach. *Hematol Oncol* 1992; **10**(1): 31–5.

Wils JA. Perspectives in chemotherapy of advanced gastric cancer. *Anticancer Drugs* 1991; **2**(2): 133–7.

Wright PA, Quirke P, Attanoos R, Williams GT. Molecular pathology of gastric carcinoma: progress and prospects. *Hum Pathol* 1992; **23**(8): 848–59.

Gastric lymphoma

Parsonnet J, Hansen S, Rodriguez L *et al.* Helicobacter pylori infection and gastric lymphoma. *New Engl J Med* 1994;**330**:1267–71.

Ruskone-Fourmestraux A, Aegerter P, Delmer A *et al.* Primary digestive tract lymphoma: a prospective multicentre study of 91 patients. *Gastroenterology* 1993;**105**:1662–71.

Gallstone disease and cholecystitis

Carey MC. Pathogenesis of gallstones. *Am J Surg* 1993 Apr; **165**(4): 410–9.

Diehl AK. Symptoms of gallstone disease. *Baillière's Clin Gastroenterol* 1992 Nov; **6**(4): 635–57.

Friedman GD. Natural history of asymptomatic and symptomatic gallstones. *Am J Surg* 1993 Apr; **165**(4): 399–404.

Goldberg HI, Gordon R. Diagnostic and interventional procedures for the biliary tract. *Curr Opin Radiol* 1991 Jun; **3**(3): 453–62.

Johnston DE, Kaplan MM. Pathogenesis and treatment of gallstones. *N Engl J Med* 1993 Feb 11; **328**(6): 412–21.

Kahng KU, Roslyn JJ. Surgical issues for the elderly patient with hepatobiliary disease. *Surg Clin North Am* 1994;**74**:345–73.

Nahrwold DL. Gallstone lithotripsy. *Am J Surg* 1993 Apr; **165**(4): 431–4.

Northfield TC. Management of recurrent gallstones. Lanzini A, *Baillière's Clin Gastroenterol* 1992 Nov; **6**(4): 767–83.

Perissat J, Huibretste K, Keane FB, *et al.* Management of bile duct stones in the era of laparoscopic cholecystectomy. *Br J Surg* 1994;**81**:799–810.

Plaisier PW, van der Hull RL, Terpstra OT, Bruining HA. Current treatment modalities for symptomatic gallstones. *Am J Gastroenterol* 1993; **88**: 633–9.

Schoenfield LJ, Marks JW. Oral and contact dissolution of gallstones. *Am J Surg* 1993 Apr; **165**(4): 427–30.

Williams LF Jr, Chapman WC, Bonau RA, McGee EC Jr, Boyd RW, Jacobs JK. Comparison of laparoscopic cholecystectomy with open cholecystectomy in a single center. *Am J Surg* 1993 Apr; **165**(4): 459–65.

Irritable bowel syndrome

Bailey LD Jr, Stewart WR Jr, McCallum RW. New directions in the irritable bowel syndrome. *Gastroenterol Clin North Am* 1991 Jun; **20**(2): 335–49.

Friedman G. Treatment of the irritable bowel syndrome. *Gastroenterol Clin North Am* 1991 Jun; **20**(2): 325–33.

Friedman G. Diet and the irritable bowel syndrome. *Gastroenterol Clin North Am* 1991 Jun; **20**(2): 313–24

Hall MJ, Barry RE. Current views on the aetiology and management of the irritable bowel syndrome. *Postgrad Med J* 1991 Sep; **67**(791): 785–9.

Talley NJ, Zinsmeister AR, Van Dyke C, Melton LJ. Epidemiology of colonic symptoms and the irritable bowel syndrome. *Gastroenterology* 1991; **101**: 927–934.

Thompson WG. Symptomatic presentations of the irritable bowel syndrome. *Gastroenterol Clin North Am* 1991 Jun; **20**(2): 235–47.

West L, Warren J, Cutts T. Diagnosis and management of irritable bowel syndrome, constipation, and diarrhea in pregnancy. *Gastroenterol Clin North Am* 1992 Dec; **21**(4): 793–802.

Whitehead WE, Crowell MD. Psychologic considerations in the irritable bowel syndrome. *Gastroenterol Clin North Am* 1991 Jun; **20**(2): 249–67.

Wingate DL. The irritable bowel syndrome. *Gastroenterol Clin North Am* 1991 Jun; **20**(2): 351–62.

Miscellaneous

Keane TE, Peel AL. Endometrioma. An intra-abdominal troublemaker. *Dis Col Rectum* 1990 Nov; **33**(11): 963–5.

2
THE ACUTE ABDOMEN
Barry Taylor

REACHING A DIAGNOSIS

The patient with acute abdominal pain presents a diagnostic challenge to the clinician, since there is little time for sophisticated investigations and the preliminary diagnosis has to be reached largely on clinical grounds. Two main questions need to be considered:

- What is the diagnosis?
- And perhaps more importantly, Does this patient need an emergency operation?

The answer to the first question is derived using a combination of clinical and laboratory criteria discussed below. The response to the second question depends almost exclusively on clinical parameters and is largely independent of the response to the first.

After a full history has been obtained a diagnosis should become apparent for 75–80% of patients. The examination and investigations are directed at confirming this diagnosis.

The history

The characteristics of the pain should be elicited, along with associated features such as vomiting and diarrhoea. Visceral pain is relatively poorly localised, but once there is peritoneal irritation, the site of the pain and maximum tenderness become good indicators of the site of underlying pathology.

Associated features may include shortness of breath or chest pain if there is a medical cause for the acute abdominal pain, such as basal pneumonia or myocardial infarction. Other features such as nausea or distension might suggest that the biliary or gastrointestinal tract is the likely source. A history of jaundice or previously documented gastro-intestinal disease, or an alteration in bowel habit are obviously important. The nature of any previous surgical intervention needs to be clarified, if possible by inspecting operation notes:

- Previous abdominal surgery is particularly relevant in small bowel obstruction.
- A 'battle-scarred' abdomen should raise a suspicion of Munchausen's syndrome.

- The possibility of mesenteric ischaemia or infarction should be an early consideration in a patient with vascular disease or atrial fibrillation.
- A patient with an obstructed kidney or bladder may have a history of previous genitourinary problems.

A complete drug history is essential. Most patients with a perforated peptic ulcer are elderly and are taking non-steroidal anti-inflammatory agents (NSAIDs), while a variety of drugs, including frusemide and azathioprine, have been implicated in the aetiology of acute pancreatitis. Anticoagulant use is particularly important if surgical intervention is a possibility. Exposure to any other drugs, including non-prescribed drugs, tobacco and alcohol, should be carefully noted.

A careful family history should always be taken. Many causes of an acute abdomen (e.g. ulcers, gallstones, vascular disease, inflammatory bowel disease) show a familial tendency, and sometimes the family history may suggest the diagnosis (e.g. acute pancreatitis or intermittent porphyria).

The examination

The physical examination of a patient with an acute abdomen aims to provide:

- A diagnosis.
- An assessment of the general condition of the patient, particularly looking for signs of peritoneal irritation, so that it can be decided whether or not an emergency operation is needed.

If these aims are not satisfactorily met after the initial examination, the examination must be repeated regularly until they are.

Powerful analgesic agents should be used sparingly until a diagnosis has been made and it has been decided whether or not a laparotomy is necessary.

It is essential to make an initial assessment of the patient's general condition, including pulse rate, respiratory rate, blood pressure and temperature, and these measurements must be repeated regularly, depending on the patient's clinical progress. It cannot be stressed strongly enough that an inexorably rising pulse rate is often the first indicator of an impending intra-abdominal catastrophe, particularly in a young fit patient, and usually occurs before any apparent changes in blood pressure. Of course, the patient with a ruptured abdominal aortic aneurysm may be significantly hypotensive from the outset, but such patients are in the minority.

The patient's hydration status should also be assessed, as any pathological process leading to unrelieved intestinal obstruction and/or peritonitis will be accompanied by some dehydration. The extracellular fluid volume should be considered to be depleted by at least three litres if dehydration is clinically apparent in an otherwise healthy, normal-sized adult. If there is proximal intestinal obstruction, dehydration is likely to be severe, since fluid is sequestered in the gut proximal to the obstructing lesion and may also be lost as vomitus. Acute pancreatitis is another cause of rapid dehydration, since large fluid shifts occur as fluid is sequestered in the peritoneal cavity.

The general physical examination should include:

- An inspection of the hands for signs of anaemia and liver disease.
- Palpation of all lymph node groups throughout the body.
- A thorough inspection of the face, mouth and tongue, noting any jaundice, conjunctival pallor, anaemia, cyanosis and dehydration, and rare signs such as the circumoral pigmentation of Peutz–Jeghers syndrome.

It is well known that acute chest conditions and myocardial infarction may be confused with acute upper abdominal conditions, and may occasionally be accompanied by guarding and even rigidity in the upper abdomen. The next step is therefore a thorough examination of the chest and cardiovascular system in an attempt to exclude conditions such as basal pneumonia, pulmonary embolism and infarction, pneumothorax, pleurisy and acute myocardial infarction. It is usually possible to exclude these conditions after the examination, but various confirmatory tests will be discussed later. The other notable intrathoracic catastrophe that may cause epigastric guarding and rigidity is Boerhaave's syndrome, or ruptured oesophagus, which is usually caused by forced vomiting against a closed glottis.

This diagnosis is sometimes considered only after a negative laparotomy has been carried out, and the importance of the physical sign of subcutaneous crepitus in the neck cannot be overstated in this situation.

Abdominal examination

Finally attention needs to be directed to the abdomen. An initial inspection should include the following:

- An assessment of the patient's ability to move the abdominal wall with or without pain. This information can be obtained by watching the patient's abdominal wall during normal breathing and coughing, and by asking the patient to sit up unaided. The general size and shape of the abdomen and any obvious masses, visible peristalsis and abdominal distension, should be noted.
- An inspection of the groins (inguinal and femoral regions) for the presence of hernias, which may have escaped the notice of the patient. The external genitalia should also be examined at this point.
- An inspection for signs of retroperitoneal bleeding. Although in general a rather late manifestation, Grey Turner's sign (bruising of the flanks) may provide useful confirmatory evidence of haemorrhagic pancreatitis in the absence of other abnormal investigations.

The abdomen should then be gently palpated in all quadrants to assess for the presence of guarding or rigidity. Palpating a rigid abdomen (a feature of an acutely perforated peptic ulcer) is rather like palpating a table top ('board-like' rigidity). If there is guarding, the patient's abdominal wall will usually move a small amount before the abdominal wall muscles contract, rendering an informative palpation impossible. Palpable masses should be sought and assessed to decide on their likely organ of origin. Patients with acute retention of urine occasionally present with severe abdominal pain and a lower abdominal mass (the bladder), with surprisingly little in the way of pre-existing genito-urinary symptoms. Moving masses will only be appreciated if the palpating hand remains still, and a failure to keep the hand still is one of the most common reasons why aortic aneurysms, however large, are missed by relatively inexperienced examiners.

▶ **Assessment of the patient with an acute abdomen**

- Repeated examination is essential when the diagnosis is in doubt
- Powerful analgesia should be avoided until a diagnosis has been reached
- Consider using prophylactic subcutaneous heparin during in-hospital investigation
- Beware the 'battle-scarred' abdomen; consider Munchausen syndrome
- If dehydration is clinically apparent in an adult the extra-cellular fluid volume is probably depleted by at least three litres
- An inexorably rising pulse rate is often the first indication of impending intra-abdominal catastrophe

The site of maximum tenderness then needs to be defined. In generalised peritonitis with rigidity any attempt at localisation is futile, but otherwise the location of maximum tenderness will often give useful clues to the underlying diagnosis, for example appendicitis, biliary pain and pelvic colon diverticulitis.

Persistent and well-localised pain with local guarding (as occurs over an ischaemic loop of bowel in small bowel obstruction) implies peritoneal irritation for whatever reason, and is usually a good indication for urgent surgical intervention.

Auscultation of the abdomen in general is not very helpful, although very high-pitched 'tinkling' bowel sounds often accompany small bowel obstruction. The presence of normal bowel sounds does not exclude generalised peritonitis, since the ileus that develops is often a rather late effect of peritoneal inflammation. Occasionally a vascular bruit will be heard in patients with mesenteric vascular stenoses or aortic disease.

Finally the importance of a digital examination of the anorectum performed by an experienced clinician cannot be overstated. To fail to carry out this part of the assessment, particularly in an adult patient, risks missing a diagnosis such as a pelvic abscess or a rectal or prostatic carcinoma.

A STEP-BY-STEP APPROACH TO ACUTE ABDOMINAL PAIN

Should the patient be referred to hospital?

If, on the basis of the clinical examination, the general practitioner feels that the diagnosis is probably a surgical condition such as acute appendicitis or cholecystitis, the patient should clearly be referred to hospital. It is difficult to set rigid rules if the diagnosis is not clear, but it is wise to refer to hospital any patient with:

- A tachycardia over 90 beats per minute.
- A fever over 37.5°C.
- Hypotension, with systolic blood pressure less than 100 mm Hg.
- Pain persisting for more than 4–6 hours.
- Pain that cannot be controlled with simple analgesic agents such as paracetamol.

The threshold for referral should be lower for children under 16 years of age and for adults over 65 years of age.

Should the patient be admitted to hospital?

Over 90% of patients referred to hospital with acute abdominal pain will be admitted for observation overnight or longer. A small number of patients with mild pain or who have symptoms that resolve during their visit to the hospital are discharged after an assessment in the emergency department by an experienced surgeon. It should be remembered however that no test is 100% sensitive for any cause of an acute abdomen: a normal full blood count does not exclude appendicitis, and a normal serum amylase on admission does not exclude pancreatitis. If there is any doubt, an admission with regularly-repeated observations is the sensible approach.

Is it appendicitis?

Patients with appendicitis typically present with central abdominal colic associated with vomiting, and this is followed by right iliac fossa pain as peritoneal irritation progresses. There may be urinary symptoms and an alteration in bowel habit in pelvic appendicitis. A fever is common, as is a foetor.

Well-localised tenderness and guarding are the cardinal signs, although the site may vary in pelvic appendicitis or pregnancy. When the appendix is situated behind the caecum or ileum, there may be surprisingly little to find on palpating the anterior abdominal wall, and a high index of suspicion is important.

There are no confirmatory tests. Radiographs will be non-specific unless the inflammatory process has progressed and the patient is presenting with small bowel obstruction, while a leucocytosis is common, but not universal.

When the diagnosis is in doubt, repeated examination is important, since the signs will usually either improve or worsen. In young women, a diagnostic/therapeutic laparoscopy may have a role to exclude gynaecological causes and, possibly, to remove the appendix without a conventional incision (**Fig. 2.1**).

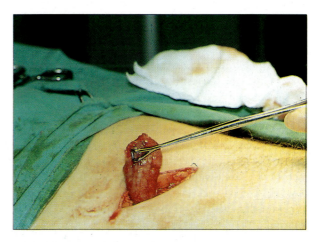

Fig. 2.1 An acutely inflamed appendix delivered through a conventional 'Lanz' incision.

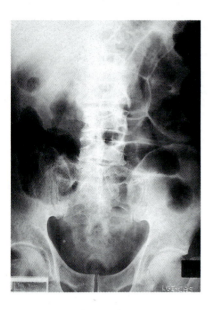

Fig. 2.2 A plain abdominal radiograph demonstrating gas in the wall of the gallbladder in gangrenous cholecystitis.

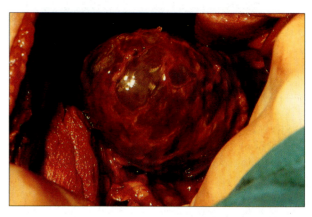

Fig. 2.3 Acute gangrenous cholecystitis: an operative photograph from the patient whose radiograph is shown in Fig. 2.2.

Is it acute cholecystitis?

The patient with acute cholecystitis, who is commonly a woman in her forties or fifties, presents with epigastric and right upper quadrant pain, which often radiates to the back and may be associated with vomiting. There may be a past history of biliary colic. There is usually a low-grade pyrexia and the white blood count may be elevated.

Clinical examination reveals marked tenderness with guarding in the right upper quadrant, and there may also be a palpable mass, although it may not be apparent when the patient is awake. A marked increase in discomfort caused by inspiration while the examining hand is in the right upper quadrant (Murphy's sign) may also be evident, and the patient may be mildly jaundiced, depending on the position of the stones. A swinging pyrexia and severe tenderness suggests an empyema, while a sudden deterioration in the patient's condition with a spreading peritonitis suggests that the gallbladder has ruptured. A combination of pain, jaundice and a fever (Charcot's triad) suggests ascending cholangitis, which is usually caused by ductal calculi and demands urgent treatment.

Plain abdominal radiography is often not particularly useful in this situation. Gallstones are radio-opaque in only approximately 10% of patients, and their presence does not necessarily implicate them as the cause of the pain, since many stones are asymptomatic. A plain radiograph may, however, demonstrate the presence of a mass in the right upper quadrant, while gas in the gallbladder wall implies impending perforation (Figs 2.2 and 2.3).

A serum amylase should be obtained as an emergency investigation to help to exclude acute pancreatitis, and if there is a suspicion of ductal calculi (jaundice or previous rigors), serum should be sent to the laboratory so that bilirubin and liver enzyme estimations can be assessed later, even if unavailable as emergency biochemical tests.

Urgent ultrasound (within 48 hours of admission) is the simplest method for confirming the presence of gallstones and will also give additional valuable information about the thickness of the gallbladder wall (Fig. 2.4), the size of the common bile duct, the appearance of the liver (particularly the presence or absence of intrahepatic bile duct dilatation) and the appearance of the pancreas.

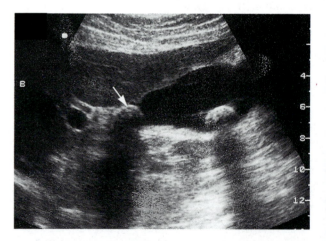

Fig. 2.4 An ultrasound scan of the gallbladder, showing multiple stones, one of which is impacted in Hartmann's pouch (arrow), and thickening of the gallbladder wall.

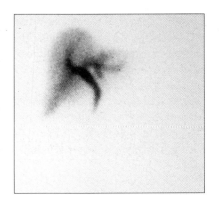

Fig. 2.5 A HIDA scan in a patient with acute cholecystitis, demonstrating normal extrahepatic biliary anatomy, but the cystic duct and gallbladder do not fill.

Oral cholecystography has no place in the management of the acute patient, but ^{99M}Tc-labelled dimethyl-acetanilide iminodiacetic acid (HIDA) scanning, when available, can help by demonstrating non-filling of the gallbladder, which is highly specific for acute cholecystitis (**Fig. 2.5**).

Is it acute pancreatitis?

Most patients with acute pancreatitis present with a relatively sudden onset of severe epigastric pain, which usually radiates to the back and is often associated with vomiting. There may be a pre-existing history suggesting biliary tract disease or a history of alcohol abuse. Easing the pain by sitting forward is a classical feature.

There are no specific signs in the acute phase except extensive tenderness and guarding in the epigastrium, usually with diminished bowel sounds. Grey Turner's sign (bruising in the flanks) indicates retroperitoneal pancreatic necrosis and haemorrhage, and is usually associated with a poor outcome, but often does not appear until the disease is well established.

Plain radiographs are not usually helpful, but pleural effusions may reflect the massive fluid shifts that accompany the process, while a sentinel loop of small bowel reflects the localised ileus produced by the inflammatory process. The serum amylase, which is characteristically higher than 1000 iu/litre, usually confirms the diagnosis. It should be remembered, however, that a relatively mild rise in serum amylase can be a feature of other upper abdominal emergencies such as visceral perforation, while patients with necrotising pancreatitis may have a normal serum amylase.

Ultrasound scanning is useful because it provides considerable information about the biliary tree (e.g. the presence of stones, the diameter of common bile duct), and may also allow visualisation of the pancreas, particularly if it is enlarged by the inflammatory process.

Is it acute diverticulitis?

A typical patient with acute diverticulitis is over 60 years of age and has acute left iliac fossa pain, a low-grade fever and marked tenderness to deep palpation in the left iliac fossa. Other features are variable: a mass may be palpable either in the left iliac fossa or pelvis. Surprisingly, a previous history of altered bowel habit is often absent, but there is usually some degree of abdominal distension and constipation during the attack. Commonly, there is a history of previous similar attacks and the patient may have been investigated for the symptoms.

There is usually a leucocytosis and there may be white cells in the urine. The chest radiograph is usually normal, but should be inspected carefully for subdiaphragmatic gas, which may be present if there is diverticular perforation. The plain abdominal radiograph is often unremarkable, but relative distension of the proximal colon with the suggestion of a mass in the left iliac fossa supports the diagnosis. If there is a mass in the left iliac fossa, an ultrasound examination will often confirm that the mass originates in the bowel (**Figs 2.6** and **2.7**) and may also demonstrate a paracolic abscess in association with the diverticular disease.

Once a clinical diagnosis of acute diverticular disease without perforation has been made, treatment is commenced with broad-spectrum antibiotics (see page 51) and further investigation is delayed for a few days to allow the inflammatory process to subside. Flexible sigmoidoscopy and a

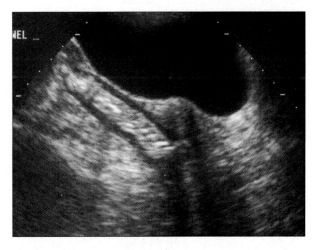

Fig. 2.6 An ultrasound scan in acute sigmoid diverticular disease showing gross thickening of the bowel wall.

barium enema can usually be deferred until after discharge. An alternative approach is to carry out an immediate water-soluble contrast study, with the specific aim of detecting any colonic leak. Other authors have advocated immediate CT scanning with both intravenous and intraluminal contrast as this should reveal paracolic abscess formation. Whatever mode of investigation is used, great care is essential, since the inflamed bowel may be easily perforated if it is over-distended.

The occasional patient with an acute problem related to a caecal or right-sided diverticulum will present with all the features of appendicitis and be explored with this diagnosis in mind. If such a patient is not explored, a subsequent contrast enema may demonstrate the abnormality (Fig. 2.8).

Is there a perforated viscus?

Most patients with a perforated viscus have severe abdominal pain and abdominal guarding or rigidity, but occasional patients, particularly frail elderly patients receiving NSAIDs, will have minimal or no signs. Conversely severe abdominal pain with guarding may occur in the absence of intrabdominal pathology in conditions such as oesophageal rupture and pulmonary embolism. Diagnosis is further complicated by the fact that few patients with a perforated peptic ulcer or diverticular disease give a previous history suggesting the diagnosis.

The systemic disturbance in patients with a perforated viscus varies enormously, from the fit young patient with little systemic effect, but severe abdominal pain, to the patient with gross septicaemia and shock on admission. The effect obviously depends on a variety of factors, including the patient's age and underlying medical problems, the duration of the perforation, the extent of contamination of the peritoneal cavity and the nature of the contaminating enteric content. A low-grade fever is common.

The peripheral white blood cell count is usually elevated, as is the serum amylase concentration (though not usually over 1000 iu/litre). Haemoglobin may be low if there has been blood loss, but is more likely to be relatively high, reflecting hypovolaemia.

The plain abdominal radiograph is likely to be normal, but an ileus is common, with gas-filled loops of normal-sized small bowel centrally. Occasional fluid levels on an erect radiograph also reflect a relative ileus, but intraperitoneal subdiaphragmatic gas on the erect chest radiograph is the most helpful radiological sign. However, up to about 30% of patients with perforated viscera will not demonstrate this sign on the initial radiograph. If clinical suspicion is high, but not sufficient to justify immediate laparotomy, a repeat chest radiograph 24 hours later may be more helpful, particularly if followed by an emergency water-soluble contrast meal (Figs 2.9 and 2.10).

Is there evidence of peritonitis?

The clinical condition here will be very similar to that described for the patient with intestinal perforation, but causes also include conditions such as mesenteric infarction and rupture of the gallbladder.

The patient with peritonitis becomes rapidly unwell over 4–6 hours, and shows increasing signs of endotoxaemia with

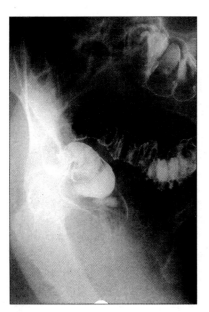

Fig. 2.7 An 'instant' barium enema confirming a short segment of diverticular disease in the sigmoid colon in the patient whose scan is shown in Fig. 2.6.

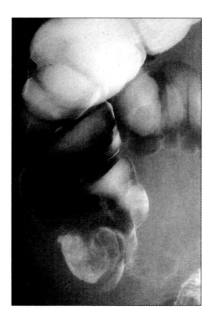

Fig. 2.8 Barium enema demonstrating a large single caecal diverticulum. The patient first presented with what was thought to be an appendix mass.

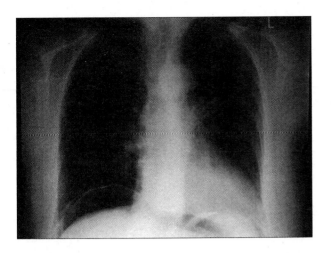

Fig. 2.9 An erect PA chest radiograph demonstrating gross pneumoperitoneum, with gas under both hemidiaphragms, secondary to a perforated peptic ulcer.

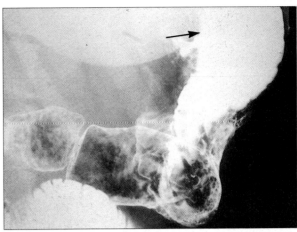

Fig. 2.10 Emergency upper gastrointestinal contrast study (using a water-soluble agent) confirming an apparently localised perforation of a proximal gastric ulcer (arrowed).

tachycardia, hypotension, oliguria and prostration. Movement of any kind worsens the abdominal pain, so the patient tends to remain very still. Involuntary guarding and rigidity of the abdominal wall on palpation are the hallmarks of the condition, and these signs alone are usually an adequate reason for recommending laparotomy.

If there remains some uncertainty about the underlying cause of the problem after the initial assessment, two investigations should be considered short of a formal laparotomy:

• The first is **peritoneal lavage**, in which one litre of warmed saline is instilled into the peritoneal cavity through a peritoneal dialysis catheter inserted under local anaesthetic. An aliquot of fluid is then withdrawn and analysed. The finding of bile, a white cell count higher than 500/ml, or a red blood cell count higher than 100,000/ml are considered to be evidence of peritonitis and may be used as an indication for surgery. A simpler technique used specifically in relation to appendicitis, involves inserting a needle into the right iliac fossa and analysing any fluid aspirated for the presence of white blood cells or bacteria.
• The second specific investigation is a **diagnostic laparoscopy** carried out under general anaesthetic with an arrangement to proceed as necessary depending on the result. Some conditions such as early appendicitis or small uncomplicated perforations may be treatable laparoscopically without the need for formal laparotomy. Laparoscopy is particularly useful for 15−45-year-old

women with lower abdominal or right iliac fossa signs, in whom the normal appendicectomy rate might otherwise approach 40%.

Is there intestinal obstruction?

A diagnosis of intestinal obstruction is based on the combination of a suggestive history and typical radiographic changes, and may be confirmed by contrast radiology.

Features in the history include colicky abdominal pain, abdominal distension, nausea and vomiting, and an alteration in bowel habit. The relative importance of each of these features depends on the level of the obstruction:

• Early vomiting is particularly prominent in high obstruction.
• Distension and constipation are more prominent in lower obstruction.

Previous abdominal surgery or the presence of a painful irreducible hernia in the groin may point to an underlying cause. Other features to look for during the clinical assessment include visible peristalsis, signs of hypovolaemia, hyperactive bowel sounds and abdominal masses.

Air−fluid levels on the erect abdominal radiograph are the hallmark of intestinal obstruction, but dilatation of small bowel loops beyond 2.5 cm or large bowel beyond 7 cm together with a paucity of intestinal gas distally, are features that improve specificity for the diagnosis.

Emergency enteroclysis (contrast small bowel series) may be used to differentiate ileus (e.g. in the postoperative period) from a mechanical small bowel obstruction. Contrast studies of the large bowel may similarly be used to differentiate pseudo-obstruction (Ogilvie's syndrome) from mechanical large bowel obstruction (**Figs 2.11–2.14**).

Is there evidence of ischaemia in association with the obstruction?

Having decided that a patient has an obstructed intestine, the possibility of ischaemia secondary to adhesive obstruction should be considered. There are no clinical features or tests that are 100% accurate in this situation. An elevated white cell count and/or fever may be present, but both are entirely nonspecific. Severe, persistent and well-localised tenderness on abdominal palpation is the most useful sign since it suggests significant peritoneal irritation and implies ischaemia of an adjacent bowel loop.

The adage "never let the sun set on an obstructed abdomen," has much to recommend it because it reduces the risk of an ischaemic segment becoming frankly necrotic and perforating with potentially severe consequences (**Fig. 2.15**).

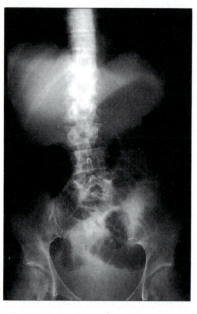

Fig. 2.11 Supine abdominal radiograph in small bowel obstruction, showing dilated small bowel loops lying centrally in the abdomen.

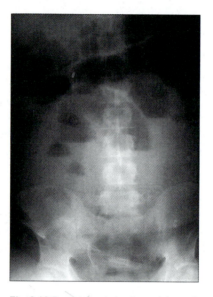

Fig. 2.12 Erect abdominal radiograph in small bowel obstruction, showing dilated small bowel loops lying centrally, with multiple air–fluid levels. Obstruction is incomplete because there is some gas in the transverse colon.

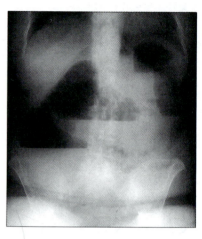

Fig. 2.13 Erect abdominal radiograph in mechanical large bowel obstruction secondary to a carcinoma of the sigmoid colon.

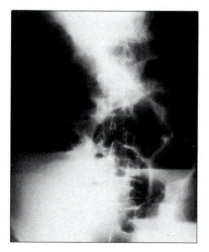

Fig. 2.14 Erect abdominal radiograph in pseudo-obstruction (Ogilvie's syndrome). The film should be compared to that shown in Fig. 2.13 to illustrate the difficulty in differentiating between mechanical and pseudo-obstruction without contrast studies.

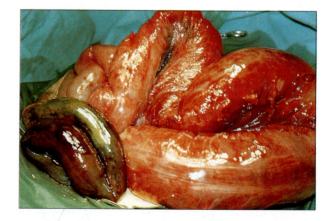

Fig. 2.15 Operative photograph of a necrotic small bowel loop discovered at the time of a laparotomy for intestinal obstruction.

Is there a leaking aortic aneurysm?

The emergency presentation of an abdominal aortic aneurysm can vary from sudden collapse and death to a patient with vague abdominal and/or back pain in whom an aneurysm is detected during a routine physical examination. More commonly, the patient, who is over 60 years of age, has a previous history of backache for a few weeks and presents with a sudden severe pain in his back and abdomen, which is followed by collapse and prostration.

In the absence of any contraindication such as known metastatic malignant disease, the finding of a tender pulsatile abdominal mass should be followed by exploration of the abdomen on the assumption that the aneurysm has ruptured. In less than 5% of patients this diagnosis will prove to be incorrect, but it is safest to explore such patients immediately rather than wait for confirmatory tests.

The diagnosis can be missed easily unless the clinician palpates the abdomen with it in mind because:

- Pulsation may be weak if there is marked hypotension.
- If back pain predominates, renal colic may be mistakenly diagnosed instead.

If the diagnosis is doubtful, the plain abdominal radiograph may demonstrate curvilinear calcification in the wall of the expanded aorta adjacent to the left border of the lower thoracic and lumbar spine (**Fig. 2.16**). Alternatively a 'shoot-through' lateral radiograph may demonstrate the front wall of the aneurysm if the plain film is inconclusive. An emergency ultrasound scan will confirm the size, and often the extent, of the aneurysm, and will also indicate the extent of intraluminal thrombus (**Fig. 2.17**). It may also detect an extraluminal leak. This can be detected more accurately, however, by an intravenous contrast-enhanced emergency CT scan, which is the investigation of choice for the stable patient in whom there is some diagnostic doubt, and is also the most accurate method for assessing the involvement of the renal and iliac arteries (**Fig. 2.18**).

Is there intestinal infarction?

A diagnosis of intestinal infarction should be top of the list of possible differential diagnoses if a patient with known arteriopathy or who is in atrial fibrillation has severe abdominal signs or symptoms. Initially there is often a discrepancy between the symptoms (which are severe, with

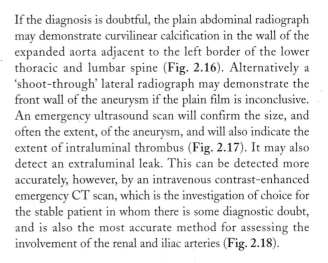

Fig. 2.16 Plain abdominal radiograph demonstrating calcification in the wall of a large abdominal aortic aneurysm (arrowed).

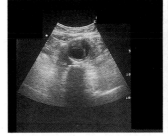 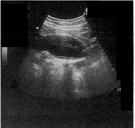

Fig. 2.17 Ultrasound scans of the. abdomen (transverse scan on the left; longitudinal scan on the right) demonstrating a large aortic aneurysm containing luminal thrombus.

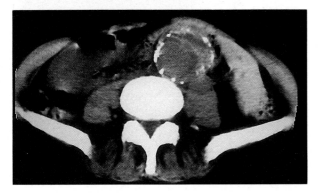

Fig. 2.18 Non-enhanced CT scan of the abdomen demonstrating calcification in the wall of the aneurysm with luminal thrombus and suggesting a leak posteriorly into the left psoas muscle.

agonising pain) and signs (which may be relatively unimpressive until the intestine infarcts and perforates). Vomiting and diarrhoea are often prominent in the early stages.

There are no reliable diagnostic tests, but neutrophilia is common. Radiographs are often surprisingly normal, though there may be an ileus. Marginal elevation of serum amylase is common. Air in the portal vein is usually a grave prognostic sign. A high index of suspicion is needed for patients at risk, with early laparotomy if there is any doubt (**Figs 2.19 and 2.20**).

Infarction due to venous thrombosis presents in a similar way, but there is often a more prolonged prodromal illness lasting a few days in which nonspecific symptoms such as vomiting and diarrhoea predominate. Haemoconcentration is common and there may be splenomegaly. Once the acute problem has been dealt with the underlying hypercoagulable state, which is usually present, will need investigation. This will include measuring antithrombin III (**Fig. 2.21**) and protein S and C levels.

Is there a gynaecological problem?

Several gynaecological conditions can cause an acute abdomen, typically in relatively young women.

Ruptured ectopic pregnancy

The most important gynaecological condition causing an acute abdomen is a ruptured ectopic pregnancy, which can be rapidly fatal if not dealt with urgently and effectively. An entirely normal menstrual history does not exclude a ruptured ectopic pregnancy, and this diagnosis must be considered in any woman of childbearing age with sudden, severe, lower abdominal pain and collapse. Shoulder tip pain suggests diaphragmatic irritation from intraperitoneal blood. A history of relative infertility is common.

The most common site for the ectopic pregnancy is in the ampulla of the Fallopian tube, so when the rupture occurs the tube is badly damaged and has to be removed. If the condition is diagnosed before it ruptures (**Fig. 2.22**), the tube can usually be reconstructed, but the primary concern of the surgeon in the emergency situation must be to control bleeding and prevent an avoidable death.

Acute salpingitis

Acute salpingitis can be caused by a variety of infecting organisms. The patient typically presents with pelvic peritonitis, which is often associated with vomiting and a high fever. There is usually marked tenderness in both iliac fossae, and pain when the cervix is moved during vaginal examination.

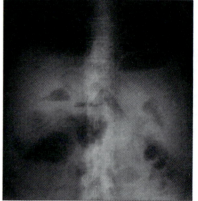

Fig. 2.20 Erect abdominal radiograph showing gas in the portal vein in a patient with mesenteric vascular occlusion and infarction.

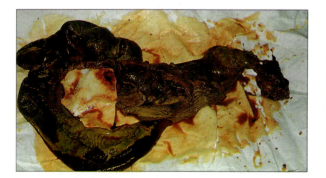

Fig. 2.19 Operative specimen from a patient with known arteriopathy showing almost total infarction of the small bowel .

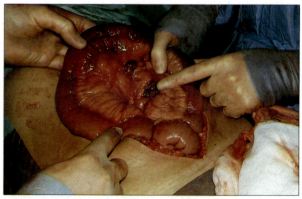

Fig. 2.21 Operative photograph demonstrating mesenteric venous thrombosis in a patient with antithrombin III deficiency.

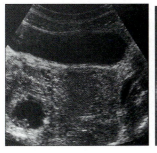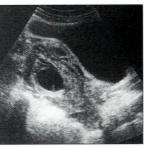

Fig. 2.22 Pelvic ultrasound scan (transverse scan left, longitudinal scan right) demonstrating an ectopic pregnancy in the right Fallopian tube.

The most important differential diagnosis is acute appendicitis, and diagnostic laparoscopy can be extremely useful in this situation.

Acute salpingitis can progress to **pyosalpinx**, which is usually bilateral and characterised by the presence of a tender, boggy swelling in the pouch of Douglas. A sudden severe deterioration with spreading peritonitis suggests an intraperitoneal rupture of a pyosalpinx.

Torsion of an ovarian cyst

Torsion of an ovarian cyst typically causes acute, severe pain and vomiting, but little systemic disturbance. A tender mass in the pelvis can usually be felt on bimanual examination. As the condition progresses and pelvic peritonitis ensues, it may become impossible to palpate the mass without a general anaesthetic due to guarding in the lower abdomen.

Occasionally, massive ovarian cysts give rise to an acute abdominal presentation, usually because of torsion or simple infarction. Although the physical signs may be difficult to interpret, the abdominal radiograph is classical.

SPONTANEOUS RUPTURE OF AN ENDOMETRIOTIC CYST

Spontaneous rupture of an endometriotic cyst, usually of the ovary, gives rise to a clinical picture that can resemble both ruptured ectopic pregnancy and acute salpingitis. In this condition irregular nodularity palpable on bimanual examination in the pouch of Douglas and in the broad ligament will suggest the aetiology.

Investigating possible gynaecological causes of acute pelvic peritonitis

If there is a possible gynaecological cause for an acute pelvic peritonitis, useful investigations include pelvic ultrasound scanning, transvaginal ultrasound scanning and laparoscopy.

In practice, abdominal or transvaginal ultrasound scanning is frequently not available or suboptimal (e.g. the patient rarely has a full bladder in this situation), and laparoscopy is the investigation most likely to provide useful information. It also offers the possibility of therapeutic intervention without resorting to a full laparotomy, though laparotomy will be ultimately necessary for some patients.

Finally, the help and advice of a gynaecological surgeon should be sought before resorting to any form of radical excisional surgery.

Is emergency laparotomy indicated?

The decision to perform an emergency laparotomy is usually based largely on clinical grounds and should not be particularly difficult to make.

- For patients with probable appendicitis, an appendicectomy should be carried out without delay, except in women of childbearing age, for whom preliminary laparoscopy may be preferable. If, however, an appendix mass has developed, surgery may be safely delayed to allow conservative management with antibiotics and a later elective appendicectomy.
- Emergency laparotomy is indicated for a probable ruptured abdominal aortic aneurysm unless there is evidence of some other life-threatening condition or terminal disease.
- A diagnosis of peritonitis, of whatever cause, based on the findings of abdominal rigidity and involuntary guarding, and usually accompanied by systemic signs such as a tachycardia and fever, is a clear indication for laparotomy.
- Impressive local signs that render adequate palpation of the whole abdomen impossible (e.g. those that might develop over an empyema of the gallbladder or ischaemic

bowel loop) should generally precipitate a laparotomy to prevent the peritonitis that may well develop otherwise.

- Patients with intestinal obstruction should generally have a laparotomy within 24 hours of presentation, but only after the diagnosis has been adequately confirmed radiologically, unless adhesions are thought to be the most likely cause and the patient's condition improves rapidly with conservative measures. It is not acceptable to wait 5–6 days for an episode of presumed adhesive obstruction to settle.
- If there is concern about a patient's progress following a laparotomy, either because of a protracted ileus or anxiety about an anastomosis, there is rarely little to be lost by a second laparotomy and occasionally much to be gained.
- Finally, if there is any question of ischaemic intestine, for example in a patient with small bowel obstruction or in a patient with known arteriopathy with abdominal pain, a laparotomy should be considered earlier rather than later.

Is there a medical cause for the acute abdomen?

Several medical conditions can present with abdominal symptoms and signs that are severe enough to precipitate an emergency laparotomy. Any acute cardiopulmonary condition may present with predominantly epigastric or upper abdominal pain. Epigastric pain, usually without tenderness is a common feature of inferior myocardial infarction, while in basal pneumonia or basal infarction due to pulmonary emboli there may be severe tenderness and guarding. Chest radiography and electrocardiography will usually resolve the problem. However linear atelectasis on the radiograph may be due either to pulmonary infarction or to a reaction to problems below the diaphragm.

A young patient with diabetes presenting with keto-acidosis may have impressive abdominal signs and if there is any suggestion of acidosis in such a patient, blood and urine glucose and arterial blood gases must be checked urgently.

Less common medical conditions that occasionally present as emergencies with abdominal pain include sickle cell disease, acute intermittent porphyria, systemic vasculitis, complement C1-esterase inhibitor deficiency and familial Mediterranean fever. Of these porphyria is arguably the most important to consider since mismanagement, particularly administration of inappropriate drugs, is likely to be fatal.

Common errors in diagnosis

- The removal of **a normal appendix** is hardly a catastrophe, but the normal appendicectomy rate should be about 10%, except in young females, among whom it should be possible to reduce this figure by introducing a policy of preliminary laparoscopy.
- Misdiagnosis of **a leaking abdominal aortic aneurysm** for left renal colic is not uncommon, and the abdomen of any patient with acute back pain must be palpated carefully for an aneurysm. A finding of aneurysmal femoral arteries on palpating the groins should alert the clinician to the possibility of an aortic aneurysm.
- A lengthy delay before carrying out a laparotomy in a patient with **intestinal obstruction and/or ischaemia** is potentially disastrous.
- Carrying out a laparotomy in a patient with **colonic pseudo-obstruction** in the belief that the obstruction is mechanical is no longer acceptable. An emergency water-soluble contrast study of the large bowel will often be therapeutic in its own right and should exclude organic obstruction.
- Carrying out a laparotomy in a patient who has **Munchausen's syndrome** is a mistake that often cannot be avoided, but if the syndrome is suspected, telephone calls to neighbouring hospitals may be helpful.
- Failing to diagnose a **femoral hernia** in a patient with small bowel obstruction is unfortunately very common, and usually delays appropriate surgical intervention.

▶ **Commoner medical causes of an acute abdomen**

- Diabetic ketoacidosis
- Inferior myocardial infarction
- Basal pulmonary emboli
- Basal pneumonia

▶ **Further points in the diagnosis of an acute abdomen**

- Intrathoracic oesophageal rupture may present as an acute abdomen
- If a ruptured aortic aneurysm is suspected, an immediate laparotomy with a small risk of a negative finding is preferable to a delay while awaiting further tests
- In intestinal infarction the signs are often unimpressive in the presence of severe symptoms, and air in the portal vein is a grave prognostic sign

CONDITIONS CAUSING ACUTE ABDOMINAL PAIN: NATURAL HISTORY AND MANAGEMENT

Acute appendicitis, appendix abscess and appendix mass

Natural history

Acute appendicitis is a common condition affecting all age groups, the current incidence being approximately 1 in a 1000 per year. It is relatively uncommon at the extremes of life, and there is a peak incidence in the second decade.

AETIOLOGY AND PATHOGENESIS

The aetiology remains unknown, but it seems to be a condition of developed societies, and the pathological process in the organ is often related to luminal obstruction, either by a faecolith or by lymphoid hyperplasia. Occasionally, patients with caecal tumours present with appendicitis after the appendiceal lumen is obstructed by the tumour.

Management

Once acute appendicitis has been diagnosed, an emergency appendicectomy should be carried out without further delay. Appendicectomy is also indicated for those patients in whom there may be some doubt about the diagnosis, but whose right iliac fossa pain and tenderness fail to resolve or worsen with time. Prophylactic antibiotics should be used (usually metronidazole only), and continued if there is considerable peritoneal contamination.

The approach used depends partly on the clinical situation:

- A classical, muscle-splitting oblique incision in the right iliac fossa is used most frequently, affords excellent access, can be extended easily and heals well (**Fig. 2.23**).
- A midline incision is probably wiser in the older patient in whom alternative, more sinister diagnoses are possible.

- In pregnancy, the incision must be sited over the position of maximum tenderness, which depends on the stage of pregnancy and may be in the right upper quadrant.

An appendix abscess should be drained at the time of appendicectomy, and which may be very difficult if the appendix is partially necrotic. The wound should be washed with a suitable antibiotic solution (e.g. tetracycline, 1g in one litre of isotonic saline).

An appendix mass, if diagnosed before the patient is anaesthetised, can be treated conservatively with broad-spectrum antibiotics (e.g. metronidazole and a cephalosporin) and close observation to ensure that it decreases in size. Signs of sepsis, such as a swinging pyrexia, indicating the development of an abscess, should lead to a rejection of the conservative approach in favour of surgery. Persistence of a mass should suggest alternative diagnoses such as Crohn's disease or a caecal tumour. If the patient is already anaesthetised when the mass is first felt, an appendicectomy should still be carried out, but in this situation it is often wise to involve a more senior surgeon because a more extensive procedure might be necessary.

A normal appendix is found in 10% of patients, but should still be removed once the incision has been made. Alternative causes of the problem (e.g. Crohn's disease, *Yersinia* infection, perforated peptic ulcer, cholecystitis, Meckel's diverticulitis or gynaecological problems, particularly on the right side) should be looked for. Some of these alternative causes can be managed conservatively or treated using the same incision, but occasionally a second, usually midline, incision will be necessary. An uncomplicated Meckel's diverticulum should not be interfered with.

Prognosis

Timely surgical intervention has a very high success rate, and usually morbidity and occasional mortality only occur when the diagnosis is delayed.

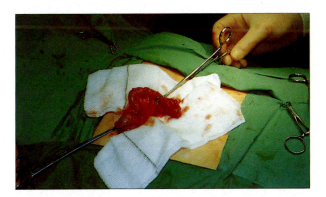

Fig. 2.23 Operative photograph showing an acutely inflamed appendix and caecal pole, delivered through a classical, muscle-splitting incision in the right iliac fossa.

▶ **Important points in the diagnosis and management of appendicitis**

- Leucocytosis is not universal
- Consider laparoscopy in women aged 15–45 years
- In pregnancy, the incision is placed at the site of maximum tenderness
- The diagnosis is most difficult if the patient is mentally subnormal, very young or very old
- If ileal Crohn's disease is discovered, appendicectomy will not affect the risk of fistula formation

Acute cholecystitis, empyema and mucocoele

Natural history

Most people with gallstones are asymptomatic. The most common presentations of patients with symptomatic gallstones seem to be recurrent attacks of biliary colic (a clinical diagnosis) leading ultimately to chronic cholecystitis (a histological diagnosis). However, a small proportion of patients with gallstones present with an acute abdomen secondary to acute cholecystitis or, more often, empyema and possible perforation.

EPIDEMIOLOGY

Gallstones are common and are present in approximately 40% of women and 20% of men by 80 years of age.

AETIOLOGY AND PATHOGENESIS

In the small proportion of patients with gallstones who present with an acute abdomen the cause is usually sudden impaction of a gallstone in the cystic duct, leading to an obstructed gallbladder containing infected bile. A few patients with acute cholecystitis have no gallstones (so-called 'acalculous cholecystitis'), and this often follows a traumatic episode such as an oesophageal resection or major burns, but may also occur in systemic vasculitis.

Management

Conservative measures including intravenous fluids, nil by mouth and (usually) intravenous antibiotics, are commenced for most patients once acute cholecystitis or empyema has been diagnosed clinically. Opiate analgesia is given to control pain until the diagnosis is confirmed. 'Liver function tests' and a serum amylase estimation should be obtained if there is any question of ductal calculi.

A small proportion of patients have signs of peritoneal irritation at presentation and fail to settle with conservative measures. The majority of such patients will require laparotomy and emergency cholecystectomy, possibly before ultrasound confirmation of the diagnosis. A simple cholecystectomy can usually be carried out in such patients because the cystic duct is blocked, but the facility for an on-table cholangiogram should be available, and used if there is any question of ductal stones at laparotomy. This type of emergency surgery (**Fig. 2.24**) can be quite difficult technically, and the technique of simple tube drainage of the gallbladder (cholecystostomy) with extraction of the stones, and formal cholecystectomy at a later date should not be forgotten in a life-threatening situation.

If the diagnosis is confirmed within 5–6 days of the onset of symptoms, there are two possible courses of action:

- Immediate cholecystectomy.
- Continuation of conservative measures with a view to elective cholecystectomy some months later.

Once 7–10 days have elapsed after the onset, urgent surgery becomes difficult and further delay is probably justified to allow the inflammatory process to settle.

In the very acute phase, the surgery is often facilitated by oedema, but it must be stressed that this type of procedure should not be undertaken by inexperienced surgeons.

▶ **Keypoints in biliary tract disease**

- Suppurative cholangitis (a high fever, usually accompanied by jaundice) is an emergency and requires urgent decompression of the biliary system
- Cholangitis is not always accompanied by jaundice (although LFTs, particularly alkaline phosphatase, are nearly always abnormal)
- If acute cholecystitis is diagnosed within 3–4 days of presentation, urgent surgery on the next available list should be considered

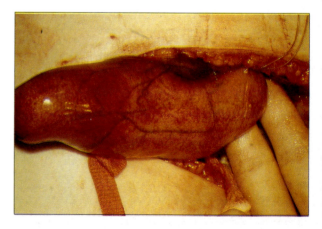

Fig. 2.24. Operative photograph of an emergency cholecystectomy carried out for empyema of the gallbladder.

In practice it is often the availability of an operating theatre and/or a suitably experienced surgeon that limits the role of urgent surgery in this situation, but reducing the number and length of admissions for an individual patient can have advantages, both for the patient and hospital.

A laparoscopic approach, either in the emergency situation or subsequently in the elective situation, has been advocated by some authors. The extent to which this technique is used will in general be dictated by the experience of the operator.

One useful tip in the emergency situation is to aspirate the gallbladder at the start of the procedure, either open or laparoscopic, to facilitate traction and dissection. Again, the extent to which cholangiography or choledochoscopy are used will depend on the individual situation, but one or other facility should be available.

Ascending cholangitis
Parenteral fluids and antibiotics are commenced early for the patient with ascending cholangitis, but the single most important aspect is drainage of the common bile duct, usually by emergency ERCP with endoscopic sphincterotomy and extraction of stones. In those few patients in which endoscopic drainage of the common bile duct is not possible, open surgical drainage may be required, but it carries a significantly higher mortality of (1–10%) than that associated with the endoscopic approach (0.5%). The requirement for later surgery to remove the gallbladder from which the ductal stones presumably originated is not universal, and generally the decision to recommend cholecystectomy in such a patient

can be taken on the basis of the presence or absence of ongoing biliary colic and/or cholecystitis.

NON-SURGICAL TECHNIQUES FOR TREATING GALLSTONES
Various non-surgical techniques have been described for treating gallstones including percutaneous removal, gallstone dissolution and extracorporeal shock-wave lithotripsy. None have a specific role in the management of the acute problem, and indeed are now used less frequently, particularly since the advent of laparoscopic cholecystectomy.

Acute pancreatitis
Natural history
Approximately 80% of patients with acute pancreatitis have a relatively mild and self-limiting illness. The remaining patients may follow a relatively stormy course with multisystem organ failure, pancreatic necrosis, pseudocyst or abscess formation, and a significant eventual mortality, which rises to 50% if a pancreatic abscess develops (Figs 2.25 and 2.26).

A combination of criteria, particularly age, hypoxaemia, hyperglycaemia, hypocalcaemia, neutrophil leucocytosis and abnormal hepatocellular enzymes provide a guide to the severity of the attack.

Gallstone-related disease may recur as acute attacks on an occasional basis, presumably as stones pass down the common bile duct, until the underlying biliary disease is corrected. Alcohol-related pancreatitis typically slips into a subacute/chronic form, which tends to be exacerbated by alcoholic binges.

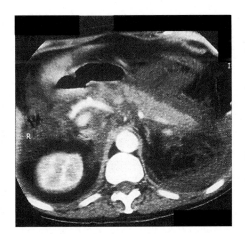
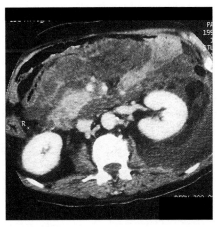

Fig. 2.25 Emergency, contrast-enhanced CT scan of the abdomen in severe acute pancreatitis, showing that most of the gland is perfused (far left), but there is extensive necrosis (arrowed) extending posteriorly to the left kidney (left).

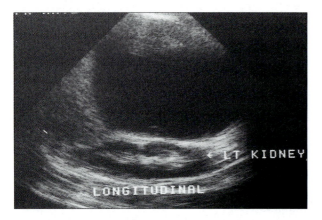

Fig. 2.26 Longitudinal ultrasound scan of the left upper quadrant of the abdomen showing a large pseudocyst (with some debris posteriorly) lying within the lesser sac, immediately anterior to the left kidney.

AETIOLOGY AND PATHOGENESIS

Causes of acute pancreatitis include the following:

- Gallstones, which are the most common aetiological factor in the UK, accounting for approximately 60% of cases.
- Alcohol, which is the cause in approximately 30% of patients.
- A variety of conditions such as certain viral illnesses (notably mumps), some drugs (e.g. corticosteroids, aza-thioprine and diuretics), hypercalcaemia, hypertri-glyceridaemia and some familial metabolic disorders are associated, usually with less severe forms of the disease.
- ERCP is complicated by a 3% risk of acute pancreatitis, which is usually mild, but may be severe, particularly if infection has been introduced.

▶ **Significant prognostic factors in acute pancreatitis within the first 48 hours**

The presence of three or more of the following factors can be considered to define a 'severe' attack (from Imrie et al. 1978)

- Older than 55 years of age
- WBC > 15×10^9/l
- Blood glucose > 10 mmol/l
- Urea > 16 mmol/l
- p_aO_2 < 8 kPa
- Serum calcium < 2.0 mmol/l
- Serum albumin < 32 g/l
- Serum lactate dehydrogenase > 600 u/l
- Aspartate transaminase/alanine transaminase > 100 u/l

▶ **Diagnosis of acute pancreatitis**

- Vomiting is common
- The pain may be eased by sitting forwards
- Serum amylase estimation is limited because:
  - It has a sensitivity of 80%
  - It has limited specificity (many other conditions cause modest elevations)
  - Associated hyperlipidaemia may interfere with the assay
  - 1–2% of the normal population have persistently high levels of serum amylase due to the presence of an abnormal protein, which is not readily excreted (i.e. macroamylasaemia)
  - Serum amylase concentration does not equate with severity of disease
- Persistent hyperamylasaemia after an attack of pancreatitis suggests pseudocyst development

It has been postulated that gallstone-related pancreatitis results from the reflux of infected bile into the pancreatic duct, but how the other forms of pancreatitis fit into this model is not clear.

Management

Management depends on the severity of the disease:

- A patient with mild acute pancreatitis may require almost no specific treatment.
- A patient with severe acute pancreatitis may require major ventilatory, circulatory and renal support.

Universal measures include bed rest, nil by mouth and an intravenous infusion with appropriate analgesia. This is followed by an assessment of severity, which will include blood tests for a full blood count, urea and electrolytes, 'liver function tests,' serum calcium, amylase, sugar and blood gases.

Blood gas estimation is particularly important because severe hypoxaemia is not uncommon and may not be easy to recognise clinically. It presumably reflects physiological shunting as part of the syndrome of acute adult respiratory distress syndrome, which is a common consequence of severe pancreatitis.

Routine monitoring is commenced and may be extended to include regular assessments of central venous pressure and pulmonary artery wedge pressure, depending on the severity of the attack. Plain films of the chest and abdomen should be obtained early. Pleural effusion and pulmonary oedema are features of severe pancreatitis.

A nasogastric tube should be inserted if the duodenal ileus is severe and vomiting is a problem. A broad-spectrum antibiotic such as ciprofloxacin may be given in what is thought to gallstone-related disease, though evidence for its efficacy is lacking. The clinical progress of the patient will dictate the need for oxygen therapy and for the infusion of potentially large volumes of both crystalloid and colloid solutions to maintain central venous pressure and urine output. Hypovolaemia may be severe and a common, but serious, error is an underestimation of fluid requirements, which may reach many litres in the first 24 hours.

Deteriorating respiratory function may require intensive care nursing and possible intubation with mechanically assisted ventilation. A labile blood pressure, cardiac output and peripheral vascular resistance may require inotropic support, while a renal dose of dopamine may be required to maintain an adequate urine output. Ultimately, dialysis may be required.

If the patient suffers a protracted ileus with ongoing obstruction to the duodenum, a period of parenteral nutrition may also be needed.

DETECTING PANCREATIC NECROSIS

Detecting pancreatic necrosis early during the course of a severe attack is not easy.

- An estimation of CRP provides a rather nonspecific marker, a level higher than 100 mg/l at 48 hours being a bad prognostic sign.
- The investigation of choice is probably an intravenous contrast-enhanced CT scan of the abdomen, since necrotic areas of the gland are not perfused and will not therefore enhance. There has, however, been recent concern that the contrast material may itself exacerbate pancreatitis, so this procedure should be used sparingly in those patients at highest risk who are most likely to benefit from surgical intervention.

Infected necrosis can be detected by ultrasound or CT-guided needle aspiration, and represents a significant worsening in the prognosis, being associated with a mortality of up to 50%. Broad-spectrum parenteral antibiotics should be commenced, and surgical intervention should be seriously considered because it offers the only real hope of survival once infection has complicated the situation.

ROLE OF SURGERY

The role of surgery in the management of acute pancreatitis is controversial. Simple peritoneal lavage with or without a formal laparotomy has produced rather negative results. The decision to abandon conservative measures in favour of an aggressive surgical approach in the patient with necrotising pancreatitis is still made largely on clinical grounds, usually when and if the patient begins to show signs of sepsis. A reasonable practice is to defer surgery as long as possible in the absence of sepsis, but to undertake a laparotomy and necrosectomy as soon as sepsis becomes apparent. Formal

pancreatic resection in the emergency situation is extremely difficult and dangerous, whereas blunt necrosectomy can be relatively straightforward if sufficient time has elapsed since the start of the illness for viable and non-viable pancreas to be delineated adequately. External drains laid into the lesser sac, through which continuous lavage can be carried out, are also considered to be important.

The treatment of pancreatic abscesses, which are an occasional late complication of a severe attack of pancreatitis (not necessarily with frank necrosis at the time), follows essentially similar lines: adequate localisation, formal drainage at laparotomy and lavage, though formal necrosectomy is not usually required.

In gallstone-related disease, a decision has to be made about the management of both the gallbladder and the common bile duct because a surgical approach for both may not be necessary. The first important factor to consider is that the gallstones responsible for pancreatitis are usually very small, and may be quite difficult to detect by conventional means such as ultrasonography. Scans negative for stones in the acute stage should be repeated at 6–8 weeks since this will detect a significant proportion of the stones that are not seen initially.

Assuming a diagnosis of gallstone-related disease, the conventional approach has been to carry out a formal cholecystectomy some weeks or even months later, risking a further attack in the interim. For the patient with mild disease that settles rapidly, semi-elective surgery (as for acute cholecystitis or biliary colic) is a reasonable option, and should include formal operative cholangiography or choledochoscopy with duct exploration if ductal stones are found.

Surgical intervention may also be required for the patient with persistent hyperamylasaemia and pain who has been shown to have developed a pseudocyst, though the majority of these can be drained adequately to the exterior under ultrasound control.

URGENT ERCP WITH ENDOSCOPIC SPHINCTEROTOMY

For patients with more severe gallstone-related acute pancreatitis who fail to settle, there is much to commend an urgent ERCP with endoscopic sphincterotomy to clear the distal common bile duct, not least because it avoids a formal laparotomy in an unstable and precariously balanced patient. Assuming endoscopic sphincterotomy cures the immediate problem, the decision to recommend further elective surgery for the gallbladder stones is one that must be made on the basis of the patient's continuing symptoms, since it may well not be necessary, particularly for elderly patients.

There is evidence that very early ERCP carried out within the first 72 hours improves the outcome in gallstone-related pancreatitis because many patients still have an impacted common bile duct stone at that time. If an impacted stone is removed early in the course of an attack the result can occasionally be dramatic, with a rapid resolution of symptoms.

Perforated viscus

Spontaneous perforation of the gastrointestinal tract is a surgical emergency that most often presents as an acute abdominal condition, though oesophageal perforation may occasionally present with predominantly cardiorespiratory symptoms and signs, and perforation below the diaphragm is sometimes entirely silent. The natural history and management will obviously vary according to the site involved, and this section has therefore been divided along simple anatomical lines.

General management

Once visceral perforation has been diagnosed or is considered to be the most likely underlying problem, initial management is similar irrespective of the suspected site of perforation. It is directed at correcting the constitutional disturbance before surgery, since surgical intervention will be recommended for all but a few patients.

Having obtained the usual baseline blood tests (i.e. full blood count, urea and electrolytes, amylase, and group and save serum), oral intake is discontinued and an intravenous infusion commenced, the rapidity of fluid replacement being dictated by the clinical situation.

Broad-spectrum intravenous antibiotics (such as gentamicin and/or cephalosporin with an anti-anaerobic agent) are started immediately (after blood has been taken for peripheral blood cultures), and a urinary catheter is placed to monitor urine output.

Routine observation of pulse, blood pressure, respiratory rate and urine output is then commenced and repeated frequently, depending on the clinical situation. The endotoxaemia and septic shock that can accompany faecal peritonitis may make it necessary to place a right heart and/or pulmonary artery catheter, particularly if there is any pre-existing cardiorespiratory disease such as valvular heart disease or congestive failure.

Pharmacological support in the form of pressor agents such as dopamine may be required to maintain urine output so that it exceeds 50 ml/hour or to sustain an adequate systolic blood pressure (higher than 100 mm Hg).

Facilities for intensive care nursing may be required, and arrangements are probably best made before operation.

Oesophageal perforation

Natural history

Non-instrumental oesophageal perforation (Boerhaave's syndrome) typically occurs in a patient who has over-indulged in food and/or alcohol and results from vomiting against a closed glottis.

A sudden severe chest pain and shortness of breath after vomiting should alert the clinician to the possibility of an oesophageal perforation, but the degree of prostration may confuse the issue and point towards alternative diagnoses such as acute myocardial infarction. Such patients may present with an acute abdomen and rigidity and the possibility of an oesophageal perforation may only be considered after a negative laparotomy. If the diagnosis is in doubt, a contrast swallow will confirm it.

The importance of the cardinal physical sign of subcutaneous emphysema, usually in the neck, but occasionally elsewhere, and also seen in the mediastinum on the chest radiograph, cannot be overstated.

Rapidly advancing respiratory embarrassment is typical, with the development of a hydropneumothorax, more often on the left side than on the right.

Management

Early recognition of oesophageal perforation is vitally important. The measures described above in 'General management' are obviously important initially, but placement of an intercostal drainage tube may also be required with some urgency because a tension pneumothorax is an occasional problem. The drainage tube will also remove some of the food debris contaminating the pleural cavity, and may be required bilaterally. At this stage a decision will have to be made about the advisability of transferring the patient to a specialised thoracic unit, depending on the availability of such a unit, the expertise of the local surgeons and the effectiveness of resuscitation.

For the surgical approach, it is best to open the left chest to approach the distal oesophagus because this is the most common site of perforation in Boerhaave's syndrome. If the perforation is recognised early and surgery is carried out within 24 hours, a primary repair may be attempted. The muscular tear must be extended and the oesophagus repaired in layers with non-absorbable material, the repair being buttressed with a patch of intercostal muscle or a 360° fundoplication.

If surgery is late, the only realistic option is to resect the partially necrotic oesophagus and to carry out an extensive debridement and lavage of the pleural cavity.

Whether or not reconstruction is attempted immediately will depend on the local surgical expertise and the condition of the patient, in the knowledge that reconstruction as a secondary procedure is likely to be difficult.

If reconstruction is attempted immediately, the intrathoracic stomach will probably be the organ of choice, but if it is attempted late, the transposed colon placed in the anterior mediastinum is most likely to be successful. In either event anastomoses placed in the neck are more likely to heal, and cause least problems if they do not heal, than those within the contaminated thoracic cavity.

A limited case can be made for aggressive conservative management using combined suction drainage of the pleural cavities and the oesophagus, but it tends to be reserved for patients whose prognosis is very poor from the outset. Furthermore, the pleural cavity obviously cannot be debrided if the chest is not opened, and such debridement constitutes a significant part of the conventional surgical approach.

PROGNOSIS

The prognosis of oesophageal perforation is relatively poor, with a mortality up to 50%, largely due to gross contamination of the mediastinum and pleural cavities.

Gastric and duodenal perforation
NATURAL HISTORY

The patient with gastric or duodenal perforation presents with sudden severe epigastric pain with involuntary guarding. Shoulder tip pain represents subdiaphragmatic irritation, while appendicitis is sometimes simulated by the leakage of gastric contents into the right paracolic gutter. The constitutional disturbance can vary enormously, from no disturbance to severe prostration with dehydration, oliguria and hypotension. Occasionally a patient has a silent perforation, and has no symptoms or signs.

AETIOLOGY AND PATHOGENESIS

Most perforations of the stomach and duodenum are due to peptic ulceration, but occasionally a gastric neoplasm presents in this way. Young dyspeptic men who smoke are still seen with an acute perforation of an anterior duodenal ulcer, but are now outnumbered by elderly women with an acute perforation of a gastric ulcer, almost all of whom give a history of taking NSAIDs.

MANAGEMENT AND PROGNOSIS

Having demonstrated a perforation of the stomach or duodenum, a surgical approach is adopted almost universally. **Conservative (non-operative) management** of perforated peptic ulcer is currently reserved for the following groups of patients:

- Patients who refuse surgery.
- Patients who are so compromised that any form of surgical intervention would be extremely hazardous.
- Patients who are well and whose perforation can be demonstrated to be well localised using contrast studies.

A non-operative approach of course risks missing an alternative diagnosis such as perforated diverticular disease.

Some knowledge of the probable natural history of the underlying problem influences the type of surgery carried out because antisecretory and proton pump-inhibiting agents are now so powerful and effective that a minimalist approach to surgery is often adopted. Simple closure of the perforation is preferred rather than a surgical procedure designed to cure the ulcer.

Which operation for perforated gastric ulcer?

Patients at greatest risk should in general receive the simplest procedure, which is usually an oversew of the perforation with a wedge biopsy if there is a gastric ulcer. In the absence of risk factors such as advanced age or coexistent major cardiorespiratory disease, definitive ulcer-curing surgery can be safely carried out. However, given the current availability of powerful and effective agents such as H_2 antagonists and proton pump blockers, many surgeons adopt a minimalist surgical approach for all patients with perforated ulcers. The elective operation of choice for gastric ulcer is a Billroth I gastrectomy, but as most patients with a perforated gastric ulcer are relatively frail and elderly, biopsies from the ulcer or even ulcer excision, plus simple closure and postoperative H_2 antagonists will be used almost universally. If malignant perforation cannot be excluded, a Billroth II gastrectomy might be more appropriate, but most patients will not be suitable for such a radical approach in the emergency setting. The prognosis for perforated gastric carcinoma is universally poor anyway because it has usually spread to the peritoneal surface and throughout the peritoneal cavity .

Which operation for perforated duodenal ulcer?

The situation for a perforated duodenal ulcer is a little more complicated, partly because most patients are younger and reasonably fit. Ulcer-curing surgery obviously takes longer, and is therefore probably associated with an increased immediate morbidity, but simple ulcer closure itself is not without morbidity, and the risks to the patient from reperforation or bleeding after closure are considerable. Up to 50% of patients with a perforated chronic ulcer (though it is not always possible to be sure that the ulcer is chronic at the time of surgery) will need long-term treatment postoperatively or even elective surgery at a later date after simple closure, and a small proportion of these patients will suffer a further life-threatening complication such as bleeding or gastric outlet obstruction.

The long-term morbidity associated with ulcer-curing surgery must also be remembered, since a proportion of patients will develop disabling symptoms such as post-vagotomy diarrhoea, dumping, or even recurrent ulceration. It is also an unfortunate truism that the less likely a particular procedure is to give rise to disabling long-term morbidity (e.g. highly selective vagotomy), the higher the rate of recurrent ulceration. However, with all this in mind, there will be some patients with a perforation due to a chronic duodenal ulcer who will benefit from an ulcer-curing operation in the emergency setting, and the important consideration then is the availability of a suitably experienced surgeon to carry out the procedure.

Some centres are now reporting encouraging results treating duodenal perforation laparoscopically, but this is still experimental.

Small bowel perforation

The natural history of small bowel perforation depends entirely on the underlying diagnosis, which can be extremely varied. The patient usually presents with diffuse abdominal pain and generalised peritonitis, with a variable degree of systemic disturbance. It should be remembered that the condition found to be causing the perforation at the initial laparotomy may affect other parts of the gastrointestinal tract to a lesser degree, and this will obviously influence the long-term outlook.

MANAGEMENT

Small bowel perforation is managed by laparotomy and intestinal resection. The extent of the resection will be determined by the operative findings, the single most important consideration being the preservation of an adequate vascular supply to the bowel ends used for the anastomosis. A conservative approach to the surgery for small bowel Crohn's disease is considered wise, with limited resection if possible (**Figs 2.27**).

Other technical points that can be useful in the surgical management of the patient with a small bowel perforation include:

- The use of defunctioning stomas as a temporary measure rather than an immediate anastomosis when the extent of peritoneal contamination is considered excessive.
- The use of a 'second-look' laparotomy at approximately 48 hours postoperatively if the initial presentation has been caused by diffuse vasculitis or ischaemia. A further resection can be undertaken if necessary before reperforation occurs.

The prognosis will depend entirely on the underlying pathological diagnosis.

Large bowel perforation

NATURAL HISTORY

Patients whose diverticular perforation is initially well-localised may present with an area of well-defined tenderness and a possible mass ('acute diverticulitis'); sudden deterioration with spreading peritonitis at a later stage suggests a communication with the peritoneal cavity. Patients with frank faecal contamination of the peritoneal cavity present with lower abdominal peritonitis and commonly a severe constitutional upset, and the decision to recommend a surgical approach is not usually difficult.

Investigations may be relatively unhelpful, but there may be a leucocytosis, and free intraperitoneal gas may be seen on an erect chest radiograph. Urgent contrast studies have

▶ **Arguments for and against definitive anti-ulcer surgery for perforated peptic ulcer**

For	Against
Lower risk of recurrence, bleeding, stenosis	Higher morbidity/mortality in sick patients
Adequate histology of gastric ulcer	Higher long-term morbidity (dumping and diarrhoea)
Avoids long-term therapy	Medical therapy highly effective
	High incidence of ulcer recurrence after highly selective vagotomy

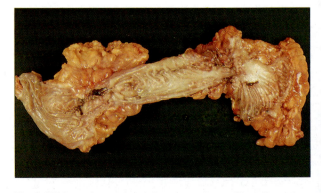

Fig. 2.27 Operative specimen of a conservative small bowel resection carried out for perforated Crohn's disease showing limited clearance of grossly involved bowel.

no role in acute perforation, but if there is some doubt about the diagnosis a water-soluble contrast study may be helpful.

Aetiology

In developed countries large bowel perforation is usually secondary to diverticular disease or a carcinoma. There may therefore be a previous history of diverticular disease or carcinoma, or even a contrast study suggesting diverticular disease or an ongoing investigation of altered bowel habit or anaemia suggesting the presence of an underlying neoplasm.

MANAGEMENT AND PROGNOSIS

The success of the therapeutic approach to large bowel perforation depends almost entirely on the ability to control the gross sepsis that usually complicates the condition. The long-term prognosis of perforated diverticular disease should be excellent if sepsis is controlled and the patient survives the initial surgical procedure, although all subsequent procedures will have their own inherent operative morbidity and mortality.

The risk of recurrent disease is high for patients with perforated carcinoma of the colon and higher than the risk for patients with non-perforated carcinoma of the colon at the same Dukes' stage. This is possibly related to the spillage of tumour cells into the general peritoneal cavity through the perforation.

However, not all colonic perforations associated with tumours occur at the site of the tumour. If there is large bowel obstruction, perforation may occur in the segment immediately proximal to the tumour ('stercoral' perforation) if it is caused by impacted faeces, or in the caecum; here the large bowel's diameter increases most rapidly in obstruction.

Other pathological processes that occasionally give rise to large bowel perforation include isolated caecal diverticulitis, which is usually indistinguishable from appendicitis, mesenteric vascular occlusion and unresolved sigmoid (or caecal) volvulus. Occasionally patients with acute inflammatory bowel disease (e.g. Crohn's disease, ulcerative colitis or psuedomembranous colitis) present with large bowel perforation, but it is rare for there not be some suggestive previous history (**Fig 2.28**).

Finally, infective causes such as amoebiasis should not be forgotten if the patient is from a developing country or has recently returned from abroad.

Acute diverticulitis

Patients presenting with an acute paracolic mass (acute diverticulitis) can usually be managed conservatively with nil by mouth and intravenous broad-spectrum antibiotics such as metronidazole and a cephalosporin, and investigated at leisure by ultrasonography and by contrast radiology using a water-soluble agent. The decision to recommend surgery is made on the basis of the patient's general condition and the

▶ **Conditions associated with small bowel perforation (from Taylor, 1992)**

Mechanical	Strangulating obstruction Foreign body Trauma (blunt/penetrating)
Idiopathic	'Non-specific' ulceration
Drug-induced	Potassium supplements NSAIDs Corticosteroids Chemotherapeutic agents
Inflammatory	Jejuno-ileal diverticula Meckel's diverticulum Crohn's disease Zollinger–Ellison syndrome Coeliac disease
Neoplastic	Primary and secondary carcinomas Lymphomas Leukaemias Carcinoid tumours
Infective	Typhoid Tuberculosis
Parasitic	Ascariasis
Vascular (arterial/venous)	Mesenteric infarction
Connective tissue disorders	Polyarteritis nodosa Systemic lupus erythematosus Wegener's granulomatosis Scleroderma Rheumatoid arthritis
Metabolic	Amyloidosis
Iatrogenic	Operative injury Radiation damage

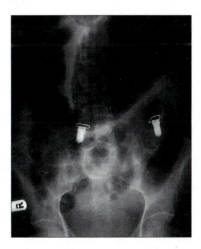

Fig. 2.28 Supine abdominal radiograph of a patient with toxic megacolon secondary to Crohn's colitis and found to be perforated at laparotomy.

degree of continuing disability: usually a simple resection and primary anastomosis will suffice, but is often not necessary.

Fistula formation will usually precipitate an earlier operation and when associated with frank sepsis, the formation of a temporary stoma might be considered safer than a primary anastomosis. If a large inflammatory mass is found at laparotomy without evidence of free perforation, simple drainage is an option, with further assessment and possible elective excisional surgery at a later date. Resection and primary anastomosis can usually be performed if sepsis and faecal loading are not prominent. Temporary stoma formation and on-table antegrade lavage (**Fig. 2.29**) are alternative techniques depending on the clinical situation.

If there is a frank perforation with purulent or faecal peritonitis, primary resection of the involved segment is the procedure of choice, with extensive peritoneal lavage using a suitable topical antibiotic solution such as tetracycline. A Hartmann's procedure with a left iliac fossa sigmoid colostomy and oversewing of the rectal stump is the procedure of choice for faecal peritonitis, but a case can be made for a primary anastomosis in purulent peritonitis. Again if faecal loading is a problem, on-table lavage can be carried out, and the anastomosis protected by a temporary loop ileostomy if necessary.

The classical three-stage approach with a laparotomy, drainage and loop transverse colostomy as the initial procedure is no longer considered appropriate because of poor overall results and the failure of many patients to progress through all three stages.

Primary excisional surgery may be technically demanding, and the availability of a suitably trained and competent surgeon is essential.

The formation of a mucus fistula through the lower end of the abdominal incision facilitates finding the rectal stump at the second procedure, but almost always requires rectal mobilisation to bring the proximal rectum to the abdominal wall, and can complicate matters enormously by forming extensive pelvic adhesions. Simple oversewing of the rectum, therefore, has much to recommend it.

Solitary caecal diverticula are adequately managed by simple excision and closure, but in the emergency situation in which the diverticulum is acutely inflamed and possibly perforated, it is often impossible to differentiate it from a caecal carcinoma. It is therefore wiser to carry out a formal right colectomy if there is any doubt about the diagnosis, with primary anastomosis between ileum and transverse colon.

Perforated colon carcinomas should be resected if at all possible. This may involve the in-continuity resection of adjacent organs such as small bowel or uterus, but the palliation achieved by resection is likely to be far superior to that achieved with lesser surgical procedures.

Perforated proximal colonic neoplasms can almost always be resected with primary anastomosis, but a Hartmann's resection is more appropriate for tumours in the sigmoid colon and rectum with extensive contamination, although on-table lavage and primary anastomosis is also a possibility.

▶ **Intestinal perforation**

- 30% of patients with upper gastrointestinal perforation have no free gas on their admission chest radiograph
- Use urgent contrast studies with water-soluble contrast when in doubt
- Subcutaneous emphysema in the neck is the cardinal sign of oesophageal perforation
- Warn patients with lower gastrointestinal perforations pre-operatively about the possible need for an intestinal stoma

▶ **Acute diverticulitis**

- Inspect the chest radiograph for subdiaphragmatic gas indicating perforation
- In the absence of perforation, treat with broad-spectrum antibiotics initially
- Care is needed if flexible sigmoidoscopy or contrast enema studies are performed as the bowel may easily perforate

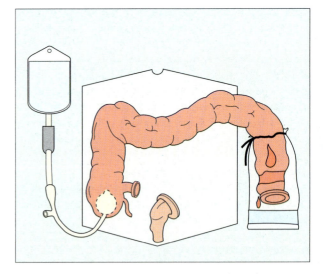

Fig. 2.29 Diagram of on-table antegrade lavage, with a catheter inserted into the caecum and warmed saline being used to flush faecal contents from the proximal colon into a collecting device. The pathological segment (containing the area of diverticular disease or an obstructing carcinoma) is resected after lavage has been completed. This technique is useful if there is possible perforation or ischaemia when conventional bowel preparation would be unsafe.

A second-look laparotomy at 48 hours is occasionally indicated if there are any doubts about the viability of the remaining colon. A subtotal colectomy and ileostomy is usually the only safe option for colonic perforation secondary to acute inflammatory bowel disease, leaving the closed rectal stump *in situ* to preserve surgical options for a later procedure.

Intestinal obstruction

The clinical approach to intestinal obstruction follows well-established lines, and may be summarised in a series of short questions, the answers providing a suitable framework for subsequent management.

A step-by-step approach to intestinal obstruction

IS THERE SYSTEMIC DISTURBANCE?

Hypovolaemia may be due to either fluid sequestration in the obstructed gut or fluid lost to the exterior as vomitus. It tends to be more marked if the obstruction is more proximal, and needs to be corrected as quickly as possible if surgical intervention is contemplated.

IS THERE ISCHAEMIC BOWEL?

There is no single investigation that is reliable in this situation. Local tenderness may be the only sign. Elevation of blood phosphate and lactate tend to be unreliable. A high index of suspicion is important because delaying surgical intervention until after an ischaemic loop has perforated is to court disaster.

WHAT IS THE LEVEL OF THE OBSTRUCTION?

Proximal obstruction can usually be distinguished from distal obstruction by carefully interpreted plain radiographs. If there is uncertainty, contrast studies, usually with barium and not water-soluble contrast, may be helpful.

WHAT IS THE PROBABLE UNDERLYING DIAGNOSIS?

Adhesions and hernias are the most common causes of small bowel obstruction, and large bowel carcinomas are the most common cause of large bowel obstruction. The precise diagnosis may be relatively unimportant in the initial management because most of these patients should have an early laparotomy and definitive surgery.

Causes of intestinal obstruction

ADHESIONS

If the patient has had previous abdominal surgery, adhesive obstruction is a probable cause of small bowel obstruction, but if the original surgery was for a malignant process, recurrent disease causing obstruction should also be considered. It is often not possible to differentiate between these two situations until the abdomen is re-opened.

If adhesive obstruction is confidently diagnosed and there are no features to suggest ischaemia, a 24-hour period of conservative measures including nasogastric aspiration, intravenous fluids and careful observation, is reasonable before re-operating if there is no improvement. Repeated plain abdominal radiographs can be helpful in this situation. The only real exceptions are:

- The patient who has had multiple previous laparotomies for adhesive small bowel obstruction and has known extensive adhesions, when procrastination beyond 24 hours may be justified.
- The patient with known peritoneal metastases for whom surgery will rarely improve the situation.

▶ **Step by step approach to intestinal obstruction**

- Is obstruction present (based on the history, examination, plain radiographs and contrast studies)?
- Is there evidence of a systemic effect (e.g. hypotension, tachycardia or oliguria)?
- Is there evidence of intestinal ischaemia?
- What is the level of the obstruction?
- What is the cause of the obstruction?

▶ **Diagnosis and initial managment of intestinal obstruction**

- Contrast studies are needed to differentiate pseudo-obstruction and mechanical large bowel obstruction
- Small bowel loops with a diameter larger than 2.5 cm or colon with a diameter larger than 7 cm together with a paucity of gas distally show a high specificity for a diagnosis of obstruction
- Erect abdominal radiographs are usually unnecessary
- It is dangerous to anaesthetise an obstructed patient without first placing a nasogastric tube
- Femoral hernia is a commonly missed cause of small bowel obstruction

HERNIAS

Hernias are the second most common cause of small bowel obstruction, and need to be actively looked for because occasionally the patient is unaware of their presence, particularly the elderly obese female with a small femoral hernia, which can be easily missed. Severe local tenderness, a lack of bowel sounds or cough impulse and a recent change in the character of the hernia such as a rapid enlargement are all features suggesting that the hernia is the cause of the problem.

Internal hernias (e.g. in the paraduodenal fossae or sacral foramina) are occasional causes of small bowel obstruction and will not become apparent until the time of surgery.

OTHER CAUSES OF SMALL BOWEL OBSTRUCTION

The patient presenting with small bowel obstruction *de novo*, who has had no previous surgery and has no obvious hernia, presents an interesting clinical challenge, which is usually resolved fairly rapidly by surgical intervention.

The range of diagnostic possibilities here is very wide, with common diagnoses being Crohn's disease, a tumour of the small bowel (e.g. a benign polyp, carcinoma, lymphoma or carcinoid) or large bowel (e.g. caecal carcinoma), or an inflammatory process involving the small bowel loops such as appendicitis, acute diverticular disease, gynaecological sepsis and endometriosis.

Therapeutic abdomino-pelvic irradiation occasionally causes significant small bowel damage, the end result often being extensive stricture formation and small bowel obstruction. This can be a difficult situation to deal with because the damage is often widespread. The combination of small bowel obstruction and gas in the biliary tree on abdominal radiography is usually caused by gallstone ileus (**Figs 2.30–2.33**).

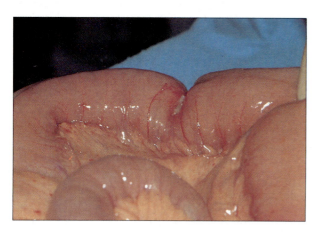

Fig. 2.30 Operative photograph of primary adenocarcinoma of the small bowel causing complete small bowel obstruction.

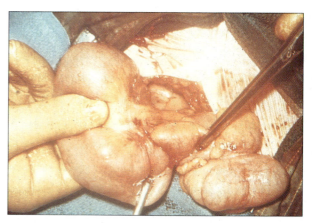

Fig. 2.31 Operative photograph showing a small bowel stricture secondary to endometriosis.

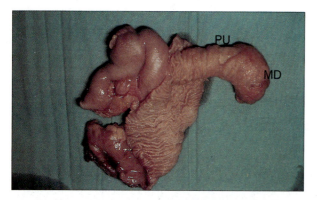

Fig. 2.32 Operative specimen of partly opened resected small bowel showing an inverted Meckel's diverticulum (MD), which had caused an intussusception and subsequent acute small bowel obstruction. The patient had previously suffered lower intestinal bleeding and a large peptic ulcer (PU) adjacent to ectopic gastric mucosa can also be seen.

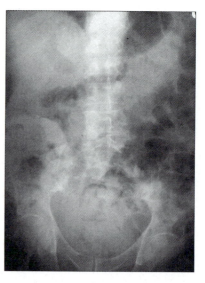

Fig. 2.33 Supine abdominal radiograph showing dilated small bowel loops and gas in the common bile duct in a patient with gallstone ileus.

COMMON CONDITIONS OTHER THAN COLORECTAL CANCER LEADING TO LARGE BOWEL OBSTRUCTION

Common conditions other than colorectal cancer leading to large bowel obstruction include volvulus (of the sigmoid or, less commonly, the caecum) and occasionally, acute diverticular disease. Once diagnosed, resection is indicated almost universally. The older procedures of operative detorsion and fixation of large bowel loops ('pexy') have fallen from favour because the results of resection are much more satisfactory. Diverticular disease causing large bowel obstruction is usually a good indication for surger (if only to exclude a co-existing neoplasm), but it may settle with conservative measures,. Occasional rarities such as colonic lipomas may present with large bowel obstruction (**Figs 2.34–2.36.**).

PSEUDO-OBSTRUCTION

Pseudo-obstruction is poorly understood and may mimic mechanical large bowel obstruction, both radiologically and clinically. A contrast study is important to confirm or refute mechanical obstruction before surgery, as surgical intervention will not help a patient with pseudo-obstruction.

Pseudo-obstruction usually occurs in elderly patients who are unwell for some other reason, such as an acute myocardial infarction or a recent orthopaedic procedure, or who have an underlying biochemical abnormality such as hypokalaemia.

Management of intestinal obstruction

Once a diagnosis of intestinal obstruction has been confirmed and the volume deficit replaced, which may require placement of a central venous line and urinary catheter depending on the extent of systemic disturbance, early surgical intervention is the mainstay of treatment, given the few exceptions discussed above. A nasogastric tube must be passed before any attempt to anaesthetise the patient because aspiration pneumonitis is a very real danger.

A midline abdominal incision is most useful for idiopathic and adhesive intestinal obstruction, particularly if this approach was used for the previous surgery. Whatever pathology is found must be dealt with on merit:

- Excisional surgery in **Crohn's disease** must be kept to a minimum and a case can be made for simply closing the abdomen and instituting maximum dose medical treatment (including steroids) in the hope that the obstructive element will settle as the inflammatory process is brought under control.

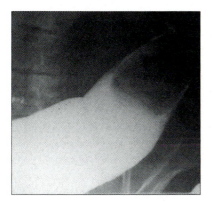
Fig. 2.34 Urgent single-contrast barium enema demonstrating a large filling defect in the sigmoid colon obstructing the passage of the barium more proximally.

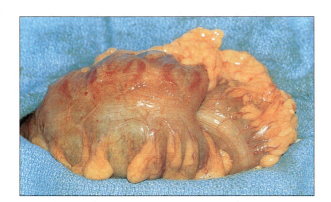
Fig. 2.35 Operative photograph of the patient whose barium enema is shown in Fig. 2.34, showing an intussuscepting tumour of the sigmoid colon causing intermittent large bowel obstruction.

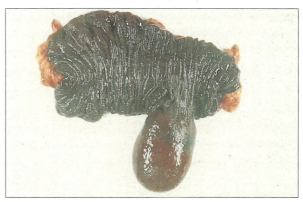
Fig. 2.36 Operative specimen from the patient featured in Figs 2.34 and 2.35, showing a large submucosal lipoma of the colon, which had been causing incomplete large bowel obstruction. The colonic mucosa also shows gross melanosis due to laxative abuse.

- In patients with **inactive Crohn's disease** in whom short fibrous strictures are the cause of the obstruction (**Fig. 2.37**), strictureplasty (i.e. a longitudinal enterotomy across the stricture, closed transversely) may be useful.
- In **adhesive obstruction** simple division of adhesions is usually all that is required, and even bowel that appears non-viable on first inspection will usually reperfuse adequately once the obstruction has been dealt with.
- Frankly **gangrenous bowel** must be resected, but is relatively uncommon.
- **Inguinal hernias** causing small bowel obstruction are generally dealt with satisfactorily using a standard groin approach and if resection becomes necessary it can usually be achieved through the same incision, simply by dilating the neck of the usually indirect hernial sac. Occasionally a second incision is needed to carry out the resection and a low midline approach is usual in this situation.
- If the problem is confidently diagnosed preoperatively as small bowel obstruction related to a **femoral hernia**, the low approach should be abandoned in favour of a midline abdominal incision from the outset, with an extra-peritoneal approach to the femoral canal. Exposure of the femoral canal (bilaterally, if necessary) is far superior from above, facilitating the performance of the repair and the bowel resection through the same incision.
- Management of obstruction related to **other pathological processes**, such as diverticular disease, volvulus or endometriosis generally involves resecting the obstructed segment, followed by a decision to defunction the bowel or an attempt at primary anastomosis. Leakage from an anastomosis can have disastrous consequences, and there may be a significant disparity between the sizes of the two lumens.

LARGE BOWEL OBSTRUCTION

The management of large bowel obstruction is a little more complicated, and depends on the site of the obstruction and the probable underlying pathology (**Figs 2.38–2.40**). The most common situation involves an obstructing carcinoma in the left colon or sigmoid. The three-stage approach involving a colostomy, a resection and a reversal as three separate stages has little to recommend it, and in general should be abandoned in favour of primary excisional surgery. Having resected the primary tumour, there are many options:

- A simple end colostomy with closure of the rectal stump (Hartmann's procedure) is usually a safe operation, but commits the patient to a second procedure to close the stoma or, indeed, to a permanent stoma.
- On-table lavage to clear the proximal colon, followed by primary anastomosis, is an alternative, but is relatively time consuming, though the advantage for the patient is the avoidance of any further surgery.

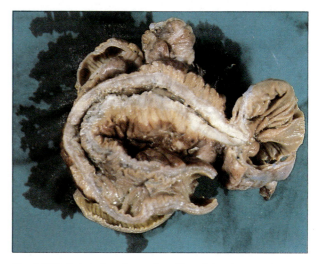

Fig. 2.37 Pathological specimen of small bowel showing a grossly stenotic segment of Crohn's disease causing acute-on-chronic small bowel obstruction.

- Usually the best approach is a subtotal colectomy, anastomosing the terminal ileum to the distal non-obstructed segment, but the functional results in terms of diarrhoea and incontinence may not be acceptable if this is carried out for distal tumours in elderly patients.
- For obstructing more proximal colonic tumours, an extended right colectomy with ileocolic anastomosis is a universally acceptable procedure.

If tumour recurrence or persistence in the pelvis is thought likely, an anastomosis to the rectum should be avoided in favour of an end-stoma, as the recurrent obstruction that often occurs in the pelvis can be difficult to manage. Colo–colic bypass is occasionally needed for totally unresectable colon cancer, but this is a relatively rare event. In sigmoid volvulus it is often possible to resolve the acute problem by passing a flatus tube (or colonoscope) through the twisted segment to deflate the sigmoid loop. Using a flatus tube at least twice as long as the rigid sigmoidoscope to allow the tube to be positioned correctly and left in place when the sigmoidoscope is withdrawn is of considerable practical importance. A primary resection and anastomosis should then be carried out once the immediate problem has resolved and formal bowel preparation has been completed.

In pseudo-obstruction surgical intervention may be required if the situation fails to resolve to the extent that caecal perforation is imminent. Therapeutic colonoscopic decompression should be attempted first, in the knowledge that the procedure is unlikely to be easy in the unprepared

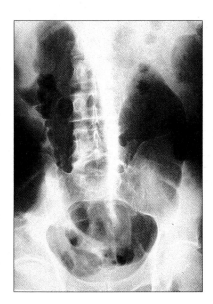

Fig. 2.38 Supine abdominal radiograph in acute large bowel obstruction showing gross dilatation of transverse colon and no gas in the left colon or rectum.

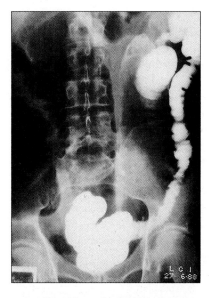

Fig. 2.39 Emergency single-contrast barium enema in the patient whose radiograph is shown in Fig. 2.30, demonstrating a stenosing carcinoma proximal to the splenic flexure.

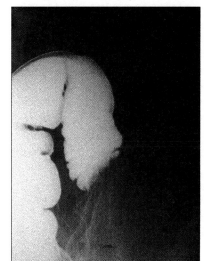

Fig. 2.40 Emergency, single-contrast barium enema showing complete obstruction in the mid-sigmoid colon secondary to a carcinoma.

bowel, and that the situation may be exacerbated by the insufflation of air (an alternative is to use carbon dioxide insufflation). Furthermore the procedure may need to be repeated if the situation still does not improve, although it is also possible to place an intraluminal tube into the colon under colonoscopic control to provide a vent. Finally, it may become necessary to decompress the colon by formal caecostomy as a last resort. Indeed, this is probably the only good indication for caecostomy in modern surgical practice.

Vascular abnormalities

Ruptured abdominal aortic aneurysm

NATURAL HISTORY

The typical patient is an elderly man with arteriopathy who presents with a sudden collapse and severe abdominal and often back pain. He may have a previous history suggesting the diagnosis and may even have a known aneurysm, which is simply being monitored.

The cardinal feature on examination is a tender pulsatile mass in the epigastrium, but this can be missed relatively easily in the hypotensive patient, and unless the diagnosis is considered early it may only become apparent at post-

mortem. A preoperative assessment of the patency of the leg and pedal pulses must be made to provide a baseline for later comparison.

MANAGEMENT

The plain abdominal radiograph may confirm the presence of an aneurysm, which shows up as a curvilinear area of calcification in the left upper quadrant, as will an ultrasound scan. Preoperative confirmation of leakage can usually only be obtained by CT scanning, and if there is any doubt about the diagnosis an urgent CT scan should be obtained. However most patients with an unexplained abdominal catastrophe or collapse with a tender aneurysm will be subjected to an emergency laparotomy on the basis that the aneurysm is leaking or has leaked. The possibility of transferring the patient to the care of a vascular surgeon, whose results for ruptured aneurysms will in general be superior to those of a general surgeon should be considered. Occasionally there may be a place for symptomatic treatment in a very elderly, unfit patient.

Once the diagnosis is made, preparation should be made for surgical intervention without undue delay. Placement of wide-bore intravenous cannulae and a urinary catheter are essential and must be completed before anaesthesia. Extras such as a right heart catheter, an arterial line and a nasogastric tube can be placed during surgery. Eight units of whole blood are cross-matched, and platelets and fresh frozen plasma are made available.

The abdomen is opened through a long midline incision after including both groins in the sterile field. Assuming the diagnosis is confirmed, the small bowel is reflected to the right and the duodeno-jejunal flexure mobilised to expose the aorta above the aneurysm. The left renal vein is reflected upwards and an arterial clamp placed above the neck to control the aorta. Both common iliacs are controlled below the bifurcation and the aneurysm is opened. Intraluminal thrombus is removed, and vessels such as the lumbar arteries and the inferior mesenteric artery are controlled, usually from within the sac. Usually, the ruptured aorta can be replaced with a straight graft, placed between the neck of the aneurysm and the aortic bifurcation, the decision depending on the degree of dilatation of the common iliacs. Alternatively an aorto–biiliac or aorto–bifemoral graft is occasionally necessary.

Mesenteric vascular occlusion

NATURAL HISTORY

The typical patient is elderly, often has a history of vascular disease, and presents with severe abdominal pain and colic, which are later associated with vomiting and diarrhoea. A contrast study of the lower bowel at this stage may show the classical sign of 'thumbprinting,' due to intense mucosal oedema in the ischaemic segment (**Fig. 2.41**). In the early stages there may a low-grade fever and an elevated white blood count.

There is often little in the way of abnormal physical signs initially. As the pathological process progresses, a combination of endotoxaemic and hypovolaemic shock follows relatively rapidly, and the outlook becomes more bleak as time progresses. The development of peritoneal irritation usually signifies full-thickness necrosis and a worsening of the prognosis.

AETIOLOGY AND PATHOGENESIS

Acute intestinal ischaemia not involving mechanical intestinal obstruction can have a variety of causes including arterial emboli and thrombosis, venous thrombosis, small vessel disease (as occurs in polyarteritis), and a low flow state (as might be seen after cardiac surgery) in an already compromised mesenteric vascular supply.

MANAGEMENT

Management before laparotomy involves aggressive resuscitation, but the longer the delay the more advanced will be the extent of damage, and early operation is important. Broad-spectrum antibiotics are administered and the patient is fully heparinised, but usually only after operative confirmation of gut ischaemia. The role of angiography is controversial, but in general is not used in the

▶ **Diagnosis and management of abdominal vascular crises**

- A patient with cardiovascular disease or atrial fibrillation and significant abdominal pain has intestinal ischaemia until proved otherwise
- Use stomas and 'second-look' surgery at 48 hours in intestinal ischaemia
- Palpate carefully for an aortic aneurysm, particularly when the femoral arteries are aneurysmal
- Investigate for underlying hypercoagulable states in mesenteric venous infarction

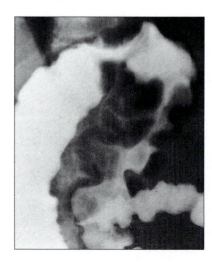

Fig. 2.41 Emergency single-contrast barium enema showing gross 'thumbprinting' in the region of the splenic flexure due to ischaemic colitis.

▶ **Arguments for and against urgent mesenteric angiography in the patient with suspected acute mesenteric ischaemia**

For	Against
May provide details of anatomical abnormality to help planning for surgery	Delays definitive treatment
Allows the use of therapeutic thrombolytic therapy	Normal study does not exclude microvascular ischaemia
	Many older patients have one or more occluded vessels without symptomatic

emergency setting because total occlusion of one or other mesenteric vessels is a common finding in asymptomatic individuals.

Once a laparotomy has been undertaken there are three surgical options:

- To do nothing (i.e. to close the abdomen and let nature take its course).
- To revascularise the gut.
- To resect.

The first option is obviously reserved for irremediable situations when the patient is extremely unwell for other reasons or because the extent of infarction is incompatible with life.

The many techniques for revascularising the gut include catheter embolectomy, formal thrombectomy, reimplantation of visceral arteries and bypass procedures. All are difficult as gaining access to the origins of the visceral arteries involves a tedious dissection, particularly in obese patients.

The usual operative finding of grossly ischaemic gut precludes any attempts at revascularisation, so a resection of all non-viable gut is the most commonly used option. In such a situation it is folly to attempt an anastomosis, and suitably-placed stomas are the safest alternative, with the possibility of reversal at a later date. Even patients who have had a massive small bowel resection can survive using long-term home parenteral nutrition, although their quality of life is often relatively poor. The chances of success with enteral nutrition are greatly increased if the ileocaecal valve can be preserved.

Mesenteric venous occlusion is rare, but important, because it occasionally complicates hypercoagulable states such as antithrombin III deficiency (**Fig. 2.42**), which must be actively and urgently searched for; further thromboses are almost inevitable unless the hypercoagulable state is adequately treated, usually with long-term anticoagulation.

Finally, as infarction is often patchy in this condition, a second-look laparotomy 24–48 hours after the first is often indicated.

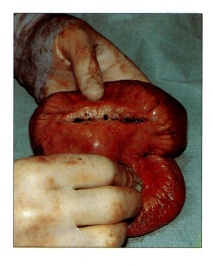

Fig. 2.42 Operative specimen showing mesenteric venous thrombosis in a patient with antithrombin III deficiency.

Acute intermittent porphyria

Natural history

The major clinical features of acute intermittent porphyria (acute abdominal pain, constipation, epilepsy, confusion, psychosis, motor neuropathy and hypertension) correlate with, but are not necessarily due to, the high porphobilinogen levels. Many of the clinical and biochemical features closely mimic those of lead poisoning.

AETIOLOGY AND PATHOGENESIS

Acute intermittent porphyria is almost unique as an example of an enzyme defect (porphobilinogen deaminase) inherited as an autosomal dominant condition. As a result of the enzyme defect there is an accumulation of porphobilinogen, which can be detected in the urine, and of its precursor delta-laevulinic acid. This in turn is synthesized from succinyl CoA and glycine. The end-products of the synthetic chain are the porphyrins, which are the precursors of haem and cytochromes.

In the liver, which is the site of the main problem in acute intermittent (or 'hepatic') porphyria, the cytochromes are the main end-products of porphyrin synthesis. Any situation that induces cytochrome enzymes, particularly drug therapy, is therefore likely to increase porphyrin synthesis and will exacerbate porphyria.

The diagnosis is readily made during an acute attack by detecting porphobilinogen in the urine, which goes dark red on standing.

Management

The first and most important step is to make an early diagnosis. Often the first case in any family is fatal because of delayed diagnosis. A common and tragic course is for acute abdominal pain to lead to laparotomy with barbiturate induction of anaesthesia, which is followed by status epilepticus and even more barbiturate therapy. Barbiturates are one of a long list of drugs that exacerbate porphyria.

A list must be obtained, if not already in the patient's possession, of those drugs that may safely be prescribed.

The main principles of therapy are:

- Pain relief with a safe analgesic (e.g. pethidine).
- Maintenance of a high carbohydrate intake, preferably enterally, but parenterally if vomiting is a problem (fasting exacerbates porphyria).
- Avoidance of hyponatraemia by careful monitoring and restricting water intake as necessary (inappropriate ADH syndrome is almost invariable).

- Treatment of hypertension, if severe, usually with propranolol.
- Controlling fits with diazepam, but *not barbiturates or phenytoin*.
- Controlling vomiting with phenothiazines if it does not settle quickly.
- Monitoring respiratory function carefully using peak flow rate or vital capacity because respiratory muscle weakness may cause dangerous hypoventilation.
- Using intravenous haem arginate or haematin therapy if the attack is not improving within about 48 hours as there is evidence that this will speed recovery.

As the condition is rare and its management is relatively complicated, an early telephone referral should be made to a centre with particular expertise (e.g. University of Glasgow Porphyria Research Unit, Tel: (0141) 339 8822 ext. 4150).

Attacks are more common in women in whom they often coincide with ovulation. Ovulation-suppressive tharapy may occasionally be necessary. The long-term prognosis is variable, but should be good with careful management.

Screening of family members is essential and needs to be done in collaboration with a major referral centre because the screening tests (usually blood porphobilinogen de-aminase estimation) are not easy to interpret.

FURTHER READING

Intestinal obstruction and perforation

Chamary VL. Femoral hernia: intestinal obstruction is an unrecognized source of morbidity and mortality. *Br J Surg* 1993; **80**(2): 230–2.

Finlay IG, Carter DC. A comparison of emergency resection and staged management in perforated diverticular disease. *Dis Colon Rectum* 1987; **30**: 929–33.

Landercasper J, Cogbill TH, Merry WH, Stolee RT, Strutt PJ. Long-term outcome after hospitalization for small-bowel obstruction. *Arch Surg* 1993; **128**(7): 765–70; discussion 770–1.

Menzies D. Postoperative adhesions: their treatment and relevance in clinical practice. *Ann R Coll Surg Engl* 1993; **75**(3): 147–53.

McGregor JR, O'Dwyer PJ. The surgical management of obstruction and perforation of the left colon. *Surg Gynecol Obstet* 1993; **177**(2): 203–8.

Ripamonti C, De Conno F, Ventafridda V, Rossi B, Baines MJ. Management of bowel obstruction in advanced and terminal cancer patients. *Ann Oncol* 1993; **4**(1): 15–21.

Taylor BA. Spontaneous perforation of the gastrointestinal tract. In: Gilmore IT, Shields R (eds). *Gastrointestinal Emergencies*. WB Saunders, London, 1992.

Acute pancreatitis

Buchler MW, Binder M, Friess H. Role of somatostatin and its analogues in the treatment of acute and chronic pancreatitis. *Gut* 1994; **35**(S):S15–19.

Buchler M, Uhl W, Beger HG. Acute pancreatitis: when and how to operate. *Dig Dis* 1992; **10**(6): 354–62.

Fernandez del Castillo C, Rattner DW, Warshaw AL. Acute pancreatitis. *Lancet* 1993; **342**(8869): 475–9.

Imrie CW, Benjamin IS, Ferguson JC. A single centre double-blind trial of trasylol therapy in primary acute pancreatitis. *Brit J Surg* 1978; **65**: 337–41 (see Table 1).

Johnson CD. Timing of intervention in acute pancreatitis. *Postgrad Med J* 1993; **69**(813): 509–15.

Malfertheiner P, Dominguez Munoz JE. Prognostic factors in acute pancreatitis. *Int J Pancreatol* 1993; **14**(1): 1–8.

Marshall JB. Acute pancreatitis. A review with an emphasis on new developments. *Arch Intern Med* 1993; **153**(10): 1185–98.

Steinberg W, Tenner S. Acute pancreatitis. *N Engl J Med* 1994; **330**:1198–210.

Thoeni RF, Blankenberg F. Pancreatic imaging. Computed tomography and magnetic resonance imaging. *Radiol Clin North Am* 1993; **31**(5): 1085–113.

Underwood TW, Frye CB. Drug-induced pancreatitis. *Clin Pharm* 1993; **12**(6): 440–8.

Acute cholecystitis and cholangitis

Kadakia SC. Biliary tract emergencies. Acute cholecystitis, acute cholangitis, and acute pancreatitis. *Med Clin North Am* 1993; **77**(5): 1015–36.

Leese T, Neoptolemos JP, Baker AR, Carr-Locke DL. Management of acute cholangitis and the impact of endoscopic sphincterotomy. *Brit J Surg* 1986; **72**: 988–92.

Laparoscopy

Cuesta MA, Borgstein PJ, Meijer S. Laparoscopy in the diagnosis and treatment of acute abdominal conditions. Clinical review. *Eur J Surg* 1993; **159**(9): 455–6.

MacFayden BV Jr, Wolfe BM, McKernan JB. Laparoscopic management of the acute abdomen, appendix, and small and large bowel. *Surg Clin North Am* 1992; **72**(5): 1169–83.

Paterson-Brown S. Emergency laparoscopic surgery. *Br J Surg* 1993 Mar; **80**(3): 279–83.

Radiology and ultrasonography

Laing FC. Ultrasonography of the acute abdomen. *Radiol Clin North Am* 1992; **30**(2): 389–404.

Nicholson DA, Driscoll PA. ABC of emergency radiology. The abdomen–I. *Br Med J* 1993; **307**(6915): 1342–6.

Acute abdomen in the elderly

Kauvar DR. The geriatric acute abdomen. *Clin Geriatr Med* 1993; **9**(3): 547–58.

Acute abdomen in pregnancy

Epstein FB. Acute abdominal pain in pregnancy. *Emerg Med Clin North Am* 1994; **12**(1): 151–65.

Intestinal ischaemia

Marston A, Buckley GB, Fiddian-Green RG, Hagland U. *Splanchnic ischaemia and multiple organ failure.* Edward Arnold, London, 1989.

Acute porphyria

Lip GY, McColl KE, Moore MR. The acute porphyrias. *Br J Clin Pract* 1993; **47**(1): 38–43.

3
DIARRHOEA

REACHING A DIAGNOSIS

Is it diarrhoea?
The patient should be asked directly whether he/she is passing liquid faeces or merely has frequent, but normally formed bowel movements.

Is the diarrhoea infective?
The duration of the diarrhoea often gives a helpful clue to the aetiology. Most infective causes of diarrhoea resolve after a few days or 2–3 weeks at the most. Exceptions that may cause more prolonged diarrhoea include pathogenic amoebae, *Giardia*, *Campylobacter jejuni* and *Yersinia* spp. Often the patient with infective diarrhoea will give a history of sudden onset of abdominal pain and vomiting and there may be a history of other family members or acquaintances who have been similarly affected.

Microscopy
Stool microscopy and culture are essential to confirm the diagnosis and allow identification of the source. If amoebic dysentery is suspected because of recent travel to endemic areas the stools should be transferred rapidly to the laboratory while still warm so that motile amoebae containing phagocytosed red cells can be identified (faeces commonly contain non-pathogenic *Entamoeba coli*, which do not ingest red cells).

Microscopy is important not only for the diagnosis of parasites such as amoebae and *Giardia*, but also for the identification of pus cells (neutrophils), which may aid in the diagnosis. Infectious diarrhoea may be classified as inflammatory or non-inflammatory according to the presence or absence of neutrophils in the faeces.

Inflammatory diarrhoea results from organisms such as *Salmonella*, *Campylobacter* and *Shigella*, which tend to infect the distal ileum and colon. The diarrhoea may then be bloody and is often accompanied by fever. In the absence of positive stool microscopy or culture inflammatory bowel disease or ischaemic colitis should be considered as differential diagnoses.

Non-inflammatory infective diarrhoea is usually more voluminous and is watery rather than bloody and contains few pus cells. It is associated with infection of the small intestine by agents such as rotavirus (particularly common in children), enteric adenovirus, *Cryptosporidium* and toxigenic *Escherichia coli*. Cholera is a classic example of this type of infective diarrhoea.

Is the diarrhoea watery or fatty?
If the diarrhoea is not infective the next step in diagnosis is to establish whether it is predominantly watery or fatty. A mistake at this stage will result in a completely inappropriate

▶ **Steps in diagnosing diarrhoea**

Initial steps

- Confirm loose consistency
- Exclude infection
- Assess whether watery, bloody or fatty

If watery:

- Check drugs
- Check diet (e.g. excessive sorbitol)
- Sigmoidoscopy
- Assess whether functional or organic
- Exclude colonic disease (colonoscopy or barium enema)
- Exclude hypolactasia (breath test)
- Exclude secretory diarrhoea (large volume persisting despite fasting and intravenous fluids)
- Exclude endocrine causes

If bloody:

- Sigmoidoscopy
- Exclude colonic disease (colonoscopy or barium enema)

If fatty:

- Exclude coeliac disease (endoscopic duodenal biopsy)
- Exclude other small bowel disease (small bowel barium meal)
- Exclude bacterial overgrowth (lactulose or ^{14}C-glycocholate breath test or trial of tetracycline)
- Exclude pancreatic disease pancreatic ultrasound)

series of investigations. The patient's description of faeces can often be misleading and it is essential to inspect the faeces. Any patient with diarrhoea that has persisted for more than a few days and negative stool cultures should have a rigid sigmoidoscopy and this allows an opportunity to inspect the faeces in addition to the rectal mucosa. Usually the history plus inspection of the faeces will give a clear guide as to whether the diarrhoea is likely to be due to malabsorption, but sometimes a further test will be required.

The standard test is the **faecal fat** estimation. This must be one of the least popular tests for patients and laboratory staff, but gives reliable information if properly carried out. Faeces need to be collected over at least a three-day period and fat intake should be at least 'average' during this time. Some authorities insist on a carefully controlled high fat intake, but a normal diet will usually produce results that can be interpreted as normal, high, or very high and this is usually adequate for clinical purposes. Alternative tests have been based on the measurement of blood lipids after oral fat (prosperol test) or on the absorption and metabolism of radiolabelled fats (^{14}C-trioleate breath test). Both these tests (and others) have proponents, but are not widely used.

Watery diarrhoea – functional or organic?

Having established that the diarrhoea is predominantly watery, the next step is to decide whether it is likely to be functional or organic. This can largely be based on the history. If the patient is under 40 years of age, gives a history of alternating diarrhoea and constipation without weight loss or bleeding and without nocturnal diarrhoea then a functional cause – the irritable bowel syndrome – is most likely. If sigmoidoscopy reveals a normal rectal mucosa (which should include rectal biopsy because of the possibility of missing microscopic colitis or Crohn's disease), faecal occult blood is negative and the full blood count and erythrocyte sedimentation rate and serum CRP are normal, then the patient can be reassured and treated symptomatically without further investigation. The irritable bowel syndrome is so common (affecting up to one in three people) that it is more appropriate to attempt a positive diagnosis, particularly in the younger patient, rather than making the diagnosis by exclusion after endoscopy and/or barium studies.

Some patients with functional diarrhoea do have more persistent diarrhoea and these require more extensive investigation, usually including colonoscopy, to exclude organic causes such as inflammatory bowel disease. Bloody diarrhoea, weight loss, nocturnal diarrhoea, continual diarrhoea that is not interspersed by normal bowel actions or diarrhoea that occurs for the first time in someone over 40 years of age should always be assumed to be due to an organic cause and thoroughly investigated.

▶ **Functional diarrhoea (irritable bowel syndrome)**

If all the following features are present a positive diagnosis of functional diarrhoea can usually be made and the patient given appropriate reassurance and symptomatic treatment (page 12) without unnecessary investigation

- First presentation under 40 years of age
- Usually intermittent
- Not nocturnal
- No weight loss/ bleeding/ anaemia
- No history of milk intolerance
- No drugs
- No family history of inflammatory bowel disease or colorectal cancer
- Normal general examination
- Normal rigid sigmoidoscopy
- Normal serum CRP and full blood count

Watery or bloody diarrhoea – drug-related?

Mistakes are often made as the result of failing to obtain a complete drug history from the patient. Many drugs occasionally cause watery diarrhoea, while others such as colchicine or magnesium trisilicate will inevitably do so if given in sufficient dosage. Any drugs that are not essential should be stopped. Drugs that commonly cause diarrhoea include methyldopa, metformin, theophylline and digoxin. Diarrhoea is common after treatment with broad-spectrum antibiotics. This is usually due to overgrowth of the bowel with the toxin-producing *Clostridium difficile*, which in its most severe manifestation results in pseudomembranous colitis. The diagnosis can be confirmed by testing for *C. difficile* toxin in faeces. Ampicillin rarely causes a haemorrhagic colitis, which is thought to be a toxic effect of the drug itself. Purgatives will of course always produce diarrhoea if taken in excess and some disturbed patients may complain of diarrhoea while going to great lengths to conceal their abuse of purgatives. Stool or urine can easily be screened for phenolphthalein by the addition of alkali (e.g. a pellet of sodium hydroxide) and most laboratories can arrange a screen for anthracine or senna derivatives.

Oral contraceptive usage is statistically associated with Crohn's disease, but there is also strong anecdotal evidence that it can cause a colitis, usually non-granulomatous, but with rectal sparing, that mimicks colonic Crohn's disease and resolves when oral contraceptives are stopped. It is thought that this occurence may be a form of microvascular ischaemic colitis.

Is it due to colonic disease?

If infection and drugs have been excluded and the diarrhoea seems unlikely to be simply functional then the colon should be investigated. A history of erythema nodosum, acute arthritis of medium-sized or large joints or anterior uveitis is suggestive of, but not specific for, inflammatory bowel disease. The perianal area should be inspected for skin tags or fistulae suggestive of Crohn's disease.

Sigmoidoscopy

Sigmoidoscopy is an essential part of the examination in a patient with unexplained diarrhoea. It can easily be done as an outpatient procedure taking only one or two minutes and allows direct inspection and biopsy of the rectal mucosa and often allows simultaneous inspection and sampling of faeces for culture and occult blood testing. Unfortunately a mystique has been built up around this technique and many doctors without gastroenterology experience are uneasy about performing it. Before fibreoptic colonoscopy or flexible sigmoidoscopy were available an attempt was usually made to negotiate the rectosigmoid junction with a rigid scope. This was often uncomfortable to the patient and as a result the procedure was sometimes performed under general anaesthesia.

In a patient with diarrhoea a view of the rectal mucosa is all that is needed initially and if the more proximal colon needs endoscopic examination (e.g. to exclude polyps or carcinoma) a flexible fibreoptic sigmoidoscopy or colonoscopy should be performed. Inspection and biopsy of the rectal mucosa can easily be performed without distress to the patient and there is no need for sedation or anaesthesia.

The normal rectal mucosa appears pale pink and shiny. In any case of chronic diarrhoea, whatever the cause, there is usually some reddening of the mucosa (and often evidence of mild inflammation on rectal histology). In ulcerative colitis the mucosa is more frankly granular with easy contact bleeding and there may be obvious mucosal ulceration in more severe colitis. Crohn's disease often 'spares' the rectum, but if it is involved there may be either small 'aphthoid' or serpiginous 'snail track' ulcers, separated by more healthy mucosa (**Figs 3.1–3.4**). In pseudomembranous

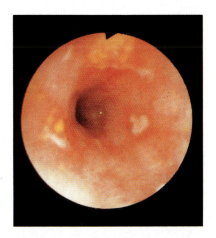

Fig. 3.1 Colonoscopic view showing frank ulceration in ulcerative colitis.

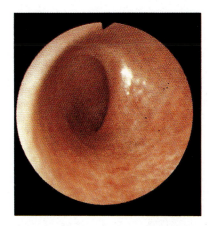

Fig. 3.2 Colonoscopic view showing granularity and contact bleeding. in ulcerative colitis

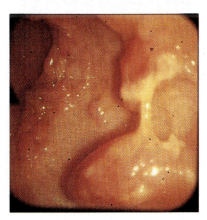

Fig. 3.3 Colonoscopic appearance of pseudopolyps. These occur in ulcerative colitis (as here) or Crohn's disease and represent islands of hyperplastic mucosa, which have been surrounded by areas of ulceration that have since healed.

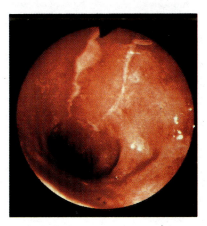

Fig. 3.4 Linear 'snail track' ulcers in colonic Crohn's disease.

colitis a characteristic yellowish membrane of sloughed-off superficial epithelium may be seen. The rectal mucosa ought to be biopsied even if it appears macroscopically normal since microscopic granulomata may be present in a normal appearing mucosa in Crohn's disease and clinically significant microscopic or collagenous colitis will also be missed without biopsy. Biopsy should probably only be carried out as a hospital (outpatient) procedure since it carries a slight risk of perforation or bleeding. This risk approaches zero if the posterior rectal wall is biopsied using sharp-edged small-cupped forceps.

Rectal histology

Rectal histology may yield one of several results (**Figs 3.5–3.11**):

- It may show diagnostic features of **Crohn's disease** (i.e. non-caseating granulomata, chronic inflammation penetrating deep to the muscularis mucosa and relative goblet cell mucus retention).
- It may be normal.
- It may show features that are highly suggestive of **ulcerative colitis** (e.g. acute and chronic inflammation,

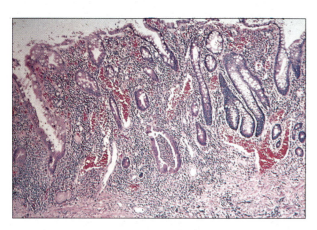

Fig. 3.5 Rectal mucosa (low magnification) showing the typical features of severe ulcerative colitis: distortion of crypt architecture with irregular and branched glands; depletion of goblet cells in the crypts; diffuse chronic inflammatory exudate in the lamina propria; and crypt abscesses. The branched glands result from hyperplasia after previous attacks and are particularly useful for distinguishing ulcerative colitis from infective colitis.

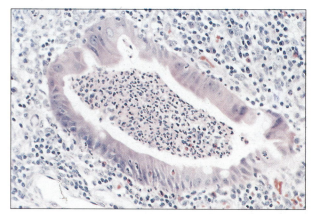

Fig. 3.6 High magnification of a crypt abscess in ulcerative colitis showing an accumulation of neutrophil polymorphs in the crypt lumen. This is typical, but not specific for acute ulcerative colitis, occurring also in Crohn's disease and in inflammatory infective diarrhoeas such as those due to *Salmonella* and *Campylobacter*.

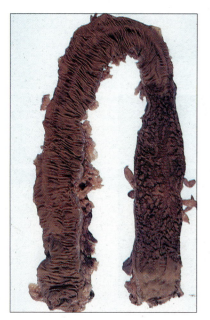

Fig. 3.7 Colectomy specimen showing a macroscopic view of ulcerative colitis. The sharp demarcation between diseased and normal bowel is typical.

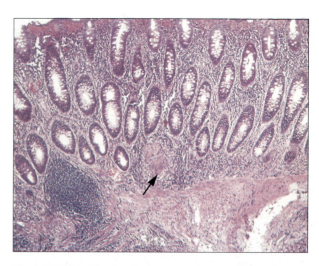

Fig. 3.8 Colonic Crohn's disease. There is inflammation throughout all layers from the luminal surface to serosa. A granuloma with a giant cell is present (arrowed) and there is a relative preservation of goblet cells despite the inflammation.

which is predominantly mucosal with crypt abscess formation, mucus depletion and sparsity or branching of crypts).

- Commonly, however, the findings will be **non-specific**: crypt abscess formation without crypt branching or sparsity, increased lamina propria mononuclear cells and mild mucus depletion. These findings will be compatible with either ulcerative colitis or an inflammatory type of infective diarrhoea such as *Campylobacter* enteritis. Patchy, focal areas of inflammation are particularly suggestive of an infective cause.

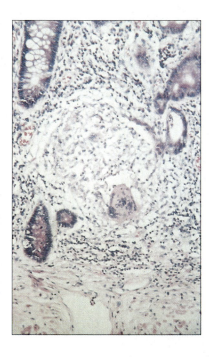

Fig. 3.9 High magnification of a granuloma in Crohn's disease, showing a giant cell. The granulomas usually originate within or adjacent to small blood vessels.

Colonoscopy or barium enema?

Colonoscopy or barium enema are necessary to study the rest of the colon if rigid sigmoidoscopy and rectal biopsy have not given a definitive diagnosis. In the investigation of rectal bleeding or anaemia, colonoscopy is the investigation of choice, but in the investigation of altered bowel habit a good case can be made for either investigation.

In most centres barium enema is more readily available, but there is little difference between the two procedures in terms of patient discomfort, cost or risk and more information (including histology) is usually obtained from colonoscopy. A double-contrast barium enema in which the colon is filled with air and the mucosa coated with a small quantity of barium will give more information about the mucosa than a single-contrast barium enema.

Neither colonoscopy nor barium enema is safe or necessary in a patient with **severe acute colitis**. If this diagnosis is suspected a plain abdominal radiograph will give valuable information: in particular whether the colon contains faeces (i.e. is relatively healthy) or is dilated. A plain abdominal radiograph in ischaemic colitis may show massive mucosal oedema reflected by the appearance of 'thumbprinting' of the colonic mucosa. Barium enema or colonoscopy should generally be deferred until the patient's condition has improved with treatment, a diagnosis having been reached on the basis of sigmoidoscopy, rectal histology and stool culture. A single-contrast 'instant' barium enema may be performed with little risk if assessment of disease extent is urgent in a patient with active colitis. Bowel preparation for barium enema or colonoscopy in patients with active colitis should be gentle (e.g. liquid diet for 48 hours and rectal washouts rather than purgatives).

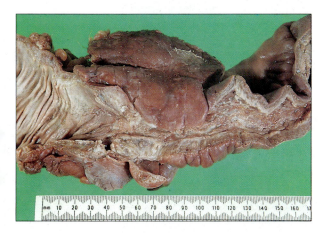

Fig. 3.10 Macroscopic view of resected ileo-caecal Crohn's disease showing marked thickening of the bowel wall and severe stricturing.

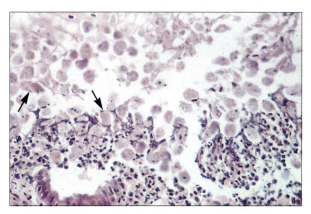

Fig. 3.11 Amoebic colitis. Many round eosinophilic amoebae are present on the surface of and within the colonic mucosa. Some amoebae have ingested erythrocytes (arrows).

Most colonic lesions are diagnosable by a combination of rigid sigmoidoscopy and double-contrast barium enema.

- **Ulcerative colitis** with superficial confluent ulceration and rectal involvement is usually readily distinguished from **colonic Crohn's disease** with deep fissure ulcers, skip

lesions and rectal sparing, but in up to 35% of patients with colitis the distinction is difficult even with histology. These patients are often labelled as having 'indeterminate colitis'. The distinction between ulcerative colitis and Crohn's disease is only of particular importance when surgery is contemplated (**Figs 3.12–3.15**).

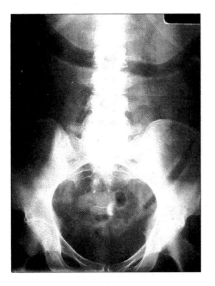

Fig. 3.12 Plain abdominal radiograph in ulcerative colitis. This is often all that is needed in the acute stage to assess the disease extent. The colon is devoid of haustra, which may be indistinct in the normal descending colon, and empty of faeces, suggesting total colitis. Colon that contains faeces is usually not severely affected. Significant dilatation with a diameter greater than 5.5 cm in the mid-transverse colon, is a grave sign and indicates toxic megacolon in a patient with active colitis.

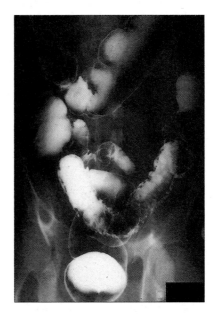

Fig. 3.13 Barium enema in a patient with active distal ulcerative colitis. The sigmoid is particularly severely affected showing 'tram lining' due to ulceration tracking along the submucosa. There is anecdotal evidence that a barium enema examination may worsen active colitis and it should generally be deferred until the attack is under control.

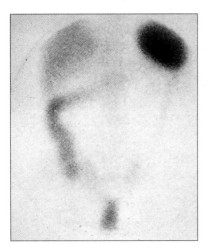

Fig. 3.14 A ¹¹¹Indium-labelled leucocyte scan showing abnormal uptake in the inflamed colon in a patient with total ulcerative colitis. This technique is also particularly useful in the assessment of small bowel Crohn's disease when radiographic appearances are equivocal. Courtesy of Dr M Critchley.

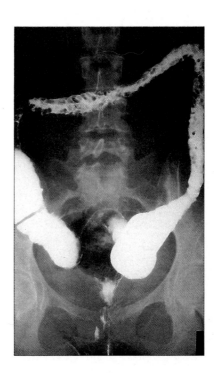

Fig. 3.15 Barium enema in colonic Crohn's disease showing the typical 'cobblestone' appearance that results from a combination of mucosal oedema and intervening ulceration. There is rectal sparing, which helps to distinguish this from ulcerative colitis.

- **Ischaemic colitis** can usually be distinguished readily. There is often (but not always) a history of a sudden onset associated with pain, the rectum is usually spared as it has a good collateral supply and marked mucosal oedema results in the characteristic thumbprinting seen on either plain abdominal radiograph or barium enema (**Figs 3.16–3.18**).
- **Behçet's disease** (oral and genital ulceration, arthritis, uveitis and venous thrombosis) can rarely cause a colitis, which mimics ulcerative colitis or Crohn's disease.

- **Colonic carcinoma** can often be confidently diagnosed on the basis of barium enema alone, but sometimes colonoscopy and biopsy is required if stricturing is equivocal or occurs in association with diverticular disease. Caecal lesions may also require colonoscopy as a prominent ileocaecal valve may mimic a carcinoma. Colonoscopy should also be performed in patients with persistent diarrhoea who have a normal barium enema. Lesions not uncommonly missed on barium enema include the serpiginous or aphthoid ulcers of colonic Crohn's disease, small carcinomas (particularly in a sigmoid colon that is affected by diverticular disease) and more rarely a villous adenoma. Occasionally colonoscopy will reveal extensive melanosis in patients with purgative abuse.
- **Irradiation enteritis** should always be considered as a possible diagnosis if there is a previous history of radiotherapy, particularly pelvic irradiation with doses greater than 40 Gray (4000 rads). Early symptoms of irradiation damage, most commonly nausea, tenesmus and diarrhoea, may occur during the first or second week of therapy, but late symptoms, due to proctitis or terminal ileitis, may occur months or even years after the irradiation. Radiological appearances can closely mimic inflammatory bowel disease in chronic disease and may show thumbprinting in the acute phase. Endoscopy may show prominent submucosal telangiectasia, and biopsy is usually helpful, characteristic features including narrowed arterioles, bizarre 'irradiation' fibroblasts and extensive fibrosis.

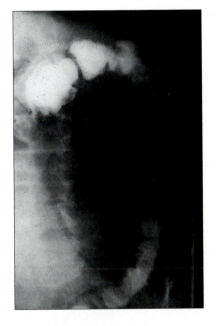

Fig. 3.16 Ischaemic colitis showing marked mucosal oedema resulting in the typical 'thumbprinting' appearance. Less dramatic thumbprinting may also be seen in Crohn's disease.

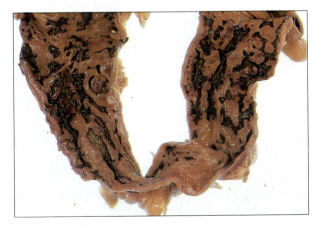

Fig. 3.17 Ischaemic colitis (resected specimen) showing severe ulceration at the splenic flexure. Rectal involvement is rare.

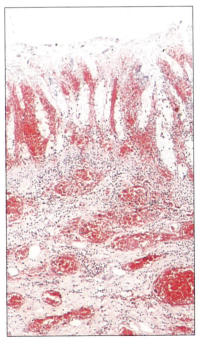

Fig. 3.18 Ischaemic colitis (low magnification). Congested vessels and an acute inflammatory exudate are seen in the submucosa and mucosa. The structure of the mucosal glands is preserved, but most of the epithelium has undergone necrosis and been lost. The submucosa is wider than normal due to oedema.

- **Pneumatosis cystoides intestinalis** is an uncommon disorder in which multiple gas-filled cysts occur in the submucosal or subserosal tissues of the small and/or large intestine. It may be diagnosed at flexible sigmoidoscopy or colonoscopy when the cysts appear as soft grape-like swellings, which may be mistaken for sessile polyps. Plain abdominal radiography will often be diagnostic. On histology the cysts may be lined either by simple cuboidal epithelium or by endothelial cells, which may coalesce to form giant cells. The cysts may be symptomless or be associated with colicky lower abdominal pain, intermittent diarrhoea and even rectal bleeding.

Is there secretory diarrhoea?

Large-volume diarrhoea of one litre or more daily usually implies active secretion of salt and water into the intestine rather than simply exudation or a failure of absorption. This suspicion can be confirmed if the diarrhoea continues at a similar rate when nothing is taken by mouth. This should only be done in hospital as intravenous fluid and electrolyte replacement will be needed. Cholera is the commonest cause of secretory diarrhoea worldwide, but unfortunately purgative abuse is probably the commonest non-infective cause in the 'civilised' world (**Fig. 3.19**).

If these conditions are excluded, rare syndromes associated with hormone or peptide-secreting tumours should be sought. These include secretion of vasoactive intestinal polypeptide (VIP) by a pancreatic tumour 'vipoma,' resulting in watery diarrhoea, hypochlorhydria and alkalosis (Verner–Morrison syndrome), and the watery diarrhoea associated with a calcitonin-secreting medullary carcinoma of the thyroid. Serum assays for VIP and calcitonin are available. Scanning and/or angiographic techniques will then be needed to localise the tumour and to assess resectability.

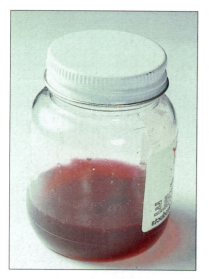

Fig 3.19 A sample of diarrhoea that has turned pink on the addition of a pellet of caustic soda, indicating the presence of phenolphthalein due to purgative abuse. Courtesy of Dr DP Jewell.

The Zollinger–Ellison syndrome (gastrin-secreting pancreatic tumour) may be associated with watery diarrhoea resulting from the massive hypersecretion of gastric acid, although some degree of fat malabsorption is commonly present.

Carcinoid syndrome (diarrhoea, flushing and wheezing due to malignant carcinoid) usually occurs only if there is considerable metastatic spread of tumour to the liver, which is usually enlarged. Urine should be screened for 5-hydroxy indole acetic acid (5-HIAA), the metabolite of 5-hydroxy - tryptamine.

Is there an osmotic diarrhoea?

Measurement of faecal osmolality may be very useful in the patient with watery diarrhoea. If the osmolality in mosmol/l exceeds the sum of the sodium and potassium (in mEq/l) multiplied by two by more than 50 mosmol/l it is likely that there is an osmotic cause for the diarrhoea. Possibilities include magnesium, lactose (in patients with hypolactasia) and sorbitol (commonly used as a filler in confectionery such as mints and also present in some packaged fruit juices).

Is there endocrine disease?

Thyrotoxicosis occasionally presents with diarrhoea, although other features will usually be present.

Diabetics sometimes get a puzzling and troublesome intermittent watery diarrhoea, which is sometimes nocturnal. Its aetiology is uncertain, but it is probably due to a combination of the effects of autonomic neuropathy on the gut and bacterial overgrowth.

Adrenal failure (Addison's disease) commonly presents with prolonged diarrhoea, vomiting and hypovolaemia. Palmar crease and buccal pigmentation should be sought and the plasma cortisol checked before and after Synacthen or adrenocorticotrophic hormone (ACTH) challenge.

Is the diarrhoea bile salt-related?

Bile salts are normally recirculated efficiently with 95% reabsorption in the distal ileum. If the ileum is diseased or has been resected conjugated bile salts will pass into the colon, causing stimulation of mucosal adenyl cyclase and resulting in a secretory diarrhoea. Since the small bowel is not involved the volume of diarrhoea is not usually as massive as with other secretory diarrhoeas, but may be considerable (500–1000 ml/day).

There is usually a clear history of surgical resection of the small intestine (e.g. for Crohn's disease), or of irradiation to the lower abdomen causing irradiation ileitis. However, some patients without any such predisposing cause may have chronic bile salt diarrhoea and this probably accounts for a small proportion of patients previously labelled as having the irritable bowel syndrome.

The diagnosis may be confirmed by measuring the absorption of an isotopically-labelled bile acid, but in practice a therapeutic trial of oral cholestyramine is a cheaper and simpler way of establishing the diagnosis. Cholestyramine is an ion exchange resin that chelates bile acids and prevents them having a stimulatory effect on colonic adenyl cyclase. Response is usually immediate if the diagnosis is correct.

Fatty diarrhoea (steatorrhoea) – which approach?

There are two possible approaches to the diagnosis of fat malabsorption: a logical approach and a practical approach:

- The logical approach is to assess the function of the systems relevant to fat absorption. A xylose absorption test can be performed to assess mucosal function, a secretin test to assess pancreatic function, and a labelled bile acid breath test to assess intraluminal deconjugation of bile salts. Although this approach is sometimes followed none of these tests will give an anatomical or pathological diagnosis and the xylose and pancreatic function tests unfortunately often give 'falsely' positive results in pancreatic and intestinal disease respectively.
- A more direct approach is to test for the presence of the disease thought most likely to be present. This approach usually leads to a diagnosis with fewer tests and is more practical even if less intellectually satisfying.

Is there intestinal disease?

Is it coeliac disease?

In a young person with iron and/or folate deficiency and steatorrhoea, coeliac disease is highly probable. Other features that suggest the diagnosis include short stature, secondary amenorrhoea and a blood film with features of hyposplenism (abnormally-shaped red cells and Howell--Jolly bodies). Hyposplenism may also occur in inflammatory bowel disease so this collection of clinical features is not specific for coeliac disease. Diagnosis requires jejunal or duodenal biopsy:

- The traditional method is jejunal biopsy using a Crosby capsule, which is a springloaded suction-activated rotating knife inside a metal capsule. This is often a tedious test to perform.
- Endoscopic duodenal biopsy is a more convenient alternative, but care then needs to be taken to ensure that adequate biopsies are taken from the distal duodenum (distal to the ampulla of Vater) otherwise the nonspecific duodenitis that is commonly present in the proximal duodenum may make interpretation difficult.

The typical findings in a duodenal or jejunal biopsy from a patient with untreated coeliac disease are villous atrophy with an increased number of lymphocytes within the epithelium and crypt hyperplasia. These findings also occur in tropical sprue and (excepting the crypt hyperplasia) secondary to vitamin B_{12} deficiency, so the diagnosis of coeliac disease cannot be confirmed until repeat biopsies have shown a return to normal architecture after gluten withdrawal.

Purists would also argue that a further gluten challenge and a repeat biopsy should then be carried out before final confirmation of the diagnosis. This is probably not necessary in adults, but should be done in children where non-gluten-related transient episodes of villous atrophy are more common (**Figs 3.20** and **3.21**).

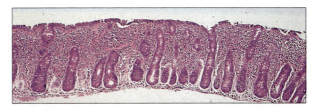
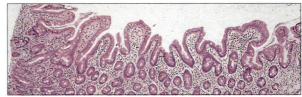

Fig. 3.20 Jejunal biopsies before (above) and after (below) three months on a gluten-free diet from a patient with coeliac disease. Before treatment there is total villous atrophy, inflammation and crypt hyperplasia, and after treatment there is almost complete recovery. The villi should normally be about three times as tall as the crypts are deep.

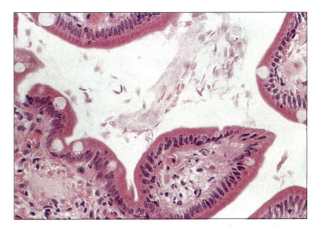

Fig. 3.21 Jejunal biopsy showing numerous *Giardia lamblia*.

Other intestinal causes of malabsorption

A duodenal or jejunal aspirate can be obtained at the same time as the biopsy and, together with the biopsy, can be examined for parasites, particularly *Giardia lamblia* and *Strongyloides*. Rarer causes of malabsorption may be diagnosed from intestinal biopsy and include Whipple's disease, intestinal lymphoma and intestinal lymphangiectasia.

GIARDIASIS AND/OR IMMUNE DEFICIENCY

Infestation with *G. lamblia* may result in either watery or fatty diarrhoea. The mechanism for the fat malabsorption is uncertain, but may simply be loss of available surface area if infestation is marked. Stool microscopy is not always positive so endoscopic duodenal aspirate, usually combined with biopsy, is a more certain way of making the diagnosis. There is usually a brisk response to treatment with oral metronidazole, 400 mg three times daily for four days.

Infestation is usually acquired by travel to areas where tap water supplies are unreliable. If no such story is obtained from the patient an underlying immune deficiency should be excluded. Deficiency of immunoglobulin A is particularly likely to result in overgrowth with *Giardia*.

Immunoglobulin A deficiency may also be associated with **nodular lymphoid hyperplasia** of the intestine. This may be found in any part of the intestine, but is particularly prominent in the distal small intestine. It is due to hyperplasia of immunoglobulin M-producing cells, presumably because secretory IgM can to some extent take the role of secretory IgA in secretions. This may be recognised on barium studies, but care needs to be taken not to over-diagnose this condition in adolescents and young adults who commonly have prominent lymphoid follicles visible on barium enema or small bowel meal examinations.

WHIPPLE'S DISEASE

Whipple' s disease is a bacterial infestation of the small intestine, which results in villous atrophy and macrophages containing Periodic acid-Schiff (PAS)-positive 'foamy' remnants of dead bacteria accumulate within the lamina propria. It typically affects middle-aged men and, as well as malabsorption, causes arthritis, usually of large joints, and central nervous system involvement, which may present as a slowly progressive encephalopathy (**Fig. 3.22**).

ALPHA CHAIN DISEASE

In patients from the Middle East or Africa with finger clubbing and malabsorption, alpha chain disease should be considered. This is a form of intestinal lymphoma in which a malignant clone of IgA-producing cells develops in the intestine. These cells produce the IgA heavy chain (alpha chain) in excess with little or no light chain. Alpha chains are shed into the plasma and excreted in urine. Diagnosis is confirmed by immunoelectrophoresis of serum or

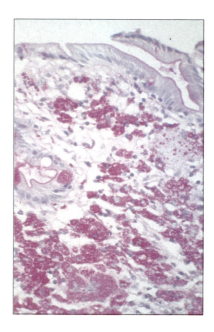

Fig. 3.22 Jejunal biopsy from a patient with Whipple's disease showing villous atrophy and numerous macrophages containing live and dead bacteria, which stain pink with periodic acid–Schiff stain.

concentrated urine and may also be made by immunohistochemistry of intestinal biopsies with staining for alpha chains and light chains.

SCLERODERMA

Scleroderma (systemic sclerosis) can affect the small intestine, resulting in severe malabsorption. Patients do not always have cutaneous manifestations of scleroderma. The bowel wall is thickened, resulting in a classical 'stacked coin' appearance on small bowel barium meal. Motility is slowed, bacterial overgrowth is common, particularly if pseudodiverticuliae have developed in the proximal small intestine. Apart from treatment aimed at the bacterial overgrowth, treatment options are very limited.

NUTRITIONAL DEFICIENCY

Nutritional deficiency can occasionally be the cause rather than the consequence of malabsorption.

Acrodermatitis enteropathica

Acrodermatitis enteropathica is a condition in which zinc deficiency results in ultrastructural abnormalities in enterocytes with resulting villous atrophy and malabsorption with diarrhoea in more than 90% of patients. The skin is affected with blistering lesions particularly the face, scalp, perineum, hands and feet. Neurological problems include lethargy and irritability and recurrent infections are common as a result of impaired T-lymphocyte function. The zinc deficiency may be inherited (rare, presenting in infancy) or acquired. A diet that is low in animal protein and high in phytates (present in unleavened bread) is likely to be low in zinc, but for clinical problems to occur there is usually also an additional malabsorptive problem such as tropical sprue, Crohn' s disease or chronic pancreatitis.

Pellagra

In developed countries pellagra, which results from deficiency of niacin, is most commonly seen in alcoholics. In developing countries, it often results from inadequate maize-based diets. It may also occur as a complication of carcinoid sydrome. There are generalised ultrastructural changes and inflammation throughout the small and large intestine, which result in diarrhoea. The classic triad of the 'three Ds' – diarrhoea, dermatitis (of light sensitive areas) and dementia – is present only in a minority of patients. There is usually a rapid response to vitamin replacement within the first week.

Barium examination of the small intestine in malabsorption

If the small intestinal biopsy is normal, barium examination of the small intestine will be necessary (**Figs 3.23–3.25**).

Conventional barium 'follow through' examinations are often unsatisfactory in patients with malabsorption because the increased small bowel secretions result in breaking up or 'flocculation' of the barium and a poor view of the mucosa. More information can often be gained by 'barium enteroclysis' or 'small bowel enema.' In this technique a naso-enteral tube is passed into the duodenum under X-ray screening and dilute barium is run rapidly into the intestine. Excellent views of the mucosa can be obtained. Diagnoses that could be made or excluded at this stage include Crohn's disease, tuberculosis and intestinal lymphoma.

Histology may be required to make the diagnosis with certainty. Gastrointestinal tuberculosis most often affects the ileocaecal region and there is sometimes, but not invariably, evidence of concomitant pulmonary disease. If the lesion can be reached by colonoscopy or terminal ileoscopy it should be biopsied and cultured for tuberculosis, but laparotomy may be necessary to obtain a tissue diagnosis.

In a Caucasian patient with typical radiological appearances of Crohn's disease, with stricturing and skip lesions separated by unaffected bowel, it may be considered reasonable to base the diagnosis and treatment solely on the radiological findings, but in patients from a population with a high incidence of tuberculosis, histological confirmation is the only safe policy if corticosteroid therapy is being considered as an option.

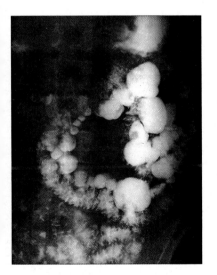

Fig. 3.23 Jejunal diverticulosis causing malabsorption of fat and vitamin B_{12} due to small bowel colonisation.

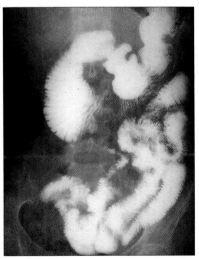

Fig. 3.24 Small bowel meal in a patient with systemic sclerosis showing the typical 'stacked coin' appearance. Cutaneous evidence of systemic sclerosis is not always present..

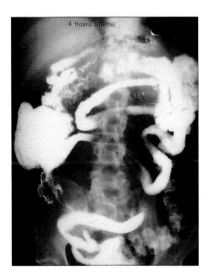

Fig. 3.25 Small bowel meal following severe mesenteric ischaemia. This patient had severe malabsorption. More usually there is either chronic mesenteric ischaemia with pain after meals, but normal radiographic appearances, or frank infarction.

Is there pancreatic disease?

A history of excessive alcohol ingestion can be obtained in at least 90% of patients with chronic pancreatitis and impaired glucose tolerance is present in 35%, so the presence of either of these factors in a patient with steatorrhoea necessitates investigation of the pancreas.

Pancreatic imaging

A plain abdominal radiograph should be performed first. Calcification of the pancreas will be visible in about 35% of patients with chronic pancreatitis and is diagnostic if present.

Further investigation of the pancreas is notoriously difficult. The 'best' test is probably endoscopic retrograde cholangiopancreatography (ERCP), which will produce a pancreatogram in approximately 90% of patients and will give a correct diagnosis in approximately 90% of these. It is however, a complicated and expensive test, carrying a 3% risk of causing acute pancreatitis, which is usually mild.

Ultrasonography in skilled hands can be a very useful way of selecting patients who need ERCP. The pancreas can be adequately visualised in about 90% of patients and a correct diagnosis reached in approximately 80%. The test however depends on the skill of the operator and the reliability of scanning may vary considerably from one centre to another.

Computed tomography (CT) scanning is marginally superior to ultrasound and less operator dependent so in centres where it is readily available it is probably preferable. In order to achieve optimum imaging of the pancreas it should be performed with contrast and with multiple small (e.g. 2 mm) sections through the pancreas.

Pancreatic function tests

Assessment of pancreatic exocrine function is useful in quantifying the problem, but will not reliably discriminate benign from malignant pancreatic disease. The standard test for pancreatic function has been the secretin test, but in routine clinical practice this has largely been superceded by 'tubeless' tests because patients never like swallowing tubes and the secretin test is time consuming for both doctor and patient. The two most widely used tubeless tests are the N-benzoly -L-tyrosyl-p-amino-benzoic acid (NBT-PABA) test and the fluorescein dilaurate test.

THE SECRETIN TEST

The secretin test requires intubation of the duodenum under X-ray screening, with a second tube aspirating the stomach to prevent contamination of the duodenal aspirate with acid. Intravenous secretin, 1 u/kg, is given, sometimes followed 30 minutes later by cholecystokinin/pancreozymin. Duodenal juice is collected in aliquots over the hour following secretin and assayed for volume, bicarbonate concentration and enzyme concentration (trypsin, lipase or amylase). Volume, maximal bicarbonate concentration and enzyme concen-

tration are usually all reduced in significant benign or malignant pancreatic disease, but in carcinoma there is a tendency for bicarbonate and amylase concentrations to be less markedly depressed than in chronic pancreatitis. This distinction however, is not reliable and the test is mainly of use either in quantifying function in patients with known pancreatic disease or in discriminating between the normal and the diseased pancreas.

OTHER TESTS

NBT-PABA is split by pancreatic chymotrypsin with release of PABA (para-amino-benzoic acid), which is then absorbed and excreted in the urine. In order to exclude the possible effects of intestinal and renal function on the test, a second part of the test involves the measurement of the absorption and excretion of PABA alone. A ratio is calculated between excretion of PABA following ingestion of PABA and following ingestion of NBT-PABA. This can be performed either as a two-day test, or in one day if ^{14}C-PABA is used to check absorption. Concurrent treatment with frusemide, thiazides, sulphonamides and paracetamol have to be avoided as these drugs interfere with the assay for PABA.

The **fluorescein dilaurate** test is similar. Pancreatic esterase splits the fluorescein from its ester and the fluorescein is then absorbed and excreted in the urine. Again a second stage is necessary to assess the handling of non-esterified fluorescein, and with this test accurate timing of urine collection is essential.

Both tubeless tests produce similar results. They are both slightly less sensitive and specific for pancreatic disease than the secretin test, but are simpler to perform and preferred by the patient. Their use in diagnosis is limited and they are of most value in excluding pancreatic disease as a cause of proven malabsorption.

Is there small intestinal bacterial overgrowth?

Overgrowth of the small intestine with anaerobic bile salt deconjugating bacteria may result in fat malabsorption. Deconjugation of bile acids results in a failure of the enterohepatic recirculation and depletion of the bile acid pool and also prevents bile acids from forming micelles with dietary fat. There may also be microscopic changes in the gut epithelium. Significant contamination of the small intestine usually only occurs if there is an anatomical abnormality, either a surgically constructed 'blind loop' such as the afferent loop of a Polya gastrectomy or if there is diverticulosis or stricturing of the small intestine. Bacterial overgrowth of the small intestine may also occur spontaneously in elderly patients without any anatomical abnormality.

The clinical presentation is either with steatorrhoea, which may be intermittent and severe, or with vitamin B_{12} deficiency. The mechanism of the B_{12} deficiency is not clearly understood. Although fat malabsorption always seem to be the result of overgrowth with anaerobic bacteria, it is thought that aerobic bacteria may sometimes cause vitamin B_{12} malabsorption. There are several possible explanations: firstly the bacteria may consume vitamin B_{12}, secondly they may break the bond between intrinsic factor and vitamin B_{12} and thirdly they may adhere to the B_{12}/intrinsic factor complex and prevent its uptake in the terminal ileum.

The most direct approach to diagnosis is by sampling the small bowel contents, but this is often unreliable as anaerobic bacteria may be difficult to culture and the siting of the sampling tube may also be critical, particularly if bacterial overgrowth is localised to a short section of the small intestine.

^{14}C-glycocholate breath test

If the main problem is fat malabsorption then the most logical test for bacterial overgrowth is the ^{14}C-glycocholate breath test. In this test a small amount of ^{14}C-labelled glycocholate is taken by mouth. The radiolabel is sited in the glycine molecule and in a healthy person approximately 95% of the ^{14}C-glycocholate is taken up intact in the distal ileum and recirculated via the liver into the bile without breakdown.

In a patient with small bowel bacterial overgrowth the glycocholate is deconjugated by anaerobic bacteria into glycine and cholic acid; the glycine is then absorbed and metabolised by the liver and one of the metabolities formed is ^{14}C-labelled carbon dioxide, which is then breathed out via the lungs.

This process is fairly lengthy and as a result the test has to be performed over seven or eight hours, but it is very simple and non-invasive apart from the small dose of radioisotope.

A known molar quantity of carbon dioxide is collected by asking the patient to breathe out through a trap containing an indicator and the proportion of the carbon dioxide that is radiolabelled is estimated by scintillation counting.

The main drawback of this test apart from its length is that patients with small intestinal disease (e.g. Crohn's disease) will fail to absorb the ^{14}C-glycocholate, which will then pass into the colon and be deconjugated by the colonic bacteria. Because of the time taken to metabolise the glycine, it is not possible to distinguish malabsorption of the ^{14}C-glycocholate from bacterial overgrowth.

The lactulose hydrogen breath test

The lactulose hydrogen breath test is an alternative test that avoids this problem. In this test 20 ml of lactulose syrup (containing approximately 8.5 g of lactulose) is taken by mouth, and breath hydrogen is sampled at 5-minute intervals for half an hour and then at 15- minute intervals for three hours.

Almost all the hydrogen in the breath comes from carbohydrate fermentation by bacteria in the intestine, and in the fasting patient, breath hydrogen levels are usually less than 20 parts/million.

In the normal patient the lactulose will pass through into the caecum with a transit time varying between 30 minutes and 120 minutes, and hydrogen will be identifiable in the breath within 5–10 minutes of the transit time. In a patient with small bowel bacterial overgrowth hydrogen can be detected in the breath in the first 10–20 minutes after swallowing lactulose (a rise of more than 20 ppm is significant).

Schilling test

If the patient has B_{12} deficiency then a Schilling test for B_{12} absorption will typically show malabsorption of B_{12} that is not corrected by addition of intrinsic factor, but this also occurs in patients with disease of the small intestine.

Therapeutic trial of antibiotics

An alternative to the performance of these tests is a therapeutic trial of antibiotics, either tetracycline or metronidazole. The breath tests are, however, very easy to perform and give a more certain diagnosis. Excretion of **indicans** into the urine as the result of bacterial metabolism of unabsorbed protein in the small intestine has been employed as a test for bacterial overgrowth in the past, but it does not discriminate from other causes of malabsorption and has been superceded by the breath tests.

Is there a protein-losing enteropathy?

Protein-losing enteropathy is a syndrome rather than a disease. It is the intestinal equivalent of the nephrotic syndrome. Some causes of protein loss from the intestine are obvious exudative conditions such as Crohn's disease or tuberculosis, but others are subtler and may present with symptoms related to the hyoproteinaemia without any intestinal symptoms. The syndrome should be suspected if there is hypoalbuminaemia unexplained by proteinuria, anorexia or an acute phase response to intercurrent illness.

The first step should be to confirm the presence of gastrointestinal protein loss. Two main techniques are used:

- Faecal chromium loss: radioactive $^{51}CrCl_3$ is injected intravenously and becomes bound to circulating albumin and transferrin. Faecal samples are then collected over several days and radioactivity counted.
- Faecal clearance of alpha-1 antitrypsin, estimated after assay in faecal and serum samples is equally effective and less invasive.

Causes of protein-losing enteropathy

Causes include any disease that causes ulceration or inflammation of the intestine, but it also occurs in other specific conditions, which include the following:

- Hypertrophic gastritis (Ménétrier's disease).
- Coeliac disease.
- Giant gastric ulcer.
- Gastric cancer.
- Intestinal lymphoma.
- Lymphatic obstruction.
- Intestinal lymphangiectasia.
- Congestive heart failure.

CONDITIONS CAUSING DIARRHOEA: NATURAL HISTORY AND MANAGEMENT

Ulcerative colitis

Natural history

Ulcerative colitis can affect patients of any age, from early childhood onwards, but the incidence is highest in early adulthood. Usually an acute attack is followed by a long period of remission, but unfortunately relapse is almost inevitable at some stage. In one series only 4% of patients remained free from attacks after 15 years of follow-up. For about 35% of patients the disease fails to go into a clearcut remission, but continues to grumble on.

The severity of attacks is very variable and is closely linked to the extent of colonic involvement. If the disease is limited to the rectum (proctitis), symptoms usually consist of passage of mucus and blood per rectum with annoying tenesmus, but little diarrhoea. More extensive ulceration causes diarrhoea, which is often bloody and if ulceration extends deeper into the mucosa pain and fever develop. In such a severe attack there is an appreciable risk of perforation and before modern surgery and corticosteroid therapy were available such attacks had a mortality of approximately 35%.

In a survey from Oxford the risks of needing colectomy during the first five years were as follows:

- 1 in 50 after the onset of proctitis.
- 1 in 20 for colitis of intermediate severity.
- 1 in 3 for severe colitis.

Another study found that the overall likelihood of needing colectomy was 15% in the first ten years.

EPIDEMIOLOGY

Surveys in Europe and the USA have shown an incidence of new cases of ulcerative colitis of 2 –8/100,000/year and a prevalence of 40–80/100,000. There is no convincing evidence of any change in frequency over the last 30 years. About 10–20% of patients have a first degree relative with inflammatory bowel disease. This will not necessarily be ulcerative colitis as there is also an increased risk of Crohn's

disease in first degree relatives of patients with ulcerative colitis (and vice versa). This has led to speculation that ulcerative colitis and Crohn's disease might represent different ends of a spectrum of inflammatory bowel disease with a common aetiology. The pattern of inheritance is unclear and no convincing link with human leucocyte antigen (HLA) type has been found in Europeans with the disease.

AETIOLOGY AND PATHOGENESIS

The aetiology of ulcerative colitis is unknown. Histologically it resembles the inflammatory types of infectious diarrhoea, but although attacks may occasionally be precipitated by gastroenteritis. there is little microbiological or epidemiological evidence to support an infective cause. Anti-colon antibodies are sometimes detectable in the serum of patients, as are lymphocytes that are cytotoxic to fetal colon cells, but there is no evidence that any of these immunological phenomena act *in vivo* as a fundamental part of the disease process. Anti-neutrophil cytoplasmic antibodies that bind in the perinuclear region (pANCA) can be found in the sera of about 60% of patients. Recently, evidence has been gathering that suggests an underlying defect in the colonic mucin glycoprotein structure, but as with the immunological studies it is difficult to be certain whether these abnormalities are occurring as a cause or as a result of the disease. There is a very striking association between nonsmoking and ulcerative colitis, up to 95% being non-smokers or ex-smokers, and there is anecdotal evidence in some patients that smoking has a beneficial effect on the colitis. Conversely there is a positive association between smoking and Crohn's disease.

▶ **Ulcerative colitis**

- Prevalence about 1/2000
- 10–20% have a first degree relative with inflammatory bowel disease
- 95% are non-smokers or ex-smokers
- 60% have circulating anti-neutrophil antibodies (pANCA)
- Over 95% have more than one attack
- Approximately 20% eventually require colectomy
- Colon cancer occurs in about 7% of patients with extensive colitis by 20 years (an 11-fold increase in relative risk)

Extra-intestinal manifestations

Ulcerative colitis and Crohn's disease both have a number of extra-intestinal manifestations (**Figs 3.26–3.28**), which occur when the bowel disease is active. These include:

- **Erythema nodosum** (painful red nodules usually on the lower legs).
- Non-erosive **arthritis,** usually of medium or large joints, particularly the knees.
- **Episcleritis** or **uveitis**.

Although troublesome at the time, they all resolve when the underlying bowel disease is effectively treated. Similar problems occur in infective diarrhoeas and it is likely that they are related to the presence of circulating immune complexes formed as a result of antigens, probably bacterial in origin, leaking in through the ulcerated intestine.

Ucerative colitis and Crohn's disease are also associated with a 20–30-fold increased risk of **ankylosing spondylitis,** which affects 2–6% of patients. It is associated with HLA B27 in approximately 65% of patients, but this association is not as strong as for ankylosing spondylitis in the absence of inflammatory bowel disease when more than 90% of the patients have HLA B27. It also bears no relation to the activity of the underlying bowel disease, which it may antedate.

Pyoderma gangrenosum is an unpleasant chronic ulcerating skin disease with lesions usually starting on the limb or trunk. It occurs in 1–5% of patients with ulcerative colitis and nearly 50% of patients with pyoderma have colitis. Its presence bears some relationship to the activity of colitis but it has occasionally developed some time after colectomy.

Finger clubbing is not uncommon in ulcerative colitis, but usually very mild. **Primary sclerosing cholangitis** is a rare chronic stricturing disease of the intra- and extrahepatic bile ducts that is associated with ulcerative colitis in over 70% of cases. The colitis may be mild or even subclinical and colectomy has no effect on the course of the liver disease, which ultimately leads to secondary biliary cirrhosis and portal hypertension. Bile duct carcinoma is also associated with ulcerative colitis and although the incidence is low (approximately 1%), the relative risk for a patient with ulcerative colitis developing this cancer is increased 22-fold compared with an age-matched control population.

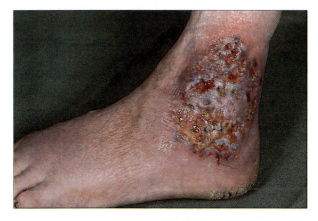

Fig. 3.26 Pyoderma gangrenosum complicating ulcerative colitis. Courtesy of Dr EL Rhodes.

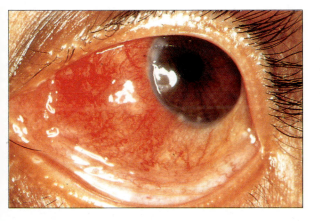

Fig. 3.27 Episcleritis complicating active Crohn's disease.

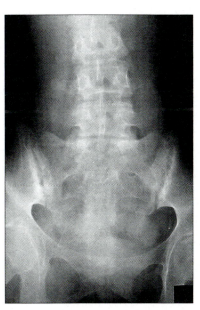

Fig. 3.28 Sacro-iliitis in a patient with ulcerative colitis.

COLORECTAL CANCER COMPLICATING COLITIS

Colonic cancer is the long-term complication of ulcerative colitis that gives most concern. The size of the increased risk correlates with the extent of the disease. Patients with disease limited to the rectum and sigmoid have little or no increase in risk, and recent data from three centres in the UK and Sweden have shown that patients with extensive colitis have a 0.6% risk of developing colonic cancer in the first ten years after diagnosis, 7.1% in the first 20 years, and 16.4% in the first 30 years.

The association with disease duration is not as simple as it seems as the age-matched relative risk remains fairly constant after the first five years, so it is possible to speculate that there may be an underlying defect that simultaneously predisposes to both ulcerative colitis and cancer rather than a simple progression from chronic inflammation through hyperplasia, dysplasia and cancer.

Management

Management is usually medical, at least in the first instance. Treatment should be started early as soon as the diagnosis is established and infective diarrhoea excluded, as there is considerable anecdotal evidence that delay in treatment reduces the chance of gaining a remission. **Corticosteroids** are the most effective treatment in the acute attack. They may be given rectally, orally or intravenously depending on the extent of the colitis. If the disease is localised to the rectum, local steroids are the best form of treatment. They may be given either as twice daily enemas or as a hydrocortisone rectal foam, which many patients find easier to manage. Topical 5-aminosalicylates as enemas or suppositories (e.g. mezalazine 500mgs/day) are also very effective. If the colitis is more extensive, in which case diarrhoea will be more prominent, systemic corticosteroids should be used. Controlled trials suggest that prednisolone, 40 mg/day, is the optimum dose in adults. The dose should be tailed down gradually over the next 6–8 weeks.

Maintenance treatment with corticosteroids has been shown to be ineffective, and should generally be avoided. In occasional patients with chronically 'grumbling'colitis alternate-day treatment with about 20 mg of prednisolone may be helpful and will not usually result in significant side-effects.

SEVERE COLITIS

If there is no convincing response to treatment within two weeks or if the patient is ill with abdominal pain, vomiting, fever or anaemia the patient should be admitted to hospital. As absorption may be unpredictable, corticosteroids should then be given intravenously (e.g. hydrocortisone, 100 mg four times daily). A plain abdominal radiograph should be performed and repeated daily if the patient is unwell or if the initial radiograph shows evidence of colonic dilatation (a diameter greater than 5.5 cm in the transverse colon).

Dilatation almost always implies that inflammation has spread through into the muscle layers of the colon and is associated with a high risk of perforation, which has a mortality of 50%. If the dilatation fails to resolve within a day or two colectomy is indicated and it may be unwise to delay even this long if the patient is toxic and tender over the colon. Blood transfusion may be necessary if the patient has become anaemic.

▶ **Extra-intestinal manifestations of ulcerative colitis**

Related to disease activity
- Non-erosive arthritis of large joints
- Erythema nodosum
- Iritis

Possibly related to disease activity
- Pyoderma gangrenosum

Not clearly related to disease activity
- Sclerosing cholangitis/ chronic active hepatitis
- Ankylosing spondylitis

▶ **Features of severe colitis**
- Pyrexia > 37.5°C
- Tachycardia > 100
- Serum albumin < 30 g/l
- Haemoglobin < 10 g/l
- Severe pain
- Severe bleeding

Severe colitis is an indication for:
- Admission to hospital.
- Plain abdominal radiography every two days to exclude dilatation.
- Intravenous corticosteroid therapy.
- Colectomy if not responding within 10 days of intensive medical therapy

Sulphasalazine and the related 5-aminosalicylates

Sulphasalazine and the related 5-aminosalicylates are the only other drugs of unequivocal benefit in ulcerative colitis. Sulphasalazine consists of a sulphonamide (sulphapyridine) linked by an azo bond to 5-aminosalicylic acid. It was first developed in the 1940s for the treatment of rheumatoid arthritis, but found fortuitously to improve colitis.

The 5-aminosalicylic acid component seems to be the active moiety, the sulphapyridine serving to carry the 5-aminosalicylic acid through into the colon in high concentration. The majority of the sulphasalazine is then split by bacteria with release of the 5-aminosalicylic acid. Its mode of action is uncertain, but seems to be unrelated to prostaglandin inhibition (and other prostaglandin inhibitors tend to make colitis worse). It has a number of immunological effects including the suppression of chemotatic leukotriene production by leucocytes. It has a mild effect in acute colitis, but is most useful as maintenance therapy to prevent relapse of the disease.

Maintenance treatment with sulphasalazine, 2 g daily, reduces the risk of relapse by 66%. Unfortunately about 20% of patients are unable to tolerate the drug in adequate dosage. The main reason for this is intolerance to the sulphapyridine, some of which is absorbed and causes nausea and headaches. This is particularly a problem in patients who are slow acetylators. The drug also causes reversible male infertility. These problems can be avoided by using one of several alternative preparations in which the 5-aminosalicylic acid is either linked to a different carrier molecule (balsalazide), dimerised via an azo-bond (olsalazine) or contained in a pH-dependent delayed-release or enteric-coated capsule (mesalazine). Occasional nephrotoxicity has been reported with these preparations so careful monitoring is essential.

Allergy is less commonly a problem and may be due to either the sulphonamide or salicylate component. In a patient with troublesome colitis it may be worth cautiously densitizing the patient by starting with very low doses, initially as a hospital in-patient.

ANTIDIARRHOEAL DRUGS

Antidiarrhoeal drugs such as codeine and loperamide should generally be avoided, first, because they may make it difficult to assess whether the colitis is responding adequately to treatment and second, because there is anecdotal evidence that they increase the risk of colonic dilatation, and third, because they have little effect on bowel frequency in colitis. Their use may be necessary in the occasional patient with chronic low-grade colitis.

OTHER DRUGS

Azathioprine has a small additional effect in patients receiving corticosteroids, but this benefit has to be balanced against the definite risk of bone marrow toxicity and its use (1–2 mg/kg/day) should be restricted to occasional patients who are responding poorly to corticosteroids. Blood counts should be monitored monthly.

Metronidazole has been shown to be ineffective in controlled trials.

Cyclosporin, for which good results have been reported in small numbers of patients, is nephrotoxic and this is likely to prevent its widespread use. It may however be useful as intravenous therapy (4 mg/kg/day) in patients with severe colitis who do not respond well to initial therapy with corticosteroids and whose colitis is not sufficiently severe or extensive to warrant immediate surgery.

Bismuth subsalicylate enemas have been found effective in steroid-resistant colitis.

Arsenic, which is one of the oldest forms of therapy, still has an occasional role in the form of **Acetarsol suppositories**. These are occasionally effective in proctitis when other treatments have failed. Although they seem safe, it is prudent to avoid them in women of childbearing age and to check for arsenic absorption in any patient receiving them for more than two months.

Oral tobramycin, nicotine patches and lignocaine enemas are other treatments that have shown promise in uncontrolled trials.

The wide variety of treatments reflects the fact that although most patients settle well with corticosteroid therapy, there are patients who do not respond well to conventional therapy. A wide range of inhibitors of cytokines and inflammatory mediators are currently undergoing evaluation and it is likely that the range of effective therapies will expand considerably in the near future.

▶ **Treatment of ulcerative colitis**

- Corticosteroids for the acute attack
- Avoid maintenance corticosteroids
- 5-aminosalycylic acid drugs for maintenance (only to be used as sole therapy for acute disease in very mild attacks)
- Avoid anti-diarrhoeal drugs
- Normal diet, but low on dairy products
- Admit if not responding within two weeks or if disease is severe

MANAGEMENT IN PREGNANCY

There is no good evidence that pregnancy makes colitis worse, and about 66% will go to term without a relapse of colitis if they were in remission at conception. The colitis should be managed as usual. There is no evidence of harm to the fetus from conventional use of 5-aminosalicylates or of corticosteroids, although the neonatalogists should be fully informed of the therapy. The fetus will be put at much greater risk if the colitis is undertreated and fails to come under control. Rigid or flexible sigmiodoscopy are safe in pregnancy if carefully performed, but should only be necessary during relapse.

DIET

Diet seems to have little effect on the course of ulcerative colitis. Bowel rest and intravenous feeding have no beneficial effect, but may be necessary in the severely ill malnourished patient. About 20% of patients will benefit from avoiding milk and it is sensible in any case to advise a low milk diet in all patients with active colitis because hypolactasia is common during attacks and milk is therefore likely to exacerbate the diarrhoea. Patients should otherwise be encouraged to eat a normal diet.

SURGERY

The main indications for colectomy in ulcerative colitis are failure of medical treatment and the development of cancer or severe dysplasia. In a patient hospitalised with severe colitis, failure to respond after one week of high-dose intravenous corticosteroid therapy should usually be taken as an indication for surgery as the chances of a useful remission being achieved if there has been no response by this time are slim. Colonic dilatation in an acute colitis that has not settled within 48 hours should also be taken as an indication for surgery. Perforation is of course an indication for emergency colectomy, but it carries a mortality of 50% and should not occur with careful and prompt medical treatment.

It is more difficult to decide when to operate on the less severe colitic who fails to go into a complete remission, but remains in good general health. Often the right side of the colon is relatively uninvolved. In such patients, a prolonged trial of alternate-day oral corticosteroids may be reasonable (in combination with a 5-ASA preparation and probably a third therapy in addition such as bismuth enemas or azathioprine), but if this fails total colectomy is the only satisfactory solution. The temptation to perform a left hemicolectomy must be avoided because colitis then inevitably develops in the residual colon and the cancer risk remains.

Colectomy is not an appropriate treatment for the extra-intestinal manifestations of colitis. Sclerosing cholangitis and ankylosing spondylitis both continue unchecked and although colectomy has been recommended for patients with intractable pyoderma gangrenosum the response is very

unreliable and there have been several reports of the skin lesion appearing for the first time after colectomy.

Types of colectomy

- The conventional operation is **total colectomy with ileostomy**. If the patient is ill many surgeons prefer to perform this as a two-stage procedure leaving behind a rectal stump at the first operation. This should not be left indefinitely however as continuing proctitis is likely to be very troublesome.
- Occasionally an **ileo-rectal anastomosis** is performed and surgeons vary considerably in their views on this. There are several published series and the proportion of patients considered suitable has ranged widely. Between 10–20% will subsequently need the rectum excising and the risk of cancer in the rectal stump has been estimated as 6% in 20 years. Most people would only consider the operation worthwhile either in the elderly or as a temporary measure in the young unmarried patient with relative rectal sparing.
- Encouraging progress has been made with the construction of a false rectum from the ileum (ileal pouch) so allowing an **ileo-anal anastomosis**. It is worth considering referring a young patient who is not severely ill to a surgeon who can offer this operation. The patient will need to be warned that it is possible that a second or even third operation might be necessary for revision of the pouch and that the hospital stay is likely to be longer. When successful, bowel frequency usually varies between three and eight times in 24 hours and most patients are normally continent, though may need to wear a pad at night. Some patients develop a recurrence of 'colitis' in the ileal pouch (i.e. 'pouchitis'), but this is usually mild and responds well to oral metronidazole.

SCREENING FOR CANCER

The increased risk of colon cancer in ulcerative colitis arguably justifies regular colonoscopic surveillance. The current practice in most units is to perform total colonoscopy with multiple biopsy at yearly or two-yearly intervals in any patients with extensive colitis of more than 7–10 years duration. The indications for colectomy (other than carcinoma) are still being defined.

Pre-malignant change (high-grade dysplasia) indicates a high risk of carcinoma, but assessment of the severity of dysplasia is subjective and panels of expert pathologists differ considerably in their grading of individual biopsies (**Figs 3.29** and **3.30**). The presence of inflammation makes dysplasia particularly difficult to interpret. The risk of cancer somewhere in the colon has been estimated at 50% if high-grade dysplasia is found on biopsy. Dysplasia in a macroscopically visible lesion, a nodule or plaque, is certainly an

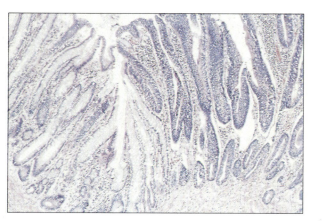

Fig. 3.29 Dysplasia in ulcerative colitis (low magnification). An area of darker, severely dysplastic crypts is seen on the right, and paler, mildly dysplastic crypts on the left.

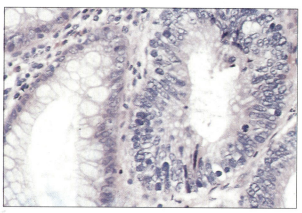

Fig. 3.30 Dysplasia in ulcerative colitis (high magnification). A contrast can be seen between severely dysplastic crypts with hyperchromatic nuclei arrranged haphazardly, and mildly dysplastic crypts with mucin-containing cells and nuclei arranged in an orderly fashion close to the basement membrane.

indication for colectomy. Dysplasia in flat mucosa should be checked by early repeat colonoscopy and rebiopsy, preferably with more than one pathological opinion, and if high-grade dysplasia is found again colectomy should be recommended.

The cost-effectiveness of such screening programmes has been questioned, but it is very difficult to stop a screening programme once started and most patients are well aware of the increased risk of colon cancer and are considerably reassured by regular screening.

Barium enema is not a suitable investigation for screening patients with long-standing ulcerative colitis for several reasons listed below:

- Cancers in ulcerative colitic mucosa usually arise as flat lesions and are unlikely to be detectable at an early stage by radiograph.
- Pseudopolyps are common in chronic ulcerative colitis. They arise from islands of hypertrophic mucosa, which have been surrounded by ulceration during previous relapse of disease. They are non-malignant, but cannot be reliably distinguished from adenomatous polyps by radiograph.
- Fibromuscular strictures are not uncommon in chronic disease, they reflect the colonic shortening and are usually not true strictures, being easily negotiated endoscopically; however, they cannot be distinguished from malignant strictures radiologically.

Crohn's disease

Natural history

The consequences of the disease depend on the site of bowel involvement and the age at onset. Ileal disease typically causes colicky pain, diarrhoea and, if untreated, weight loss, while colonic disease causes diarrhoea and sometimes rectal bleeding, usually with relatively little pain.

As with ulcerative colitis, active disease may be associated with 'reactive' inflammation outside the intestine in the form of acute arthritis, anterior uveitis or erythema nodosum. Crohn's disease may actually present with one of these extraintestinal manifestations in the absence of symptoms of intestinal disease. Pyoderma gangrenosum may occur, but is much more commonly associated with ulcerative colitis. Significant liver disease is also uncommon as a complication of Crohn's disease and there are very few convincing cases of sclerosing cholangitis reported in association with Crohn's disease. Pericholangitis, the accumulation of inflammatory cells around small bile ducts within the portal tracts is common, but of little or no clinical significance.

Amyloidosis may rarely complicate Crohn's disease and may occasionally present early in the course of the disease. It is probably linked with the very marked 'acute phase response' associated with active Crohn's disease. One of the acute phase proteins produced by the liver as part of this response is the amyloid A protein. Other proteins produced in increased quantity include orosomucoid (serum acid glycoprotein) and CRP, measurement of which gives a useful guide to the activity of the Crohn's disease.

EPIDEMIOLOGY

Crohn's disease occurs with a similar frequency to ulcerative colitis. Reported incidence of new cases averages about 4/100,000/year in the UK with a prevalence about 50/100,000. The disease almost never affects black Africans and the risk for black Americans is only about 20% of that for white Americans.

AETIOLOGY AND PATHOGENESIS

Genetic and environmental factors are probably both important in the aetiology. Approximately 10% of patients have a relative with inflammatory bowel disease, which in about 35% of cases is ulcerative colitis rather than Crohn's disease. This has led to speculation that Crohn's disease and ulcerative colitis may represent opposite ends of a spectrum of one inflammatory bowel disease rather than being separate diseases.

Dietary surveys have shown that patients with Crohn's disease tend to have a high pre-illness intake of refined sugar and a low intake of vegetable fibre. A controlled trial of a high-fibre, low-sugar diet has however failed to show benefit and it may be that some other aetiological factor correlates with a sugary, low fibre 'modern' diet. For whatever reason the disease seems to have become increasingly common over the last 30 years, although recent data suggests that the incidence may now be 'plateauing' out.

Other aetiological theories for Crohn's disease include immunological abnormalities and infectious agents, but there is as yet no conclusive evidence to support these hypotheses. There is probably an association between oral contraceptive use and a form of colitis that mimics Crohn's disease and this may account for a small proportion of colonic Crohn's disease.

PATHOLOGY

Although Burrill Crohn and his colleagues described only terminal ileal disease and its complications in 1922, it is now known that the disease can affect any part of the gastrointestinal tract from mouth to anus. The commonest site for disease is the ileo-caecal region followed by the colon alone, small intestine alone and much more rarely stomach, mouth and, very rarely, oesophagus. Inflammation runs deep into the layers of the intestine in distinction to ulcerative colitis, where it rarely breaches the muscularis mucosa. As a consequence, strictures, fissures and fistulae are hallmarks of the disease. Fistulae are particularly disabling and may lead from one segment of intestine to another, and from intestine to bladder, vagina or skin. Malabsorption is common and if the disease occurs in childhood, growth is likely to be inhibited, and this may even be the presenting symptom if intestinal symptoms are mild.

Histologically the hallmark of the disease is the occurrence of non-caseating granulomas. All layers of the mucosa contain increased chronic inflammatory cells. Crypt abscesses occur in colonic disease, but mucus is usually retained even in the presence of inflammation unlike ulcerative colitis where mucus depletion is marked.

Management

Much of the management of Crohn's disease has until recently been empirical and in no other condition can the Hippocratic principle 'if you can't do any good at least do no harm' be more appropriate. Common mistakes in clinical management have in the past included inappropriate maintenance corticosteroid therapy with all its inherent risks, excessive resection of diseased intestine and inadequate attention to nutrition.

SUPPRESSION OF ACTIVE DISEASE: DRUG THERAPY

Corticosteroids

Until the cause of Crohn's disease is known, the treatment inevitably remains empirical. Corticosteroids are effective at suppressing symptoms, but there is no evidence that they improve the prognosis. It is reasonable to treat active disease with short courses of corticosteroids starting with prednisolone, 20–30 mg/day in an adult, and tailing off over 2–3 months. Unfortunately the symptoms frequently recur when the corticosteroids are tailed off. Maintenance corticosteroid therapy should be avoided if at all possible. Alternate-day corticosteroid therapy reduces the risk of side-effects and should be used, particularly in children with Crohn's disease if prolonged therapy proves unavoidable. Rectal Crohn's disease may be treated with limited success by corticosteroid enemas, but corticosteroid therapy in Crohn's disease that affects other sites needs to be systemic. It is important to treat the patient and not the radiographs. Severe radiological abnormalities can sometimes persist for several years in association with minimal symptoms.

Sulphasalazine and other 5-aminosalicylates

Sulphasalazine is of doubtful value in Crohn's disease. Trials have shown conflicting results in both small intestinal and colonic Crohn's disease. It probably has a mild beneficial effect and is worth trying in patients with troublesome disease. The results of trials with mesalazine and olsalazine are similarly mixed, but encouraging results are being reported with enteric coated mesalazine (Pentasa), 2 g/day. in patients with distal ileal disease.

Metronidazole

Metronidazole is valuable in the treatment of colonic Crohn's disease (in contrast to ulcerative colitis in which it has no effect) and perianal disease. Treatment usually has to be prolonged (eg. 400 mg three times daily orally for 2–3 months). More lengthy courses carry a high risk of drug-related peripheral neuropathy.

Immunosuppression

Azathioprine (2 mg/kg/day) or its active metabolite 6-mercaptopurine are sometimes used in the treatment of chronically 'grumbling' Crohn's disease, particularly if steroid withdrawal is proving difficult. There is a considerable risk of marrow suppression even with careful monitoring so these drugs should only be used for occasional patients under very careful supervision. Controlled trials have shown a beneficial effect in active Crohn's disease and there have been several anecdotal reports of fistula closure.

DIETARY THERAPY

Good results have been reported with various forms of dietary therapy. These are used not just to improve nutrition, but also to suppress active disease. Three main forms of dietary treatment have been used:

- Intravenous feeding.
- Enteral feeding with an amino acid-based 'elemental' feed.
- Exclusion diet therapy.

Enteral elemental feeding with an amino acid-based liquid feed (e.g. EO28) as the sole feed has been shown to be as effective as corticosteroids in suppressing active disease. Subsequent studies have shown equally good results with some whole-protein liquid feeds (e.g. Triosorbon), but there are interesting discrepancies between some of these studies, and further studies are required to determine what essential features are required in an enteral feed to obtain a remission of Crohn's disease. There is some evidence that feeds containing very little long-chain fat give better results.

Intravenous feeding may be necessary in occasional patients with intestinal obstruction or severe malabsorption, but is several times more expensive and carries the risks of central venous line sepsis and pneumothorax. It is no more effective than enteral feeding and should only be used when enteral feeding is impossible (e.g. because of fistula formation or obstruction).

It is at present not clear which patients are most likely to benefit from dietary therapy or how this form of therapy should be continued. The great advantage of enteral feeding is that it is almost totally without risk to the patient. It is particularly useful in the short-term therapy of the ill patient with extensive Crohn's disease. Unfortunately the disease tends to relapse when normal food is introduced (50% relapse within six months). In one interesting study this problem was avoided by stepwise reintroduction of foods with exclusion of any that were subsequently found to induce symptoms (**Figs 3.31 and 3.32**). Not all units seem to have had such good results with exclusion diets, however, and further studies are needed.

The mechanism for the therapeutic effect of dietary treatment is quite unclear. Possibilities include the avoidance of antigenic material or potentially harmful food additives (carrageenan E407 has been suspected), or simply that the lower residue and low fat content either result in a reduction in intestinal bacteria or reduce the 'strain' on the supposedly ischaemic mucosa. Some studies have shown similar benefit

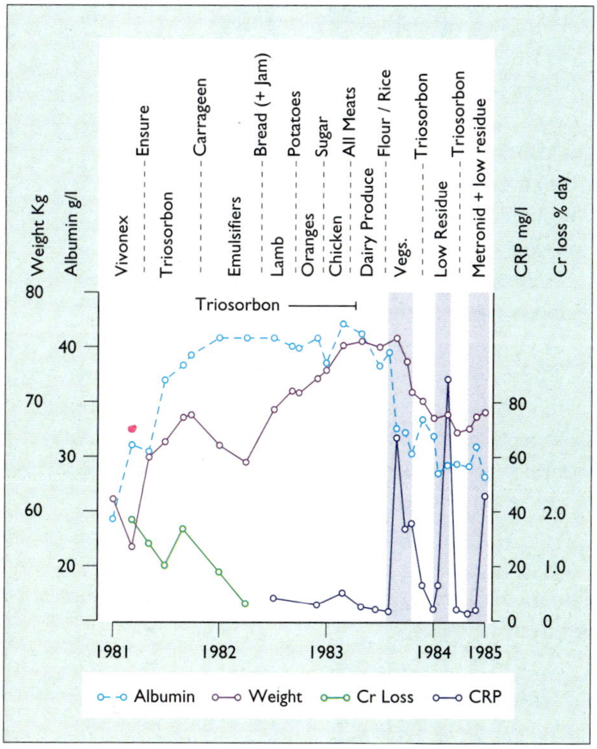

Fig. 3.31 Effect of long-term enteral feeding in a patient with extensive small bowel Crohn's disease. Remission (indicated by a gain in weight and serum albumin and a fall in faecal protein loss estimated using radiolabelled chromium) is achieved initially with an amino-acid-based feed (Vivonex) and maintained with a whole protein feed (Triosorbon), while various food substances are reintroduced. Relapse eventually occurs when fruit and vegetable fibre is introduced, and is indicated by a marked rise in serum CRP. Two further relapses correspond to further attempts to reintroduce food. (With permission from Raouf et al., Gut 1991; **32**: 702.)

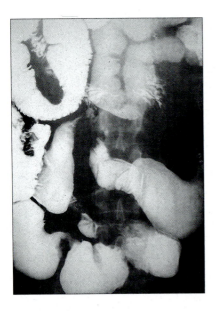

Fig. 3.32 Multiple small bowel strictures due to Crohn's disease (same patient as featured in Fig. 3.31). These were eventually treated with multiple stricturoplasty without a significant loss of small intestine.

from supplementing an otherwise normal diet with enteral feeds and it has been shown that improved nutrition produces changes in the immune response, particularly enhanced cellular immunity, that might also be responsible for a therapeutic response.

▶ **Enteral therapy as therapy for Crohn's disease**

- As effective as corticosteroids for inducing remission in small bowel disease
- No side-effects
- Requires a stoical well-motivated patient
- Takes 3–4 weeks to induce a clinical remission in 67% of patients
- Approximately 50% of patients relapse within six months of returning to a normal diet
- Not all enteral feeds are equally effective

SURGERY

Surgery for Crohn's disease is never curative. In patients treated by surgery the median interval between resections is about 15 years. There has therefore been a trend for surgery in Crohn's disease to be increasingly conservative. This has been reinforced by the recognition that anastamoses may be made successfully in diseased bowel providing any distal obstructions have been relieved.

The main indications for surgery in Crohn's disease are strictures, fistulae and colonic disease that are not responding to medical therapy.

▶ **Common mistakes in the management of Crohn's disease**

- Inappropriate maintenance corticosteroid therapy
- Excessive resection of diseased small intestine
- Inadequate attention to nutrition

Strictures

Most Crohn's disease lesions are stricturing and the decision whether to resect is often difficult. Symptoms often correlate poorly with the radiological appearance, and medical treatment, either corticosteroids or dietary should usually be tried in the first instance. Different units vary considerably in their threshold for surgery although overall rates for surgery are remarkably similar (i.e. it is the delay before surgery that varies rather than the proportion of patients operated on). The extent of the disease is an important factor.

- If there is only a single short ileal stricture surgery may well be preferable to prolonged corticosteroid therapy.
- If there is extensive involvement surgery may result in resection of unacceptable lengths of bowel.

This problem has been reduced by the introduction of stricturoplasty, a procedure first used in tuberculous intestinal strictures. This is a plastic operation to widen the lumen in a way analogous to pyloroplasty.

Fistulae

Fistulae in Crohn's disease may be entero-enteral, entero-vesical, enterovaginal or enterocutaneous.

- Entero-enteral fistulae can often be ignored if they do not bypass sufficient intestine to cause clinically significant malabsorption.
- Small entero-vesical fistulae may cause surprisingly few problems, but frequent urinary infections will necessitate surgery.
- Enterovaginal fistulae and enterocutaneous fistulae almost always require surgery.

There are anecdotal reports of fistula closure with azathioprine and its metabolite 6-mercaptopurine, but these are exceptional. Fistulae often dry up when the patient is fed enterally or intravenously, but usually break down when normal food is reintroduced.

Colonic disease

The medical treatment of colonic Crohn's disease tends to be unsatisfactory.

- Sulphasalazine is of doubtful benefit, most studies showing only marginal benefit compared with placebo.

▶ **Treatment of Crohn's disease**

For most patients with acute disease there are three alternative therapies

	Advantages	Disadvantages
Surgery	50% free from recurrence for five years	50% recurrence in five year
	Avoidance of steroid therapy	Shortens intestine
	Tissue diagnosis	Usually requires laparotomy (occasionally laparoscopy-assisted)
Corticosteroids	Easy for doctor and patient	No effect on long-term prognosis
	Good symptomatic relief	Difficult to withdraw without relapse
		Side-effects sometimes worse than disease
		Ineffective in fibrous strictures
Dietary (enteral feeding)	Totally safe	Requires stoical patient
	Good response in 67%	Relapse common on return to normal diet
	'Buys time' for the sick patient	Relatively expensive

- Corticosteroids are helpful and should be given rectally, preferably as a steroid foam or enema if the disease is limited to the distal colon, or systemically if the more proximal colon is involved.
- Metronidazole, 400 mg three times a day, has been shown to be effective, but normally has to be continued for 2–3 months. Longer courses of treatment are precluded by the risk of peripheral neuropathy.
- 'Resting' the bowel by elemental diet or surgical short circuiting of the colon ('split' ileostomy) often improves colonic Crohn's disease, and may allow time for the nutritional state to improve in a sick patient before definitive surgery, and occasionally produces a more sustained remission.

Ultimately about 50% of patients with colonic Crohn's disease will need surgery. The nature of the operation will depend on the site of the disease. A partial colectomy is occasionally an acceptable option (contrary to ulcerative colitis); the rectum can sometimes be spared if little involved.

Perianal disease
Perianal Crohn's disease occurs in up to 70% of patients with Crohn's disease and may be very distressing.

- Surgery should be kept to the minimum as a conventional approach to fistula excision will often result disastrously in a non-healing ulcer with recurrence of fistula and incontinence. Likewise skin tags should be treated by local hygiene rather than excision. (See also page 155.)
- Perianal abscesses may require drainage, but this should be achieved simply without excision.

- Metronidazole 400 mg three times a day for up to three months, may be useful probably because secondary infection contributes considerably to the morbidity. Longer term therapy with metronidazole carries an unacceptably high risk of drug-related neuropathy.

MANAGEMENT IN PREGNANCY
About 60–70% of mothers with inflammatory bowel disease will pass through pregnancy uneventfully if in remission at the time of conception. Metronidazole should be avoided but relapse should otherwise be treated conventionally. Corticosteroid therapy during pregnancy has not been shown to harm the fetus providing that neonatologists are fully informed. Attention to nutrition is particularly important during pregnancy and the puerperium.

Microscopic colitis
A normal-looking colon at colonoscopy, may show inflammation on biopsy, with an increase particularly in lamina propria lymphocytes. The condition is then usually termed 'microscopic colitis' and is usually a pancolitis. Patients are typically middle-aged or elderly women with watery diarrhoea, usually of fairly high output (> 500 ml/day). At least 50% of reported patients have also had small intestinal abnormalities (partial villous atrophy with lymphocytic infiltration), but usually with little or no response to a gluten-free diet. Laxative and non-steroidal anti-inflammatory drug (NSAID) use should be considered as possible causes of microscopic colitis. The majority of patients improve with sulphasalazine, but there is often little response to corticosteroids.

Collagenous colitis

This condition overlaps with microscopic colitis and some workers regard them as variants of the same condition. It is defined by an increase in the thickness of the subepithelial collagen band (**Fig. 3.33**). Normally this is up to 7 µm thick whereas in patients with the condition it is usually more than 10 µm thick. The patients also have chronic watery diarrhoea and associations have been reported with coeliac disease, scleroderma, and rheumatoid arthritis, but there is also some evidence that it may result from chronic use of non-steroidal antiinflammatory drugs, which could explain some of these associations.

NSAIDs should be stopped, a small bowel biopsy performed to exclude coeliac disease and, if negative, a trial of therapy with sulphasalazine started.

Ischaemic colitis

The colon is relatively prone to ischaemic damage, particularly in the region of the splenic flexure, which is a 'watershed' area between supplies from the middle colic and left colic arteries. Most patients are over 50 years of age. Presentation is typically with acute onset of left iliac fossa pain, rectal bleeding and subsequent diarrhoea. The rectum is almost never involved, which is a helpful diagnostic point. Right-sided colonic ischaemia occasionally occurs in younger people, sometimes in association with oral contraceptive usage. Barium enema will show characteristic mucosal oedema, 'thumb printing,' which is often visible on plain abdominal radiography.

For over 90% of patients the condition resolves spontaneously with bed rest, analgesia, intravenous fluids and broad-spectrum intravenous antibiotics. Laparotomy is indicated if there are signs of peritonitis or persistent bleeding. Resolution may be either complete or partial with resulting stricturing that usually requires no further treatment.

Irradiation enteritis

The **early phase of irradiation enteritis** can usually be managed with symptomatic treatment. Nausea can be effectively controlled with agents such as metoclopramide, domperidone and ondansetron. Watery diarrhoea may respond well to cholestyramine. Stool-bulking agents and a lactose-free diet may also be helpful. If there is a frank proctitis resulting in tenesmus, frequency and rectal bleeding, treatment with 5-ASA preparations or rectal corticosteroids is usually started, although there is little objective evidence of benefit in this situation.

Occasionally rectal bleeding may be severe, necessitating transfusion and some form of local therapy. Success has been reported with a variety of local treatments including laser therapy and diathermy cautery.

Later problems occurring months or years after the radiotherapy may include stricture formation. Rectal stricturing may necessitate defunctioning colostomy, which may be reversible after 6–12 months. Ileal stricturing may require resection, but symptomatic treatment should first be tried with cholestyramine or tetracycline (in case of bacterial overgrowth due to stasis). Occasionally rectovaginal fistulae may heal spontaneously, but most enterovesical and enterocolic fistulae eventually need surgical repair.

Pseudomembranous colitis and antibiotic-associated diarrhoea

Antibiotic-associated diarrhoea is commonly the result of overgrowth by toxin-producing *Clostridium difficile*. This may occur up to 3–4 weeks after antibiotic therapy. Any broad-spectrum antibiotic may be the precipitant, but clindamycin and lincomycin are particularly prone to this problem. The resulting illness can range from a mild watery diarrhoea to life-threatening pancolitis with toxic dilatation. Diagnosis is made in severe illness by seeing 1–2 mm diameter yellowish plaques at sigmoidoscopy, biopsy of which shows focal areas of mucosal necrosis (**Figs 3.34** and **3.35**).

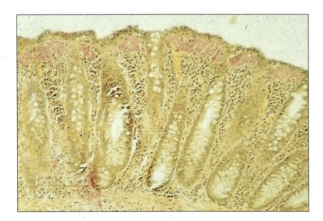

Fig. 3.33 Collagenous colitis. The subepithelial band of pink-staining collagen is clearly seen.

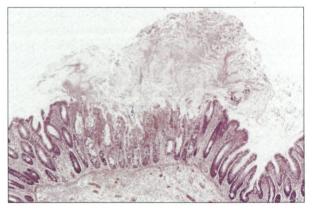

Fig. 3.34 Pseudomembranous colitis (low magnification). The superficial part of the colonic mucosa is inflamed and damaged, with overlying slough and inflammatory exudate forming a 'pseudomembrane'.

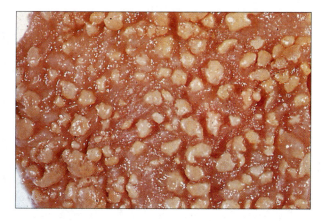

Fig. 3.35 Pseudomembranous colitis (resection specimen). The mucosal surface of the colon is covered by pale plaques of inflammatory exudate, each about 5 mm in diameter.

Management

Stool samples should be tested for the *C. difficile* toxin and cultured for *C. difficile*. Treatment is with either metronidazole, 400 mg three times daily for one week, or vancomycin, 125 mg four times daily for one week. Vancomycin is considerably more expensive, but its effectiveness is not significantly superior. Recurrence is a major problem (10–20%), probably due to a persistence of spores since antibiotic resistance does not occur. It can be treated by a further course of either antibiotic, followed by oral cholestyramine, 3 g four times daily for two weeks.

Ampicillin is occasionally associated with a specific colitis, sometimes haemorrhagic, which is a direct side-effect of the drug and stops when the drug is withheld. This is much less common than *C. difficile*-associated colitis.

Lactose intolerance

The most important aspect to the management of lactose intolerance is the need to exclude any significant underlying small intestinal disease. Acquired hypolactasia is usually idiopathic or the result of viral gastroenteritis (in which case the brush border disaccharidase activity usually recovers within a few weeks or months). Occasionally however hypolactasia may be the presenting feature of coeliac disease or Crohn's disease. An endoscopic duodenal biopsy should therefore be performed in any adult who develops persistent hypolactasia. Dietary advice is fairly straightforward, but patients who are keen to continue taking milk can either obtain lactose-free milk or a lactase preparation for pre-treatment of milk. It is important to note that many drug tablets contain lactose as a filler.

It should be noted that only people of Western European extraction retain lactase activity into adult life. In other races, hypolactasia is normal in adults.

Diabetic diarrhoea

Idiopathic diarrhoea in people with diabetes is a mysterious condition. It is generally assumed to be due at least in part to autonomic neuropathy, but its sudden onset, sometimes equally sudden response to tetracycline, and tendency to occur at night, are not well understood. Although it can be very troublesome the prognosis is generally good. It is important to exclude other causes of diarrhoea, particularly drugs. Metformin-induced diarrhoea is probably the commonest cause of diarrhoea in diabetics.

Infective diarrhoea

Natural history

The nature of the illness depends partly on whether the infection causes an inflammatory enteritis or has a predominantly secretory effect. Inflammatory infective diarrhoeas such as those caused by *Salmonella*, *Campylobacter* and *Shigella* tend to cause more systemic upset with a higher fever (38°C or more) and considerable abdominal pain. Median duration of symptoms is about 10 days. Secretory diarrhoeas such as that caused by enterotoxigenic *E. coli* ('travellers diarrhoea') usually cause a milder illness with less pyrexia. Usually they also have a shorter median duration (about five days) with the notable exception of cholera. The degree of debility depends very much on the success with which hydration is maintained.

EXTRA-INTESTINAL MANIFESTATIONS

Extra-intestinal manifestations of infective diarrhoea may be due to disseminated infection or immunological reaction.

- *Salmonella* septicaemia is often associated with minimal gastrointestinal symptoms and may result in abscess formation in any part of the body with a particular tendency to cause empyema of the gallbladder.
- Patients with sickle cell disease are unusually liable to develop *Salmonella* osteomyelitis.
- Patients with gallstones often fail to clear *Salmonella* even if they avoid empyema, and cholecystectomy is then the only way to eradicate the organism.
- Patients with HLA B27 are particularly prone to develop a transient reactive non-erosive arthropathy following *Salmonella*, *Campylobacter* or *Yersinia* enteritis.
- Erythema nodosum may also occur and cause confusion with inflammatory bowel disease. Both the reactive arthritis and erythema nodosum are assumed to be immune-complex-mediated and to reflect antigen leakage through an inflamed gut.

AETIOLOGY AND PATHOGENESIS

The causes and consequences of infective diarrhoea vary widely and depend on who is infected and where they are at the time. Adults infected in Europe or North America are most likely to have a *Campylobacter* or *Salmonella* infection; travellers in hotter countries are morely likely to acquire enterotoxigenic *E. coli*, while children are particularly prone to infection with rotavirus.

The type of infection sometimes depends on host resistance. Classic examples of the relationship between host resistance and infection include *C. difficile* infection (pseudomembranous colitis) following the use of broad-spectrum antibiotics, giardiasis in patients with immunoglobulin A deficiency, and cryptosporidiosis in patients with the acquired immune deficiency syndrome (AIDS).

Management

Most types of infective diarrhoea resolve spontaneously and much the most important part of treatment is the replacement of water and electrolytes. This has been revolutionised by the discovery that sugars will enhance salt and water absorption by the intestine, which has allowed even patients with very severe diarrhoea to be given adequate replacement therapy by mouth without the need for intravenous infusion. Effective treatment is now therefore much more readily available in the developing world and has had a major impact on the mortality from infectious diarrhoea. The formula recommended by the World Health Organization comprises:

- Sodium chloride, 3.5g/l.
- Trisodium citrate dihydrate, 2.9g/l.
- Potassium chloride, 1.5g/l.
- Glucose, 20g/l.

Cruder mixtures of salt and sugar are effective providing a simple measure (such as a double-ended spoon with appropriately sized ends, one for sugar and one for salt) is used to obtain the correct ratio of sugar to salt.

ANTIDIARRHOEAL DRUGS

Antidiarrhoeal drugs such as loperamide are useful in mild diarrhoea, but have little or no effect in more severe diarrhoea and may prolong the course of the illness. Suspensions of bismuth subsalicylate (Pepto-Bismol) 30 ml every 30 minutes until diarrhoea settles are effective and have an inhibitory effect on some *E. coli* toxins.

ANTIBIOTICS

The standard teaching has been that antibiotics should generally be avoided as they normally have little effect on the course of the illness and may actually prolong the duration of faecal excretion of bacteria. The situation has changed somewhat since the introduction of 4-quinolones such as ciprofloxacin, which do not have the disadvantage of prolonging excretion, and to which resistance is fortunately uncommon. It is now becoming increasingly accepted practice to take prophylactic ciprofloxacin if travelling for a few days only to a hot country, or to travel with a small supply so that treatment can be initiated immediately any symptoms appear. Patients should be warned that it potentiates the effects of alcohol.

There are certain specific indications for antibiotics:

- Systemic salmonellosis with a high fever, chills and general malaise (usually responsive to cotrimoxazole or ciprofloxacin).
- Severe *Shigella* dysentry (culture and sensitivity needed to decide on antibiotics).
- Prolonged *Campylobacter* enteritis (erythromycin).
- *Yersinia enterocolitica* (usually cotrimoxazole, but also sensitive to other antibiotics).

Hypolactasia is a common sequel of severe gastroenteritis and may last several months, so a reduction in milk intake is often advisable.

▶ **Treatment of infective diarrhoea**

- Fluid and electrolyte replacement is the main aim
- Antibiotics if there is a systemic illness (high fever, tachycardia, hypotension), if there is immunocompromise, or if there is underlying inflammatory bowel disease

PARASITIC CAUSES OF DIARRHOEA

Parasites infest most of the world's population, but frequently cause no symptoms. Symptoms vary according to the parasite and the degree of infestation.

Amoebic dysentery

Natural history

SYMPTOMS

The main consequence of amoebiasis is a colitis that mimics ulcerative colitis. Symptoms include diarrhoea with blood and mucus and lower abdominal pain. If the disease is untreated perforation may ensue and the overall mortality is about 3%. Colonic ulcers tend to be discrete rather than confluent, but distinction from ulcerative colitis depends on finding the amoebae in faeces. Chronic amoebiasis may lead to stricturing mass lesions (amoeboma) that mimic carcinoma. Approximately 1% of patients will subsequently develop an amoebic hepatic abscess, sometimes many years later.

AETIOLOGY AND PATHOGENESIS

In tropical areas it has been estimated that over 50% of the population harbour the pathogenic amoeba *Entamoeba*

variable. Amoebae seem to act synergistically with colonic bacteria and this may explain why previously asymptomatic carriers can suddenly develop symptoms. Infection first occurs as a result of eating food that has been contaminated by faeces containing *E.histolytica* cysts. Each cyst divides into eight amoebae. On stool microscopy these are distinguished from non pathogenic amoebae by the presence of phagocytosed red cells. For the management of amoebic dysentery see page 90.

Giardiasis

Natural history

SYMPTOMS

Diarrhoea results and may be watery or fatty. Its mechanism is unclear, although sometimes infestation may be so severe as to obscure a considerable porportion of the surface absorptive area. Hypolactasia commonly ensues and contributes to the diarrhoea. Extraintestinal disease does not occur.

AETIOLOGY AND PATHOGENESIS

Giardia lamblia infestation is extremely common, but the development of symptoms depends on the dose of infection and the host immunity. In some parts of the world, notably the Rocky Mountains and Leningrad, water is heavily contaminated and clinically important infection is a common cause of travellers' diarrhoea. In other places such as the UK where *Giardia* are much less prevalent in water, symptomatic giardiasis raises a suspicion of immunodeficiency -particularly secretory IgA deficiency such as is found in common variable immunodeficiency and in nodular lymphoid hyperplasia.

Cysts are swallowed, usually in contaminated water, and change into the mature trophozoites in the intestine. Invasion of the mucosa may occur, but most of the trophozoites are found adhering to the mucosal surface. For the management of giardiasis see page 90.

Schistosomiasis

Schistosomiasis affects over 200 million people and in Egypt the prevalence is higher than 80%. Three principal species are involved: *Schistosoma mansoni, Schistosoma japonicum* (in the Far East) and *Schistosoma haematobium*. The cercarial forms are secreted into water by the snail intermediate host. Humans become infected by wading barefoot through streams or mud. The cercariae penetrate the skin and are transmitted via the venous system, right heart and lungs and eventually reach the liver and mature into adult worms. They swim upstream in the portal system, *S. japonicum* typically ends up in the small intestine and ascending colon, *S. mansoni* in the descending colon, and *S. haematobium* in the bladder and rectum.

The worms then mate and produce thousands of eggs, which migrate into the surrounding tissues as a result of enzymatic digestion. Multiple small intestinal ulcers develop and a severe dysentery may rarely result. More typically there is diarrhoea or rectal bleeding due to chronic inflammation of the intestine, which may result in polyp formation. Some ova may be carried back in the portal system and become trapped in the portal tracts of the liver where the ensuing inflammatory and granulomatous reaction results in portal hypertension. For the management of schistosomiasis see page 90.

Strongyloidiasis

This parasite also gains entry via the skin. Infective larvae in contaminated soil penetrate the skin, pass via the circulation to the lungs and develop into worms about 2 mm long within the alveoli. Itchy rashes and a pneumonitis lasting about two weeks result. The worms are then coughed up and swallowed and invade the intestinal mucosa. Symptoms depend on the extent of infestation. Chronic nausea or abdominal pain and, more rarely, severe diarrhoea may result. Fatal dissemination may occur in immunosuppressed patients. Self-infection may perpetuate the disease indefinitely.

Ascariasis (round worm)

Eggs are ingested in faecally contaminated food and hatch into larvae in the small intestine. They invade the mucosa and travel via the portal system and the liver to the lungs where they develop further, are coughed up, swallowed and develop into mature worms up to 20 cm long in their second trip through the intestine. Diarrhoea may occur, but obstructive symptoms are common. Migration into the bile ducts or appendix may result in jaundice or appendicitis. Pneumonitis occurs during the pulmonary stage.

Trichuris (whipworm)

The adult whipworm is 3–5 cm long and shaped like a whip, with a thin anterior portion containing its oesophagus and a thick posterior portion. Eggs ingested in contaminated food or water hatch into larvae, which mature into adult worms within the colon. Abdominal pain, diarrhoea and anaemia are the chief symptoms and in severe infection rectal prolapse may occur.

OTHER CAUSES OF DIARRHOEA

Intestinal tuberculosis

Aetiology and pathogenesis

Gastrointestinal tuberculosis used to be due mainly to infection with *Mycobacterium bovis* contracted from infected

▶ **Management of parasitic intestinal infections (None of these drugs are of proven safety in pregnancy, and metronidazole and mebendazole are teratogenic in rats. Their use should therefore be avoided in pregnancy, particularly in the first trimester unless the parasite infestation is severe.)**

Parasite	Therapy (adult dosage)
Amoebae (*E. histolytica*)	Metronidazole (800 mg tds for five days)
Giardia lamblia	Metronidazole (400 mg tds for ten days)
Schistosomiasis	
S. mansoni, S. haematobium	Praziquantel (40 mg/kg, single oral dose)
S.japonicum	Praziquantel (20 mg/kg, three doses in one day)
Strongyloides stercoralis	Thiabendazole (25 mg) or mebendazole (2 mg/kg bd for three days, repeated after two and four weeks)
Ascaris lumbricoides	Piperazine (75 mg/kg as a single dose on two consecutive days) or pyrantel pamoate (10 mg/kg as a single dose)
Trichuris trichiuria	Mebendazole (100 mg bd for three days)

milk, but this route of infection has now been abolished in developing countries by tuberculin testing of cattle. The disease is however still not uncommon particularly in Asian immigrants. It is now almost exclusively due to *Mycobacterium tuberculosis (hominis)*, which has usually spread from the lungs via swallowed sputum.

Any part of the intestine may be affected, but in approximately 60% of patients it is the ileo-caecal region. The radiological, macroscopic and histological appearances closely mimic Crohn's disease, and skip lesions may occur.

Management

Treatment is with triple chemotherapy for 18–24 months unless culture and sensitivity results are available, in which case the treatment may be reduced to two appropriate drugs after three months.

When the differential diagnosis is in doubt a trial of antituberculous chemotherapy should always precede a trial of corticosteroids for presumed Crohn's disease, as the results of inappropriate corticosteroid therapy in tuberculosis may be disastrous with rapid dissemination. If uncertainty

remains and corticosteroid therapy is felt necessary for presumed active Crohn's disease antituberculous cover should be given concurrently. Corticosteroid therapy is sometimes used intentionally in combination with antituberculous therapy to reduce the risk of permanent stricturing from tuberculosis.

Approximately 50% of patients with intestinal tuberculosis require surgery at some stage, particularly for the treatment of strictures or fistulae. Sometimes this can be accomplished without resection by means of a plastic surgical approach to strictures (stricturoplasty) in which the stricture is incised longitudinally and then the incision closed transversely as in a pyloroplasty. Perforation through a tuberculous ulcer may also occur and carries a mortality of 30–50%.

Coeliac disease

Natural history

Coeliac disease has a prevalence of about 1 in 1000, and about 35% of patients present in childhood. The mode of presentation is variable. It may be subtle (e.g. growth

▶ **Intestinal tuberculosis**

- Among UK Asians with radiological ileo-caecal disease, approximately 50% have tuberculosis and 50% have Crohn's disease
- Radiological and endoscopic features of tuberculosis cannot be readily distinguished from those of Crohn's disease
- Only a minority of patients with intestinal tuberculosis have an abnormal chest radiograph
- Chemotherapy should be for 18–24 months
- 50% require surgery at some stage for strictures or fistulas

▶ **Coeliac disease**

- Prevalence is 1 : 1000
- Only 33% present in childhood
- May present with growth retardartion, anaemia, tetany, bruising, nonspecific gastrointestinal complaints

retardation or anaemia) or more obvious with fatty diarrhoea and features of deficiency of fat-soluble vitamins.

Diagnosis requires the demonstration of duodenal or jejunal villous atrophy plus resolution of these changes with gluten withdrawal. In children a further challenge with gluten should usually be given after resolution since transient villous atrophy due to causes other than coeliac disease (particularly following viral gastroenteritis) is common.

Striking splenic atrophy is not uncommon. Its mechanism is uncertain, but may be due to constant bombardment of the reticulo-endothelial system with foreign antigens penetrating a leaky intestinal barrier. Changes in the peripheral blood then include abnormally-shaped red cells, and Howell–Jolly bodies and marked thrombocytosis may occur. There is also an increased risk of sepsis, particularly pneumococcal, which should be remembered if the patient requires surgery for any reason.

AETIOLOGY AND PATHOGENESIS

Gluten is a mixture of water-insoluble cereal proteins, which give bread its elastic springy consistency. Bread made from gluten-free flour unfortunately tends to be bland and crumbly. The gluten can be further subdivided into toxic gliadin fractions, and IgA antibodies to gliadin are commonly present in the peripheral blood of coeliac patients. The damage to the epithelium is almost certainly cell-mediated rather than humoral however. This is reflected by an increase in intraepithelial lymphocytes (predominantly T lymphocytes) and an increase in lamina propria mono-nuclear cells. There is a strong association with the HLA DR3 antigen, and presence of this antigen also correlates with known autoimmune diseases.

There is a close link with the skin condition **dermatitis herpetiformis**. Itchy vesicles characteristically occur on extensor surfaces of the forearms and other pressure areas. The majority of patients have some degree of small intestinal villous atrophy, and in about 50% there is a good therapeutic response to gluten withdrawal. IgA deposits are found at the dermo-epidermal junction.

Management

Toxic gluten is contained in all foods made from wheat, barley or rye, and probably oats. Rice and maize are free from toxic glutens. Patients vary considerably in their susceptibility to gluten. In some patients, very small amounts of gluten such as are present in communion wafers are enough to precipitate a relapse, while others seem able to eat gluten-containing foods for several years before relapsing. There are anecdotal reports of patients failing to go into remission following subsequent lapses in diet, and the only practical and safe advice to the patient is to avoid gluten indefinitely once the diagnosis is made.

Patients should be advised to contact a patient group such as the Coeliac Society (P.O. Box 181, London NW2 2QY), which is able to give invaluable support and help with recipes and advice about the safety of foods. Gluten-free flour, bread and biscuits are available on prescription in the UK.

Remission should be confirmed by repeat jejunal or distal duodenal biopsy after about three months of gluten avoidance. Occasional patients who have otherwise typical features of coeliac disease fail to respond to gluten withdrawal. Some of these patients are found to be taking gluten inadvertently, for example in beer. It has recently been shown that occasional 'non-responsive coeliacs' may respond to avoidance of soy protein. In others there is no explanation, but the combination of continued gluten avoidance and corticosteroid therapy may produce a remission.

Patients should usually be followed up in a gastro-enterological clinic indefinitely, even if only at annual intervals, so that they can be kept up to date with developments and have the need for continued gluten avoidance reinforced, even when they remain well.

The increased risk of malignancy (up to 15% over eight years in one study) is worrying, but it has not been sufficiently high to justify screening. Any unexplained deterioration should however suggest the possibility of small bowel malignancy, either lymphoma (**Fig. 3.36**) or carcinoma, which should be investigated by high quality radiology of the small intestine and will usually necessitate intubation of the small intestine (i.e. small bowel barium 'enema' rather than 'follow through').

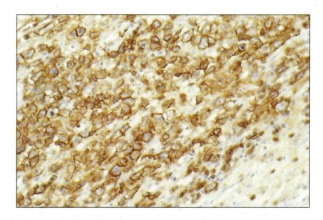

Fig. 3.36 Ileal lymphoma. This has been immunostained using an antibody against T lymphocytes, and is the lymphoma that usually complicates coeliac disease. Intestinal lymphomas not associated with coeliac disease are usually of B-cell origin.

Prognosis

The prognosis is excellent once the diagnosis of coeliac disease has been made and treatment by gluten withdrawal initiated. The increased risk of carcinoma, particularly of the small intestine also includes other sites, particularly the oesophagus, and an increased risk of an unusual form of intestinal lymphoma. This was thought to be of histiocytic origin, but subsequent studies using cell specific monoclonal antibodies showed that it is a **T cell lymphoma** and that the histiocytes that are frequently seen in this tumour are probably reactive. Fortunately the incidence of these tumours as a complication of coeliac disease seems to be declining. It is not certain why this should be because the link between the risk for these tumours and the degree of control of the coeliac disease is disputed.

Occasionally patients fail to respond to gluten withdrawal. **Ulcerative jejuno-ileitis**, which is arguably a severe form of coeliac disease, has a very poor prognosis, though some patients will respond to a combination of corticosteroid therapy and gluten withdrawal. **Collagenous sprue** is another very rare cause of villous atrophy and malabsorption without response to gluten withdrawal. Dense collagen deposition occurs in the lamina propria. The aetiology is unknown and prognosis poor.

Tropical sprue

Tropical sprue presents in much the same way as coeliac disease with features of fat and folic acid malabsorption, glossitis and anaemia in a patient who has recently been in a hot country. Small intestinal biopsy shows partial or, occasionally, severe villous atrophy. The aetiology is unclear, but is thought to be due to a combination of bacterial contamination of the small intestine and folate deficiency. Other infections such as giardiasis and strongyloidiasis should be excluded by small bowel sampling. If left untreated the condition may persist for months or even years.

Oral tetracycline, 1 g daily should be given for two weeks, and oral folic acid, 10 mg daily until asymptomatic. Vitamin B_{12} supplementation may also occasionally be needed. Hypolactasia is inevitable and a low milk intake will help to reduce diarrhoea.

Whipple's disease

This unusual disease most commonly affects middle-aged men. Partial villous atrophy and malabsorption result in diarrhoea and pigmentation, and about 65% of patients have joint symptoms, typically an intermittent migratory arthritis affecting large or small joints. Fever and lymphadenopathy are common. A chronic encephalitis with altered behaviour, memory loss and cranial nerve lesions may occur and can be the dominant feature.

Small bowel biopsy shows diagnostic macrophages within the lamina propria that are packed with foamy PAS-positive material, the remains of ingested dead or dying bacteria. The bacterium has been identified as a Gram-positive actinomycete, *Tropheryma whippelii*. The condition occurs sporadically and infectivity is presumably very low.

Management

Untreated, the disease is usually fatal, but fortunately there is usually a good response to antibiotics such as tetracycline, cotrimoxazole or penicillin, but treatment may have to be continued for several months with monitoring by repeated intestinal biopsy (endoscopic duodenal biopsies should suffice). Even with effective antibiotic therapy, it may take a year before all the intestinal macrophages are free of the bacteria. Supplementation with fat-soluble vitamins and calcium will also be necessary for patients with severe malabsorption.

Intestinal lymphoma

Lymphoma of the intestine may be either primary or secondary to lymphoma elsewhere. Obstruction, bleeding, perforation, malabsorption and weight loss may all occur.

Short primary lymphomatous lesions, which have the best prognosis, usually present with obstructive symptoms or as a mass. More extensive involvement is likely to cause malabsorption and anaemia. Any part of the intestine may be involved, but the distal small intestine is the commonest site followed by the stomach.

▶ **Intestinal lymphoma**

- Mostly B cell origin (T cell if complicating coeliac disease)
- Primary Hodgkin's disease is rare
- Resection is the best therapy
- 75% five-year survival if resected

The cell of origin is often difficult to ascertain with certainty, but modern cell marker techniques are beginning to clarify this situation. The majority of primary lymphomas of the intestine are B-cell lymphomas, the main exception being the lymphomas that complicate coeliac disease, which are T-cell lymphomas. Hodgkin's disease only rarely involves the intestine.

Management

Short primary intestinal lymphomas are best treated by surgical resection and the prognosis is then good with up to 75% five-year survival. More extensive primary lymphomas have a worse prognosis, but may respond well to chemotherapy. The prognosis in this group is at present very unpredictable. Secondary involvement of the intestine by lymphoma elsewhere has a poor prognosis with a five-year survival of about 10%; chemotherapy may be useful.

Alpha chain disease (Mediterranean lymphoma)

Alpha chain disease is arguably only pre-malignant in its early stages and should probably be considered separately from other intestinal lymphomas. There is hyperplasia followed by frank neoplasia of IgA-producing cells within the intestine, possibly as a result of chronic antigenic stimulation. The malignant cells produce IgA heavy chains (α chains) in excess, without light chains. The α chains can be detected in blood and urine. There is a consequent defect in secretory IgA function, and bacterial overgrowth or giardiasis, villous atrophy and malabsorption ensue.

Patients present with severe malabsorption, anaemia and abdominal pain, and often have severe clubbing. The disease occurs predominantly in young men in countries around the Mediterranean, in Africa, South America and the Far East. It is thought that poor hygiene and chronic intestinal infestation predispose to it.

Management

In its early premalignant phase improvement and even cure may result from tetracycline therapy, but when invasive lymphoma has developed, cytotoxic chemotherapy is usually necessary and the prognosis is poor.

Nodular lymphoid hyperplasia

Nodular lymphoid hyperplasia may present with watery diarrhoea or malabsorption. Some degree of lymphoid hyperplasia is normal in childhood and early adult life and may cause diagnostic confusion when seen on barium examinations. Prominent lymphoid follicles seen in the duodenum on endoscopy or in the colon at colonoscopy or barium enema are usually abnormal after 25 years of age.

Usually there is underlying immunoglobulin deficiency, either selective IgA deficiency or common variable immuno-deficiency. The prominent follicles often contain a predominance of IgM-containing cells, presumably because secretory IgM can, to some extent, take the place of secretory IgA (**Figs 3.37 and 3.38**). Giardiasis is common and should be sought as symptoms can be improved with appropriate treatment (metronidazole). The prognosis is good, but there is a small risk of subsequent intestinal lymphoma.

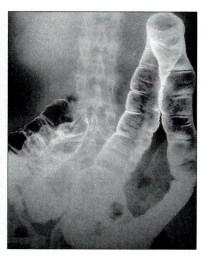

Fig. 3.37 Nodular lymphoid hyperplasia. This is a normal finding in children and young adults, but in older adults is associated with immune deficiency, usually either selective IgA deficiency or combined immunoglobulin deficiency. Small intestinal overgrowth with *Giardia lamblia* is common.

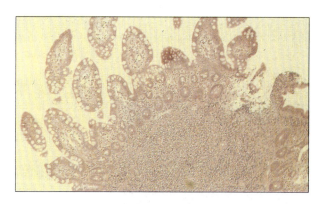

Fig. 3.38 Histological appearance of nodular lymphoid hyperplasia. In selective IgA deficiency the nodules consist mainly of IgM-producing plasma cells (secretory IgM is to some extent able to take the place of secretory IgA).

Pneumatosis cystoides intestinalis

In this unusual condition, multiple gas-filled cysts may occur at any site in the small or large intestine (**Fig 3.39**). About 20% of the patients have chronic airways obstruction and analysis of the gas has shown that its composition usually approximates that of air. In these patients the gas has presumably tracked down from the mediastinum following rupture of emphysematous bullae. Resolution may then occur if the patient is treated with oxygen therapy. In these patients the condition follows a very benign course. A more sinister situation may result when intramural gas results from anaerobic infestation of the bowel wall as in necrotising enterocolitis or mesenteric ischaemia. Other cases may occur in association with a wide range of underlying conditions which include intestinal ulceration or perforation, intestinal infections such as tuberculosis, malabsorptive states such as cystic fibrosis and Whipple's disease and intestinal lymphoma.

The pneumatosis will often need no specific treatment providing the underlying condition resolves. The response to antibiotics such as metronidazole is variable and the most consistently successful therapy is prolonged breathing of oxygen at high concentration (60–70%). Surgical resection is only rarely necessary and should usually be avoided as recurrence may occur at any site of the intestine.

Intestinal amyloidosis

Intestinal involvement occurs in approximately 70% of patients with amyloidosis. Initially, amyloid protein is laid down around submucosal vessels, but as the disease progresses the muscle layers and then the mucosa become infiltrated (**Fig. 3.40**). In primary amyloidosis the proteins deposited are immunoglobulin light chains while in secondary amyloidosis the protein is an acute phase reactant, usually amyloid A protein, that has been produced in excess during chronic inflammation or infection.

Because of the muscle involvement motility problems are common, particularly diarrhoea. If involvement is extensive malabsorption and protein losing enteropathy may occur. Bleeding, perforation and ischaemic damage are further complications of this condition.

Management

The treatment is unsatisfactory. Amyloid protein has a β-pleated sheet structure, which mammalian proteases cannot digest, so once laid down it tends to be undegradable. Occasionally primary amyloidosis responds to cytotoxic drugs such as melphalan, and if the cause of secondary amyloidosis can be removed, regression sometimes occurs.

Chronic pancreatitis

Natural history

The majority of patients have pain, which may be severe and intractable. It is typically epigastric and radiates to the back. Duration of pain and association with eating is variable. Weight loss is usual and is often marked if malabsorption is present. Fat malabsorption implies a greater than 90% reduction in pancreatic exocrine function since the healthy pancreas has a large functional reserve. Glucose tolerance tests are abnormal in about 65% of patients, but clinical diabetes, which is usually mild, occurs only in about 35%. Jaundice may result from biliary obstruction, and if untreated can progress to secondary biliary cirrhosis.

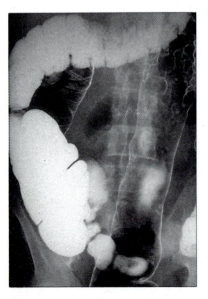

Fig. 3.39 Barium enema showing pneumatosis. Associated chronic obstructive airways disease is common.

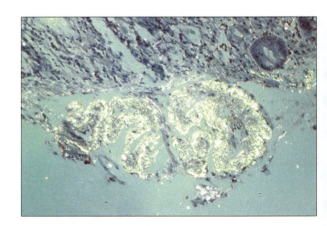

Fig. 3.40 Intestinal amyloidosis in long-standing rheumatoid arthritis. The amyloid protein (amyloid A protein, which forms β-pleated sheets) is birefringent in polarised light. Here deposition is seen mainly around the submucosal vessels, but there may be more extensive infiltration resulting in malabsorption.

PANCREATIC ASCITES

Pancreatic ascites is a rare problem and develops insidiously, particularly in patients with alcoholic chronic pancreatitis, and presumably results from rupture of a dilated side duct or pseudocyst. Diagnosis is confirmed by finding a very high concentration of amylase in the ascitic fluid.

CLASSIFICATION

The definitions and classification of chronic pancreatitis have caused confusion. Two clinical patterns are recognisable:

- A gradual inexorable deterioration in pancreatic function and ductular damage, which may be associated with pain.
- Recurring attacks of acute pancreatitis accompanied by a gradual (and often mild) deterioration in pancreatic function.

The first pattern is recognisable unequivocally as chronic pancreatitis. The second pattern is often difficult to distinguish from recurring attacks of acute pancreatitis (e.g. due to gallstones), with return to normal function between attacks ('relapsing acute pancreatitis').

AETIOLOGY AND PATHOGENESIS

Gallstones are much the commonest cause of relapsing acute pancreatitis and almost never produce chronic pancreatitis. Alcohol is much the commonest cause of the recurring acute pancreatitis that is associated with deteriorating pancreatic function and sometimes called chronic relaping pancreatitis. Approximately 50% of alcoholics have evidence of chronic pancreatitis at postmortem or on testing pancreatic function.

Other predisposing factors for chronic pancreatitis include hyperparathyroidism (which carries a 5–10% risk of chronic pancreatitis), cystic fibrosis, severe protein malnutrition (kwashiorkor) and a rare hereditary (autosomal dominant) form of chronic pancreatitis that presents in childhood or early adult life.

PATHOLOGY

The ductular system becomes dilated and irregular. Proteinaceous plugs may block side branches or even the main pancreatic duct and subsequently calcify. Acinar tissue atrophies and is replaced by fibrous tissue.

Management

The most important step is to remove the underlying cause, usually alcohol. If the patient manages to stop drinking there may be a surprising improvement in symptoms and even in the radiological appearance of the pancreatic duct system. Pain relief is often difficult and patients frequently become addicted to opiates. Oral pancreatic supplements can sometimes be helpful in reducing pain by suppressing pancreatic secretion. Coeliac plexus blocks often produce temporary relief, but are not without risk and the pain usually returns within a year or less.

SURGERY

The role of surgery is uncertain. If a patient is still in pain after one year's abstinence from alcohol it is worth performing an ERCP to look for stricturing of the main pancreatic duct with proximal dilatation. Occasionally partial pancreactectomy may be helpful in this situation. Various other operations have been tried including laying open ('filleting') the main pancreatic duct and anastomosing it to jejunum, and subtotal or even total pancreatectomy. Opinions vary widely as to their efficacy. The relationship (if any) between intraductal pressure (or calculi) and pain is unclear, and patients left with any residual pancreas often have recurrent pain, while total pancreactectomy usually results in very 'brittle' diabetes, often in a patient who is already addicted to opiates. The least unsatisfactory course is often a more conservative medical approach emphasizing alcohol abstinence above all else, as this carries the only significant hope of long-term improvement.

MALABSORPTION DUE TO CHRONIC PANCREATITIS

Malabsorption is much more readily manageable than the pain of chronic pancreatitis. Oral preparations of pancreatic lipase, amylase and protease are readily available. They are rapidly inactivated at low pH, so are more effective if taken either in an enteric-coated form or preceded by an H_2 antagonist. With adequate dosage (up to 3–4 capsules with each meal) it is usually possible to achieve a reduction in faecal fat excretion of at least 50%. The diet should be high in protein and carbohydrate, and low in fat.

▶ **Bacterial overgrowth**

- May present as weight loss, B_{12} deficiency, osteomalacia
- Serum folate typically high (bacteria synthesize folate)
- May occur in the elderly without anatomical abnormality

Bacterial contamination of the small intestine (blind loop syndrome)

Aetiology and pathogenesis

Intestinal stasis is the main factor in the development of clinically important bacterial overgrowth of the small intestine. The commonest causes of this are surgical blind loops (e.g. the afferent loop of a Polya gastrectomy), small bowel diverticulosis, stricturing (e.g. Crohn's disease) and, more rarely, a motility disorder, as in scleroderma. It has also been shown that elderly patients without any anatomical blind loop may develop bacterial overgrowth without any clear reason except possibly reduced gastric acidity.

The two main consequences are B_{12} deficiency and fat malabsorption.

- B_{12} deficiency may be sufficiently severe to cause megaloblastic anaemia or neurological defects (subacute combined degeneration of the cord, peripheral neuropathy or dementia).
- Fat malabsorption may be constant or intermittent and complicated by hypoproteinaemia and hypocalcaemia.

Bile salts are deconjugated by anaerobic bacteria and subsequently dehydroxylated by bacteria to secondary bile acids (deoxycholic acid and lithocholic acid). These free acids cannot form micelles and do not take part in the enterohepatic circulation, so are not reabsorbed in the distal ileum and cause impaired absorption of salt and water from the colon, thus contributing to the diarrhoea. The bile salt pool becomes depleted. Mild to moderate inflammatory changes and villous atrophy may occur in the small intestine and also contribute to the malabsorption.

Management

Treatment consists of correcting nutritional deficiencies with vitamin B_{12} and fat-soluble vitamin supplements. Tetracycline, 250 mg four times daily orally, is the traditional antibiotic of choice, and is usually highly effective. Metronidazole should theoretically be as effective since the offending bacteria are almost exclusively anaerobes, but long-term or recurrent therapy is often necessary, and tetracycline is therefore preferable because of its lower risk of side-effects in long-term use. If calcium supplements are needed they should be taken at a different time of day to prevent binding with tetracycline.

Surgical correction of the blind loop is not usually necessary or appropriate unless there is stricturing with proximal stasis.

SECRETORY DIARRHOEA

Cholera

Aetiology and pathogenesis

Cholera is the classic cause of secretory diarhoea and knowledge of its pathophysiology has led to a better understanding of fluid and electrolyte handling by the small intestine.

The cholera vibrio causes no structural damage to the mucosa, but its toxin binds irreversibly with a receptor on the epithelial surface. The active component of the toxin then enters the epithelial cell where it stimulates adenylate cyclase. This increases the intracellular concentration of cyclic AMP, which stimulates secretion of salt and water from the crypt cells and inhibits absorption by the villous cells, resulting in a

devastating change in the large fluxes of salt and water that normally occur in the small intestine so that up to 25 litres/day of watery diarrhoea may result. This is not solely due to a secretory effect because the healthy small intestine can absorb up to 20 litres/day (**Fig. 3.41**). As with most other examples of secretory diarrhoea there is an absorptive defect as well.

Management

If fluid replacement is adequate the diarrhoea resolves within a few days and is usually only massive for the first 24 hours. In cholera and all other examples of massive diarrhoea the

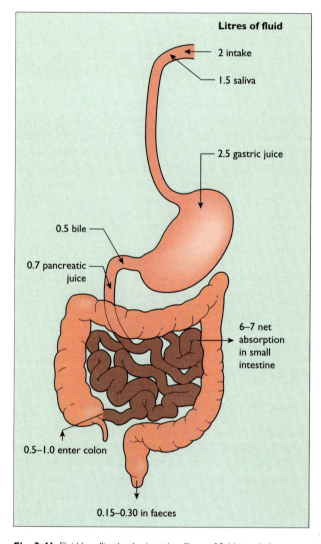

Fig. 3.41 Fluid handling by the intestine (litres of fluid per day).

most essential aspect of treatment is fluid and electrolyte replacement. This may need to be given intravenously, but a huge advance has been made in the management of cholera by the realisation that sugar/salt solutions, given enterally usually achieve successful rehydration. This is because glucose (and neutral amino acids such as glycine) enhances absorption of sodium. The World Health Organisation recommends an oral rehydration solution consisting of sodium chloride 4 g/l, sodium acetate 6.5 g/l, potassium chloride 1 g/l and glucose 9 g/l. With adequate rehydration mortality from cholera approaches zero whereas it may otherwise be rapidly fatal.

Peptide-secreting tumours

Aetiology and pathogenesis
Other diarrhoeas usually classed as secretory because of a high stool volume (greater than 300 ml/day) in the fasting state include diarrhoea associated with the following peptide-secreting tumours:

- Vipoma of the pancreas.
- Medullary carcinoma of the thyroid.
- Carcinoid syndrome.

In these conditions other mechanisms, particularly altered motility also contribute to the diarrhoea.

VIP (vasoactive intestinal peptide) can be produced in excess by neuroendocrine tumours of the pancreas, neural tissues (ganglioneuroblastoma) or lung (oat cell carcinoma). This results in a syndrome, described by Verner and Morrison in 1958, of watery diarrhoea, hypokalaemia and achlorhydria. Diarrhoea is typically massive (greater than one litre/day). VIP does not cause sufficient inhibition of adenyl cyclase for this to be its main mechanism of action, and it is likely that some other mechanism, and possibly also another peptide, contributes to the diarrhoea. With vipomas, as with other pancreatic endocrine tumours such as gastrinomas and insulinomas, the possibility of one of the hereditary **multiple endocrine neoplasia, type 1 (MEN1)** syndromes should be considered. This syndrome includes the 'three Ps': pituitary, parathyroid and pancreas. Hypercalcaemia due to hyperparathyroidism and hyperprolactinaemia should be excluded. In the MEN1 syndrome, tumours are invariably multiple and surgery is unlikely to be curative.

Diarrhoea associated with **medullary carcinoma of the thyroid** is usually less massive (300 ml/day or so). Calcitonin levels are greatly increased in the plasma, but do not seem to be responsible for the diarrhoea, which is probably postaglandin-mediated.

Carcinoid syndrome results from excessive release of a wide group of peptides and other factors including 5-hydroxytryptamine (which is probably the cause of the

diarrhoea), bradykinin, histamine, catecholamines, prostaglandins and other peptide hormones. The syndrome may include flushing attacks, wheezing, abdominal pain, diarrhoea and right-sided valvular heart lesions. Pellagra may result from niacin deficiency that results from diversion of tryptophan to serotonin rather than niacin synthesis.

Management

Pancreatic cholera due to a VIP-producing tumour
Pancreatic cholera due to a VIP-producing tumour can be treated successfully by resection of the tumour in about 60% of patients. If metastases have already developed, symptomatic relief and sometimes tumour shrinkage may be achieved with streptozocin or somatostatin. Corticosteroids or the somatostatin analogue octreotide, sometimes improve the diarrhoea.

Carcinoid syndrome
Carcinoid syndrome usually implies the presence of hepatic metastases, but these are slow growing, and if confined to one lobe of the liver, prolonged remission may be achieved by resection.

Pharmacological treatment is complicated and not always successful. Methysergide (which can cause severe retroperitoneal fibrosis) and methyldopa may alleviate the diarrhoea, and antihistamines occasionally relieve flushing. If hepatic metastases are too extensive for resection then palliation may be achieved by embolisation via the hepatic artery. Before this is performed the patient should be given a 'cocktail' of inhibitors to prevent problems due to the sudden release of carcinoid products into the circulation. This consists of:

- *p*-chlorophenylalanine, 500 mg four times daily orally for 48 hours before embolisation and continued afterwards.
- Cyproheptadine, 4 mg three times daily for 24 hours before and continued afterwards.
- Nicotinamide, 250 mg four times daily.
- Methylprednisolone, 1 g intravenously at the start of embolisation.
- Aprotinin (Trasylol) 50,000 units hourly as an intravenous infusion, given one hour before embolisation and for 48 hours after.
- Intravenous hydralazine as required for hypertension.
- Albumin or plasma for hypotension.

An acceptable alternative to this cocktail is the use of subcutaneous octreotide, the somatostatin analogue, supplemented if necessary with additional intravenous octreotide.

Medullary carcinoma of the thyroid
Medullary carcinoma of the thyroid occasionally produces diarrhoea when metastases have developed, but survival is

often remarkably good with little progression over several years. Diarrhoea may respond to prostaglandin antagonists including indomethacin and ground nutmeg! Recently good results have been reported with somatostatin or its long-acting synthetic analogue, octreotide.

Unresectable peptide-secreting tumours

Unresectable peptide-secreting tumours have been treated with various forms of chemotherapy. Cure is unfortunately rare, but response rates of about 50% have been reported with combinations such as adriamycin and 5-fluorouracil. Occasional impressive tumour regression has also been reported with somatostatin and somatostatin analogues and as these generally cause fewer side-effects than conventional chemotherapy, they should probably be used in preference.

Purgative abuse

Purgative abuse can be notoriously difficult to diagnose. Clinical features if it is severe can include severe malabsorption, clubbing, hypogammaglobulinaemia and tetany. Diagnosis requires a high index of suspicion.

Management

Although the doctor may feel a great sense of personal triumph when the diagnosis is established the trouble is usually only just beginning. Direct confrontation of the patient will often produce complete denial or a switch to another self-induced disease, which may even lead to a suicide attempt. An air of tolerance and understanding needs to be conveyed rather than victory. Psychiatric help should be sought, but there is no clear consensus about the optimal treatment, and the prognosis in severe cases is poor.

Bile acid diarrhoea

Bile acid diarrhoea most commonly follows resection or irradiation damage to the distal small intestine where 95% of secreted bile acids are normally reabsorbed for re-circulation. Unabsorbed bile acids stimulate adenyl cyclase in the colonic epithelium, resulting in a net loss of salt and water into the lumen. It has been suggested that a small proportion of patients with the irritable bowel syndrome, particularly those with chronic watery diarrhoea, may also suffer from bile salt malabsorption. In some instances of post-vagotomy diarrhoea, particularly if combined with cholecystectomy, bile salt diarrhoea also seems to be an important mechanism.

Treatment with oral cholestyramine, the ion exchange resin, is usually dramatically effective and the dose, usually one to two sachets daily, can be adjusted according to the response. Care should be taken to avoid taking other drugs simultaneously that might be adsorbed by cholestyramine.

Short bowel syndrome

The small intestine has remarkable powers of adaptation following resection:

- Up to 1.5 m of mid-small intestine may be resected in the adult without necessarily causing any clinical evidence of malabsorption.
- Resection of up to 100 cm of distal ileum will cause malabsorption of vitamin B_{12} and bile salts, resulting in watery diarrhoea (see above), but without significant fat malabsorption.
- With more extensive resection, fat malabsorption occurs, partly as a result of reduced absorptive area, but also because of a reduced bile acid pool.

Diarrhoea may be most marked immediately after resection, but gradually reduces over the following weeks as adaptation takes place. It is important to realise that this adaptation will not occur unless the patient is fed enterally.

The most devastating resections are usually those required when mesenteric infarction has occurred. So long as the duodenum, part of the jejunum and the ileo-caecal valve are intact there is a good chance of achieving adequate absorption in the long term, although intravenous supplementation may be required for some time while adaptation occurs.

Management

Management includes:

- Early intravenous feeding.
- Early enteral feeding with a medium-chain triglyceride-based feed.
- H_2 antagonists because there is often gastric hypersecretion.
- Liberal use of antidiarrhoeals such as loperamide.
- Vitamin, calcium, zinc and magnesium supplementation.

FURTHER READING

Inflammatory bowel disease (epidemiology)

Calkins BM. A meta analysis of the role of smoking in inflammatory bowel disease. *Dig Dis Sci* 1989; **34**(12): 1841–54.

Mayberry JF. Recent epidemiology of ulcerative colitis and Crohn's disease. *Int J Colorectal Dis* 1989; 4(1): 59–66

Rhodes JM, Cocke R, Allan R, *et al.* Colonic Crohn's disease and the contraceptive pill. *Br Med J* 1983;**288**:595–6.

Inflammatory bowel disease (aetiology)

Fiocchi C. Immune events associated with inflammatory bowel disease.*Scand J Gastroenterol Suppl* 1990; **172**: 4–2.

Hellers G, Bernell O. Genetic aspects of inflammatory bowel disease. *Med Clin North Am* 1990; **74**(1): 13–9.

Hodgson HJ. Immunological aspects of inflammatory bowel diseases of the human gut. *Agents Actions* 1992; Spec No: C27–31.

MacDonald TT, Murch SH. Aetiology and pathogenesis of chronic inflammatory bowel disease. *Baillieres Clin Gastroenterol* 1994;**8** :1–34.

North CS, Clouse RE, Spitznagel EL, Alpers DH. The relation of ulcerative colitis to psychiatric factors: a review of findings and methods. *Am J Psych* 1990; **147**(8): 974–81.

Podolsky DK. Inflammatory bowel disease (1). *N Engl J Med* 1991 Sep 26; **325**(13): 928–37.

Tsai HH, Rhodes JM. Mucus glycoprotein alterations in inflammatory bowel disease. *Europ J Gastroenterol Hepatol* 1993; **5**: 214–218.

Inflammatory bowel disease (miscellaneous)

Brostrom O. Prognosis in ulcerative colitis. *Med Clin North Am* 1990; **74**(1): 201–18.

Farmer RG. Infectious causes of diarrhea in the differential diagnosis of inflammatory bowel disease. *Med Clin North Am* 1990; **74**(1): 29–38.

Madden MV, Farthing MJ, Nicholls RJ. Inflammation in ileal reservoirs: 'pouchitis'. *Gut* 1990 Mar; **31**(3): 247–9.

Rankin GB. Extraintestinal and systemic manifestations of inflammatory bowel disease. *Med Clin North Am* 1990; **74**(1): 39–50.

Shepherd NA, Hulten L, Tytgat GN, *et al.* Pouchitis. *Int J Colorectal Dis* 1989; 4(4): 205–29.

Cancer risk and screening

Albert MB, Nochomovitz LE. Dysplasia and cancer surveillance in inflammatory bowel disease. *Gastroenterol Clin North Am* 1989; **18**(1): 83–97.

Gyde S. Screening for colorectal cancer in ulcerative colitis: dubious benefits and high costs (see comments). *Gut* 1990; **31**(10): 1089–92.

Winawer SJ, Schottenfeld D, Flehinger BJ. Colorectal cancer screening. *J Natl Cancer Inst* 1991; **83**(4): 243–53.

Inflammatory bowel disease (treatment)

Alexander Williams J. Inflammatory bowel disease revisited: surgery today and tomorrow. *Scand J Gastroenterol* 1990; **175**(Suppl): 107–12.

Allgayer H. Sulfasalazine and 5 ASA compounds. *Gastroenterol Clin North Am* 1992; **21**(3): 643–58.

Carpani de Kaski M, Hodgson HJF. Rolling review: Inflammatory bowel disease. *Alimen Pharmacol Ther* 1993; **7**: 567–579.

Cole AT, Hawkey CJ. New treatments in inflammatory bowel disease. *Br J Hosp Med* 1992; **47**(8): 581–90.

Geier DL, Miner PB Jr. New therapeutic agents in the treatment of inflammatory bowel disease. *Am J Med* 1992; **93**(2): 199–208.

Hodgson HJ. Cyclosporin in inflammatory bowel disease. *Alimen Pharmacol Ther* 1991; **5**(4): 343–50.

Kozarek-RA. Review article: immunosuppressive therapy for inflammatory bowel disease. *Alimen Pharmacol Ther* 1993; **7**(2): 117–23.

Mulder CJ, Tytgat GN. Review article: topical corticosteroids in inflammatory bowel disease. *Alimen Pharmacol Ther* 1993; **7**(2): 125–30.

O'Donoghue D. Current treatment of ulcerative colitis. *Br J Hosp Med* 1992; **48**(5): 226–31.

Sagar PM, Taylor BA. Pelvic ileal reservoirs: the options. *Br J Surg* 1994:**81** : 325–32.

Silk DB, Payne James J. Inflammatory bowel disease: nutritional implications and treatment. *Proc Nutr Soc* 1989; **48**(3): 355–61.

Thomson AB. Review article: new developments in the use of 5 aminosalicylic acid in patients with inflammatory bowel disease. *Alimen Pharmacol Ther* 1991; **5**(5): 449–70.

Coeliac disease

Ferguson A, Arranz E, O'Mahony S. Clinical and pathological spectrum of coeliac disease—active, silent, latent, potential. *Gut* 1993; **34**(2): 150–1.

Holmes GK, Prior P, Lane MR, Pope D, Allan RN. Malignancy in coeliac disease—effect of a gluten free diet. *Gut* 1989; **30**(3): 333–8.

Howdle PD, Blair GE. Molecular biology and coeliac disease. *Gut* 1992; **33**(5): 573–5.

Kagnoff MF Celiac disease. A gastrointestinal disease with environmental, genetic, and immunologic components. *Gastroenterol Clin North Am* 1992; **21**(2): 405–25.

Kelly CP, Feighery CF, Gallagher RB, Weir DG. Diagnosis and treatment of gluten-sensitive enteropathy. *Adv Intern Med* 1990; **35**: 341–63.

Report of Working Group of European Society of Paediatric Gastroenterology and Nutrition. Revised criteria for diagnosis of coeliac disease. *Arch Dis Child* 1990; **65**(8): 909–11.

Marsh MN. Gluten, major histocompatibility complex, and the small intestine. A molecular and immunobiologic approach to the spectrum of gluten sensitivity ('celiac sprue'). *Gastroenterology* 1992; **102** (1): 330–54.

Michalski JP, McCoombs CC. Celiac damage: clinical features and pathogenesis. *Am J Med Sci* 1984; **307**:204–11.

Trier JS. Celiac sprue. *N Engl J Med* 1991; **325**(24): 1709–19.

Chronic pancreatitis

Banks PA. Management of pancreatic pain. *Pancreas* 1991; **6**(Suppl 1): S52–9.

Beglinger C. Relevant aspects of physiology in chronic pancreatitis. *Dig Dis* 1992; **10**(6): 326–9.

Fink AS. Endoscopic intervention in pancreatitis. *Pancreas* 1991; **6**(Suppl 1): S23–30.

Geenen JE, Rolny P. Endoscopic therapy of acute and chronic pancreatitis. *Gastroint End* 1991 **37**(3): 377–82.

Gooszen HG. Surgical treatment of painful chronic pancreatitis: an unresolved problem? *Dig Dis* 1992; **10**(6): 345–53.

Muench R. Etiology and natural history of chronic pancreatitis. *Dig Dis* 1992; **10**(6): 335–44.

Parikh NJ, Greenen JE. Current role of ERCP in the management of benign pancreatic disease. *Endoscopy* 1992; **24**(1-2): 120–4.

Tuberculosis of the gut

Marshall JB. Tuberculosis of the gastrointestinal tract and peritoneum. *Am J Gastroenterol* 1993; **88**: 989—999.

Travellers diarrhoea

Arduino RC, DuPont HL. Travellers' diarrhoea. (Review.) *Baillières Clinical Gastroenterology* 1993; **7**(2):365–85.

Chak A, Banwell JG. Traveller's diarrhea. (Review.) *Gastroent Clin N Am* 1993 **22**(3): 549–61.

DuPont HL, Ericsson CD. Prevention and treatment of traveller's diarrhea. *N Engl J Med* 1993; **328**(25): 1821–7.

Farthing MJ. Review article: prevention and treatment of travellers' diarrhoea. *Alimen Pharmacol Ther* 1991; **5**(1): 15–30.

Miscellaneous

Basser RL, Green MD. Recent advances in carcinoids and gastrointestinal neuroendocrine tumors. *Curr Opin Oncol* 1991; **3**(1): 109–20.

Bjarnason I, Hayllar J, MacPherson AJ, Russell AS. Side effects of nonsteroidal anti-inflammatory drugs on the small andlarge intestine in humans. (Review.) *Gastroenterology* 1993; **104**(6): 1832–47.

Buller HA, Rings EH, Montgomery RK, Grand RJ. Clinical aspects of lactose intolerance in children and adults. (Review.) *Scand J Gastroent* 1991; **188**(Suppl): 73–80.

Doyle MP. Pathogenic *Escherichia coli*, *Yersinia enterocolitica,* and *Vibrio parahaemolyticus*. (Review.) *Lancet* 1990; **336**: 1111–5.

Farthing MJ. Octreotide in dumping and short bowel syndromes. (Review.) *Digestion* 1993; **54**(Suppl 1): 47–52.

Gurgui Ferrer M, Prats Pastor G, Mirelis Otero B. *Yersinia enterocolitica*: intestinal features. (Review.) *Dig Dis* 1990; **8**: 313–21.

Kingham JGC. Microscopic colitis. *Gut* 1991; **32**: 234–5.

Marshall JB, Bodnarchuk G. Carcinoid tumors of the gut. Our experience over three decades and review of the literature. *J Clin Gastroenterol* 1993; **16**(2): 123–9.

Nightingale JM, Lennard–Jones JE. The short bowel syndrome: what's new and old? *Dig Dis Sci* 1993; **11**(1): 12–31.

Nussbaum ML, Campana TJ, Weese JL. Radiation enteritis. Radiation-induced intestinal injury. (Review.) *Clin Plast Surg* 1993; **20**(3): 573–80.

Ogbonnaya KI, Arem R. Diabetic diarrhea. Pathophysiology, diagnosis, and management (see comments). (Review.) *Arch Int Med* 1990; **150**(2): 262–7.

Papiris SA, Moutsopoulos HM. Rare rheumatic disorders. A. Behçet's disease. (Review.) *Baillières Clin Rheum* 1993; **7**(1): 173–8.

Rader DJ, Brewer HB Jr. Abetalipoproteinemia. New insights into lipoprotein assembly and vitamin E metabolism from a rare genetic disease (clinical conference). (Review.) *JAMA* 1993; **270**(7): 865–9.

Riddell RH, Tanaka M, Mazzoleni G. Non-steroidal anti-inflammatory drugs as a possible cause of collagenous colitis: a case control-study. *Gut* 1992; **33**: 683–6.

Saebo A, Lassen J. A survey of acute and chronic disease associated with *Yersinia enterocolitica* infection. A Norwegian 10-year follow up study on 458 hospitalized patients. (Review.) *Scand J Infect Dis* 1991; **23**: 517–27.

Vinik AI, McLeod MK, Fig LM, Shapiro B, Lloyd RV, Cho K. Clinical features, diagnosis, and localization of carcinoid tumors and their management. *Gastroenterol Clin North Am* 1989; **18**(4): 865–96.

4
CONSTIPATION

REACHING A DIAGNOSIS AND MANAGEMENT

What is constipation?
Constipation covers a range of symptoms, which include:

- Anxiety that bowels are evacuated infrequently.
- Painful defecation as a result of hard stools.
- Bloating or abdominal pain attributed to infrequent defecation.
- The necessity of straining on defaecation.
- A feeling of incomplete evacuation.

None of these symptoms correlate closely with the frequency of evacuation. Some patients will feel well with only one or two evacuations a week whereas others will evacuate several times a day yet feel constipated. The 'normal' range of evacuation is quoted as being between three times daily and three a week, but young healthy women often defaecate less frequently without symptoms.

In the absence of a significant change in bowel habit it is therefore reasonable to reassure without investigation any patient whose only worry is the infrequency of bowel actions, but who has no other symptoms.

There is a better correlation between symptoms and the appearance of the stool rather than the frequency of evacuation. The passage of separate round lumps or pellets or a sausage-shaped conglomerate of such lumps can be taken to indicate constipation. Enthusiastic researchers have developed a 'penetrometer,' a pointed weight that is dropped onto the stool from a height, to measure this objectively.

A small number of patients exaggerate their problem, claiming to defecate extremely infrequently (e.g. once a month). The simplest way to sort this out is to measure whole gut transit time by giving the patient 50 segments of radio-opaque polyvinyl tubing within gelatin capsules and

▶ **What is constipation?**

> Symptoms of constipation correlate better with the appearance of the stool than with the frequency of evacuation

performing a plain abdominal radiograph five days later. The test is abnormal if more than 20% of the markers are retained after five days.

Pathophysiology
Constipation may arise from:

- A generalised abnormality of colorectal motility.
- Disordered anorectal physiology.
- Voluntary overriding of normal physiology (i.e. failure to respond to need to defecate).
- Inadequate fluid or fibre intake.

Passage of faeces around the colon occurs mainly as a result of two types of activity:

- Haustral contraction, where the contents of one or a group of haustra are transferred to the next haustra or group of haustra.
- Peristalsis.

In addition, once or twice daily, often at the time of defecation, there may be a mass propulsion in which contraction of several haustra propels colonic contents from the transverse colon down to the pelvic colon.

The arrival of stool in the rectum cause the rectum to contract, the internal anal sphincter to relax, and the external anal sphincter and puborectalis to contract. Stool then passes into the anal canal and the urge to defecate is created. If this is ignored the external sphincter and puborectalis remain contracted and faeces may eventually reflux back into the sigmoid colon, and the desire to defecate then passes. If this process is repeated faecal impaction will eventually result.

Defecation is achieved by voluntary relaxation of the external sphincter and puborectalis combined with contraction of the abdominal muscles. Straining against a contracted external sphincter and puborectalis produces the type of constipation (much commoner in women) known as anismus. Prolapse of rectal mucosa into the anal canal induces a desire to defecate, which is part of the solitary rectal ulcer syndrome.

Approach to diagnosis

The approach to the diagnosis depends on the age of the patient. An organic cause is more likely if constipation is occurring for the first time in someone over 40 years of age.

A careful history and general examination should pay attention to excluding endocrine problems such as **hypothyroidism** and **hypercalcaemia, neurological disorders** and **drug therapy**.

A barium enema should be performed to exclude neoplasm and to assess the diameter of the colon (**Fig. 4.1**).

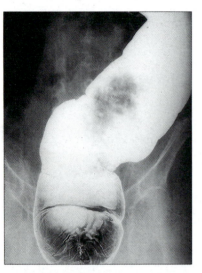

Fig. 4.1 Barium enema showing typical appearances of idiopathic megacolon. A lateral view showed that dilatation extended down to the upper end of the anal canal, thereby helping to exclude short segment Hirschsprung's disease.

All patients should have rigid sigmoidoscopy, which allows a careful look for evidence of a solitary rectal ulcer. If this is suspected (e.g. if there is a history of tenesmus and a sense of incomplete evacuation), a defecating proctogram may be useful by demonstrating anterior rectal mucosal prolapse.

Patients who give a history of having to strain excessively may benefit from having rectal manometry to confirm a failure of relaxation of the external sphincter (anismus) (**Figs. 4.2 and 4.3**).

A diagnosis of short segment Hirschsprung's disease should be excluded if a young patient has been constipated since childhood and has a dilated colon. This requires a full thickness or suction (mucosa plus submucosa) biopsy taken at least 3 cm from the dentate line. The diagnosis is confirmed if there is a complete absence of ganglion cells in the myenteric and submucosal plexuses (**Figs. 4.4 and 4.5**).

Is it the irritable bowel syndrome?

Most young to middle-aged patients with constipation have the irritable bowel syndrome. An attempt should be made to make a positive diagnosis on the basis of the history and physical examination to avoid unnecesary investigation, particularly since it has been shown that at least 20% of the population suffer from this syndrome. Typical features include bloating, colicky pain, which may be in any quadrant of the abdomen, but is more commonly in the lower abdomen, relief of pain with defecation and alternating constipation and diarrhoea. Rectal bleeding, weight loss, persistent diarrhoea and nocturnal pain all

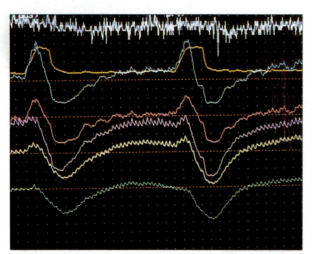

Fig. 4.2 Normal anorectal manometry. Pressure recordings are made simultaneously at six sites. The lowest trace shows recordings 0.5 cm above the anal verge and the upper traces show recordings at 0.5 cm intervals up to 4.0 cm above the anal verge. The top recording shows the ano-rectal electromyogram. A 30 ml balloon has been inserted into the rectum and the patient has been asked to strain. The consequent rise in pressure in the rectum (upper traces) is accompanied by appropriate relaxation of the anal sphincter (lower trace). Courtesy of Tracy Norris.

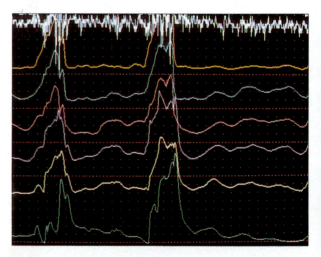

Fig. 4.3 Anismus. Straining with a 30 ml balloon in the rectum results in a simultaneous pressure rise in the rectum and inappropriate contraction of the anal sphincter. Courtesy of Tracy Norris.

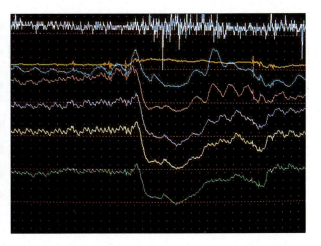

Fig. 4.4 Normal recto-anal inhibitory reflex. An 80 ml balloon has been inflated in the rectum and elicits involuntary relaxation of the anal sphincter. Courtesy of Tracy Norris.

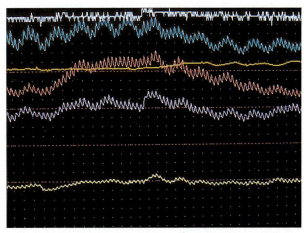

Fig. 4.5 Absent recto-anal inhibitory reflex. This recording is from a patient with paraplegia, but a similar appearance would be expected in Hirschsprung's disease. Courtesy of Tracy Norris.

require further investigation. Manometric studies have shown that patients with irritable bowel syndrome have an increased frequency of non-propagated contractions and the rectum is more sensitive to distension.

Management
The most important aspect of treatment is reassurance and explanation of the nature of the syndrome. Instruction booklets are extremely helpful. It is not helpful to tell the patient that there is 'nothing wrong' as their symptoms are real enough and they will then be inclined to seek a second opinion and start all over again with increasing anxiety and probably a worsening of their symptoms as a result.

A high cereal fibre intake or bulking agents such as bran or ispaghula may help, but many patients already have a normal fibre intake. Antispasmodic drugs such as mebeverine, 135 mg three times daily, may then be more helpful. Irritable bowel syndrome is discussed earlier in Chapter 1.

Severe constipation in young women
There is a group of patients, nearly all women, whose main complaint is severe diet-resistant constipation, sometimes associated with abdominal pain or bloating, but without the alternating diarrhoea that typifies the irritable bowel syndrome. Manometric study of these patients usually demonstrates inability to relax the external sphincter and puborectalis during straining (**anismus**). These patients have difficulty in expelling a simulated stool or barium from the rectum and may need to assist defecation by digital pressure in the vagina or rectum. However, the rectum is often empty on rectal examination and barium enema shows no colonic dilatation. Some of the patients also have difficulty in initiating micturition and have cold hands, blackouts and gynaecological problems more commonly than controls.

Management
Treatment of this group of patients is extremely difficult. They are often already taking considerable dietary fibre and tend to have very little response to conventional laxatives. A variety of drastic surgical manoeuvres have been tried including subtotal colectomy and division of the puborectalis with unpredictable results ranging from no effect to incontinence. The most promising results so far have been obtained with biofeedback, a technique that uses a self-applied electromyograph, which allows the patient to see the response of her external sphincter during straining so that she can train herself to relax the sphincter.

Is there megacolon?
This has been defined as an area of rectal shadow on barium enema that exceeds 115 cm^2 and when the diameter of the rectum at the pelvic brim exceeds 6.5 cm. Megacolon is rare among people with constipation, but conversely all patients with megacolon have constipation. The condition may be:

- **Primary** due to abnormal innervation as in Hirschsprung's disease.
- **Acquired** as a consequence of any condition producing chronic faecal loading.

Patients have slow transit times and reduced rectal sensation. Acquired megacolon is frequently associated with a history of faecal impaction and soiling dating back to childhood and is common in patients with mental subnormality. Both sexes are equally affected.

Patients with severe neurological disease such as parkinsonism, demyelination or spinal cord lesions may develop megacolon. Patients with spinal cord lesions require regular suppositories or enemas to induce reflex defaecation.

▶ **Diagnostic features of conditions causing constipation**

Irritable bowel syndrome

- No megacolon
- Manometry shows increased rectal sensitivity to distension and increased non-propagated contractions

Anismus

- Commonest in young women
- Rectum usually empty on examination
- No megacolon
- Manometry shows failure to relax external sphincter on straining

Solitary rectal ulcer syndrome

- Ulcer 5–10 cm proximal to the anal canal with typical histology
- Severe tenesmus
- Rectum usually empty on examination
- No megacolon
- Defecating proctogram likely to show rectal mucosal prolapse, usually anterior wall

Impaction

- Rectum full
- Commonly in elderly or mentally subnormal
- Megacolon common

Hirschsprung's disease

- Rectum empty
- Megacolon usual
- Manometry shows failure of internal sphincter to relax in response to rectal distension
- Submucosal biopsy shows absence of ganglion cells

Hirschsprung's disease must be excluded. If the patient is presenting as an adult this would be short segment disease and the characteristic narrowed segment between dilated proximal colon and narrow distal colon will therefore not usually be seen on barium enema. The rectum will typically be empty in contrast to the rectum in acquired megacolon. Manometric testing will show failure of relaxation of the internal sphincter in response to rectal distension. A conventional rectal biopsy 3 cm proximal to the dentate line may be useful to exclude the diagnosis if it includes muscularis with ganglia, but if negative a deeper biopsy will be required, either suction biopsy if available or full thickness biopsy under general anaesthetic.

Management

Treatment of acquired megacolon is often very difficult. The patient has often been taking stimulant laxatives for many years and this in itself results in degeneration of ganglion cells. Dietary manipulations and osmotic purgatives should certainly be tried, but subtotal colectomy and ileoproctostomy may eventually be required.

Is it the solitary rectal ulcer syndrome?

Solitary rectal ulcer syndrome is due to prolapse of the rectal mucosa. The prolapsed mucosa enters the anal canal stimulating the urge to defecate. Attempts to defecate then produce no satisfactory result and often rectal bleeding followed by rectal pain. The diagnosis can be confirmed by visualisation and biopsy of a rectal ulcer 5–10 cm proximal to the anal canal. Histology shows extensive replacement of the lamina propria by fibroblasts running at right angles to the muscularis. A defecating proctogram may demonstrate prolapse of the rectal mucosa.

Treatment is by surgical fixation of the posterior wall of the rectum, usually with good results.

Faecal impaction in the elderly

Faecal impaction in the elderly usually results from failure to respond to the call to defecate, either as a result of confusion, immobility or depression. Rectal examination reveals an impacted mass of faeces. Reduced anal sensation may also be a factor and the problem is often exacerbated by constipating drugs such as tricyclic antidepressants or phenothiazines. Paradoxical diarrhoea and incontinence due to seepage around the faecal mass is common.

Manual fragmentation and evacuation of the faecal mass with the aid of local anaesthetic jelly is indicated followed by small volume enemas. Sodium phosphate enemas are usually satisfactory providing the patient is not in renal failure when phosphate should be avoided. Regular use of suppositories may then be helpful in preventing recurrence.

FURTHER READING

Christiansen J. Surgical treatment of severe constipation. *Scand J Gastroenterol* 1991; **26**(3): 225–30.

Camilleri M, Thompson WE, Fleshman JW, Pemberton JH. Clinical management of intractable constipation. *Ann Intern Med* 1994; **121**:520–8.

Clayden GS. Management of chronic constipation. *Arch Dis Child* 1992; **67**(3): 340–4.

Fleshman JW, Fry RD, Kodner IJ. The surgical management of constipation. Bailliere's *Clin Gastroenterol* 1992; **6**(1): 145–62.

Gattuso JM, Kamm MA. Review article: the management of constipation in adults. *Aliment Pharmocol Ther* 1993; **7**: 487–500.

Kamm MA. Idiopathic constipation: any movement? *Scand J Gastroenterol Suppl* 1992; **192**: 106–9.

Kamm MA, Stabile G. Management of idiopathic megarectum and megacolon. *Br J Surg* 1991; **78**: 899–900.

Moriarty KJ, Irving MH. ABC of colorectal disease. Constipation. *Br Med J* 1992; **304**(6836): 1237–40.

Preston DM, Lennard-Jones JE. Severe chronic constipation of young women: 'idiopathic slow transit constipation.' *Gut* 1986; **27**: 41–48.

Wrenn K. Fecal impaction. *New Engl J Med* 1989; **321**: 658–62.

Read NW, Sun WM. Disordered anorectal motor function. *Clin Gastroenterol* 1994; **5**: 479–503.

West L, Warren J, Cutts T. Diagnosis and management of irritable bowel syndrome, constipation, and diarrhea in pregnancy. *Gastroenterol Clin North Am* 1992; **21**(4): 793–802

Williams JG, Kumar D. Recent advances in anorectal physiology. *Surg Annu* 1994; **26**: 27–47.

5
ANORECTAL PROBLEMS

REACHING A DIAGNOSIS

Rectal bleeding

It is important to obtain a careful history with the aim of distinguishing:

- Blood spotting on toilet paper only, which is almost always due to minor local trauma and occurs in most people at some time.
- Blood in the pan that is separate from faeces.
- Blood that is on the surface or mixed in with faeces.

The diagnostic approach to bleeding and anaemia is discussed in Chapter 6, but it is worth remembering that any patient presenting with rectal bleeding as the main problem should at least undergo rigid sigmoidoscopy even if it is just spotting.

At the same occasion the anal canal should be carefully inspected. Gentle parting of the anal canal will reveal the presence of a fissure and the patient should be asked to strain to allow detection of rectal prolapse or engorgement of the external venous plexus. No further investigation is required if the sigmoidoscopy is normal, if there is never any blood in the pan or on the faeces, and if there are no other symptoms.

Blood in the pan or faeces needs more thorough investigation. If the blood is separate from the faeces then flexible sigmoidoscopy is sufficient providing preparation is adequate to allow a clear view. If the nature of bleeding is difficult to establish with certainty from the history or if there is a clear history of blood mixed with faeces then full colonoscopy should be performed.

- Blood seen on paper only is usually due either to small haemorrhoids, minor local trauma usually associated with pruritus, or anal fissuring.
- Blood separate from faeces is most commonly due to haemorrhoids, but may also be due to a variety of other causes including rectal carcinoma and proctitis, which is usually also associated with the passage of mucus.

► **Investigation of rectal bleeding**

- Colonoscopy is superior to barium enema in the investigation of active rectal bleeding
- Flexible sigmoidoscopy plus barium enema is a reasonable compromise if bleeding has settled

- Blood mixed with faeces may be due to carcinoma, vascular abnormalities (e.g. angiodysplasia), inflammatory bowel disease, either ulcerative proctitis or Crohn's disease, but bleeding without diarrhoea in a patient with previous extensive ulcerative colitis should always be carefully investigated.

Polyps are often a chance finding when bleeding is investigated, but are rarely the cause of bleeding unless very large or frankly malignant. Diverticula can occasionally give rise to brisk arterial bleeding when inflamed, but do not usually cause recurrent low-grade blood loss. Brisk upper gastrointestinal bleeding (e.g. due to duodenal ulceration), may be rapidly passed rectally as bright red blood, but this will invariably be associated with haemodynamic signs of bleeding.

Barium enema is not a very satisfactory examination when rectal bleeding is the only symptom. Vascular lesions will be missed, and for most patients a cause for the bleeding will not be found and they will need to be referred on for colonoscopy. If colonoscopy lists are under pressure, the combination of flexible sigmoidoscopy and barium enema is a reasonable compromise that should detect all serious disease, but will miss angiodysplasia.

Faecal occult blood testing is of little help. If positive it merely confirms the presence of bleeding and if negative just implies that the bleeding is intermittent, but in no way reduces the need for further investigation.

Pain

A careful history is needed to determine whether pain is:

- Anal.
- Rectal.
- Pelvic.

Anal pain is most commonly due to either fissuring or thrombosed haemorrhoids (**Fig. 5.1**) and careful inspection will usually give an immediate diagnosis.

Rectal pain is more difficult. It is rarely due to organic disease, the commonest form being proctalgia fugax (i.e. intermittent severe rectal pain that is not associated with defaecation and may even wake the patient). In men, acute prostatitis may be associated with perineal pain and rectal pain that is worse on defaecation. Rectal examination will then reveal a tender prostate.

Pelvic pain is much commoner in women. Gynaecological conditions such as ovarian pathology, endometriosis, uterine or cervical cancer and ectopic pregnancy may all need exclusion, but in many patients no obvious cause is found. Often the pain may be a variant of the irritable bowel syndrome. There has been disconcerting evidence that a high proportion of the patients in whom no organic cause is found have been subjected to previous sexual abuse. Pelvic abscess, most commonly due to diverticulitis, but also due to Crohn's disease, salpingitis or local perforation due to ingestion of animal bones, for example, may present with vague symptoms of malaise and low-grade pyrexia without clear localising signs. A careful rectal examination is mandatory, but a high index of suspicion combined with pelvic ultrasound or CT scanning may be necessary to make a correct diagnosis.

Tenesmus

Tenesmus is a feeling of incomplete evacuation or frequent sensation of the need to evacuate. It is a usual accompaniment of diarrhoea whether this has an organic or functional cause, but is particularly prominent when there is rectal disease. Any mass lesion in the rectum such as a tumour or large polyp may cause tenesmus and it is often the most unpleasant symptom in ulcerative proctitis.

The **solitary rectal ulcer** syndrome is a cause of tenesmus that is often misdiagnosed. Although it is associated with rectal mucosal prolapse a clear history of this is often lacking; moreover when the ulcer is seen on sigmoidoscopy it is sometimes wrongly assumed to indicate some form of inflammatory bowel disease. The ulcer is on the anterior rectal wall in about 65% of patients and histology is characteristic (**Fig. 5.2**), with marked fibromuscular hyperplasia. Carefully performed defaecating proctography will usually confirm mucosal prolapse. Tenesmus is usually accompanied by urgency although urgency alone is a common feature of the irritable bowel sydrome and is then not commonly associated with tenesmus.

Discharge

Spontaneous discharge of pus indicates anal or rectal disease. Careful anal inspection should reveal any anal or perianal pathology such as anal tumours or fissuring, perianal fistula or perianal infections such as herpetic ulceration, syphilitic chancre or perianal warts. In the absence of obvious fissuring, rigid sigmoidoscopy should then be performed. If proctitis is present a rectal swab should be taken for gonococcal culture in addition to rectal biopsy for routine histology.

▶ **Tenesmus**

- Solitary rectal ulcer syndrome may be the cause of tenesmus

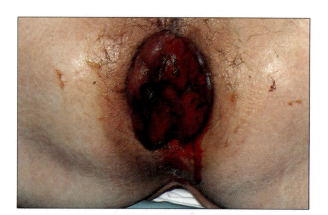

Fig. 5.1 Thrombosed prolapsed haemorrhoids.

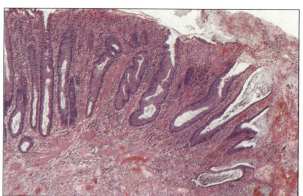

Fig. 5.2 Histology of a solitary rectal ulcer showing characteristic fibromuscular hyperplasia underlying the ulcer. Although clinicians are often suspicious that the rectal ulcer may be the result of self-digitation it is probably almost invariably due to mucosal prolapse on straining.

Incontinence

Few problems are as unpleasant, as poorly understood, and as poorly treated as faecal incontinence. Incontinence can occur in the presence of a normal sphincter if there is severe diarrhoea, but it is more commonly due to poor sphincter function. It is much commoner in women and is then often related to previous obstetric trauma, which may have passed unnoticed at the time. Diagnosis depends on an assessment of sphincter function. There are three main components of the sphincter:

- The puborectalis sling, which is the inner component of the levator ani and which maintains an acute angle between the anal canal and rectum.
- The internal sphincter consisting of involuntary muscle fibres, which are a continuation of the circular muscle coat of the rectum.
- The external sphincter, which surrounds the internal sphincter, consists of voluntary muscle fibres and is attached to the coccyx posteriorly and the perineal body anteriorly.

The external sphincter, can be assessed crudely by voluntary contraction during rectal examination, but facilities should now be available in every health region to allow proper objective measurement of sphincter function before any consideration of corrective surgery. This assessment should include assessment of:

- Resting pressure (normally 60–100 mm Hg until the sixth decade after which it falls progressively).
- Squeeze pressure (normally 100–220 mm Hg).

Barium enema examination should also be performed to allow measurement of the anorectal angle (the angle between the posterior wall of the rectum and the longitudinal axis of the anal canal, which should be approximately 90°. Transanal ultrasound examination is invaluable for diagnosis or exclusion of defects in the sphincter due to previous trauma.

Anal lesions

There are two components to the normal anal mucosa:

- Anal skin distal to the dentate line.
- Columnar epithelium between the dentate line and the anorectal junction.

Malignant tumours may of course cross the dentate line, but tumours arising above the line are more commonly adenocarcinomas, while those below the line are skin tumours and therefore include squamous and basal cell carcinomas and melanomas.

Sexually transmitted diseases need consideration in anal ulceration. Herpetic ulcers usually cause severe pain and tenesmus, while syphilitic ulcers are characteristically painless. Anal warts (condylomata acuminata) are usually easily recognised by their papilliferous appearance. Condylomata lata, the mucosal lesions of secondary syphilis, are flatter.

Macular, fissured or ulcerated anal lesions should always be biopsied particularly since the malignant conditions Bowen's disease (squamous carcinoma *in situ*) and Paget's disease (intraepithelial mucous adenocarcinoma) can only be diagnosed with histology (**Fig. 5.3–5.11**).

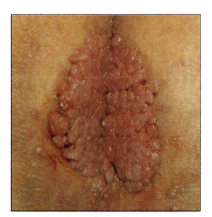

Fig. 5.3 Condylomata acuminata, which are anal warts due to human papillomavirus infection. They are nearly always sexually acquired.

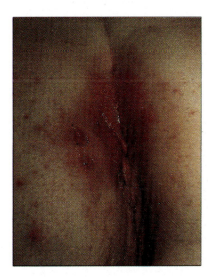

Fig. 5.4 Perianal skin tags and fistulae in Crohn's disease.

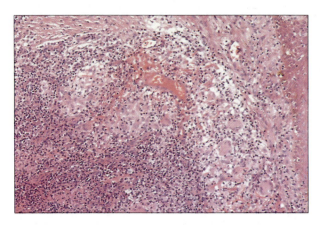

Fig. 5.5 Histology of a Crohn's disease skin tag showing typical giant cell granulomas.

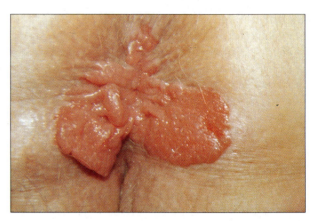

Fig. 5.6 Squamous cell carcinoma of the anus. Such tumours are commoner in homosexuals and may complicate condylomata acuminata. Treatment with local radiotherapy is often effective.

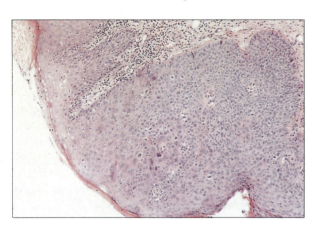

Fig. 5.7 Histology of early (in situ) squamous cell carcinoma of the anus. There are numerous mitoses and most of the cells are dysplastic with large irregular nuclei and a high nucleus to cytoplasm ratio.

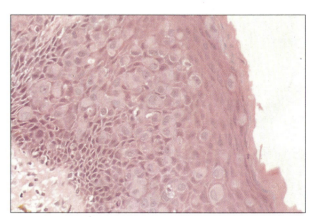

Fig. 5.8 Paget's disease of the anus. This is an intraepithelial mucinous adenocarcinoma, probably arising from subepidermal apocrine glands. Treatment is local excision.

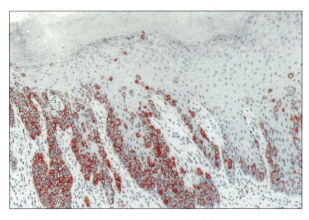

Fig. 5.9 Paget's disease: immunohistochemistry using a marker (CAM 5.2) for cytokeratin.

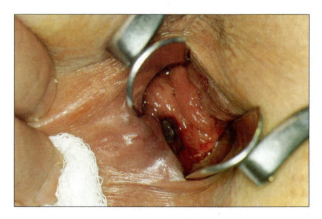

Fig. 5.10 Malignant melanoma of the anal canal. This is a very aggressive tumour and requires wide excision if secondary spread has not already occurred.

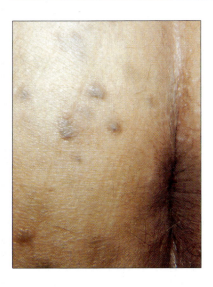

Fig. 5.11 Kaposi's sarcoma affecting the buttocks in a patient with AIDS.

Perianal abscess and fistula

Diagnosis of the lesion itself is usually obvious, but there are two main traps:

- Failing to recognise the presence of underlying Crohn's disease.
- Failing to make a correct assessment of the extent of the fistula.

The presence of thickened skin tags, usually of a dusky purple colour, should alert to the possibility of Crohn's disease. This should be excluded not only by assessment of the colon, but also by small bowel barium meal to exclude terminal ileal Crohn's disease. It is particularly important not to miss an underlying diagnosis of Crohn's disease since traditional treatment of a fistula or abscess by surgical debridement and laying-open will often be disastrous with very poor healing and further fistulation. Direct injection of radiographic contrast through the fistula (fistulogram) is often helpful to determine the extent of the fistula, and it is particularly important to determine whether or nor it extends proximal to the internal sphincter before surgical excision is considered.

Pruritus

Pruritus ani is a very common condition and is most commonly associated with poor local hygiene, which in turn may be associated with some degree of faecal incontinence. This may not be obvious from the history and if the problem is persistent then anorectal physiological studies will be indicated.

The anal area should be carefully inspected to exclude any local skin conditions such as eczema or Paget's disease, and a stool sample should be microscoped for ova or parasites. Rigid sigmoidoscopy should also be performed to exclude rectal pathology, and also because it may allow rapid diagnosis of threadworm infestation.

▶ **Pruritus ani**

> Pruritus ani is usually due to poor local hygiene

ANORECTAL CONDITIONS: NATURAL HISTORY AND MANAGEMENT

Haemorrhoids

Natural history

Bleeding most commonly occurs at the end of defaecation, but may occasionally be retained in the rectum to be passed on the next defaecation as dark blood. Such a history always necessitiates further investigation by flexible sigmoidoscopy or colonoscopy. Uncomplicated haemorrhoids are impalpable, but painful thrombosis is a common complication. This may occasionally be extensive, involving the whole circumference, but is more commonly localised, typically as a thrombosed venous saccule (previously called perianal haematoma).

PATHOLOGY

Haemorrhoids are usually formed as a result of enlargement of the normal anal cushions, which consist of areas of venous dilatation covered by smooth muscle, elastic and fibrous tissue. These venous cushions are found in three characteristic positions:

- Left lateral (3 o'clock).
- Right posterior (7 o'clock).
- Right anterior (11 o'clock).

The presence of arteriovenous communications explains the typical bright red colour when they bleed, and why portal hypertension is associated with rectal varices, but not enlarged haemorrhoids.

Although it is essential to exclude rectal carcinoma as an alternative diagnosis it is no longer thought that rectal carcinoma itself predisposes to haemorrhoids. Haemorrhoids are traditionally classified into:

- First degree (non-prolapsing, but bleeding).
- Second degree (prolapse, but reduce spontaneously).
- Third degree (require manual reduction).
- Fourth degree (irreducible prolapse).

Management

Many patients have only minor intermittent bleeding and when other causes of the bleeding have been excluded they may require no further treament other than dietary advice or possibly a bulking agent to relieve constipation.

Vigorous anal dilatation under general anaesthetic used to be commonly performed, but is now much less often used because of the unpredictable results and an appreciable risk of incontinence, particularly in elderly patients. Small haemorrhoids are usually treated by injection sclerotherapy (usually 5 ml of 5% phenol in arachis oil injected sub-mucosally into the haemorrhoid at the anorectal junction).

Injection is usually ineffective for prolapsing haemorrhoids, which are treated either by rubber band ligation or if this fails, by excision. Band ligation usually results in pain, which persists for about one week and secondary haemorrhage may occur in up to 10%. Approximately 10% patients will require surgical excision, particularly those with irreducible prolapsed haemorrhoids.

Other techniques in use in some centres include cryo-surgery and infrared coagulation, but these are mainly used for small non-prolapsing haemorrhoids.

Anal fissure

Anal fissures (**Fig. 5.12**) present with severe pain during defaecation associated with bright rectal bleeding. Diagnosis can usually made by direct inspection after parting of the buttocks. Rectal examination is likely to be very painful and should be deferred until symptomatic treatment or spon-taneous healing has had a chance to take effect and may then require preliminary administration of local anaesthetic ointment. Chronic anal fissures are commonly identifiable by the presence of a classical triad consisting of:

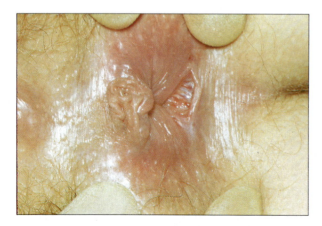

Fig. 5.12 Anal fissure

- 'Sentinel' external tag or 'pile'.
- The fissure.
- Hypertrophied anal papillae at the upper end of the fissure.

More than 90% are posterior and midline. There is ulceration down to the transverse muscles of the internal sphincter muscle with associated fibrosis.

Aetiology and pathogenesis

Acute anal fissures consist of a break in the anoderm with-out surrounding fibrosis. They are usually the result of passage of a large constipated stool.

Management

Acute anal fissures can usually be treated conservatively with bulking agents. Local anaesthetic suppositories or ointment are also commonly used, but are of uncertain benefit.

Conservative treament of a chronic anal fissure is usually ineffective. Although the pathophysiology of chronic fissuring is poorly understood it is thought to result generally from a constant high pressure at the internal sphincter. It is successfully treated by surgical lateral internal sphincterotomy. Published results are variable, but this procedure is probably associated with a lower risk for incontinence (1%) than the previous standard procedure of anal stretch.

Multiple or lateral fissures should raise the possibility of alternative diagnoses such as traumatic damage, Crohn's disease, leukaemia, syphyllis or tuberculosis and biopsy should be taken after injection of local anaesthetic. These 'secondary' fissures require treatment of the underlying condition, but should not themselves be treated by sphinc-terotomy.

Anal tags

Anal tags do not themselves cause symptoms or require treatment, but may be a clue to important underlying conditions. They commonly occur as the end result of a thrombosed external plexus haematoma ('thrombosed external pile'), but also mark the external end of chronic anal fissures.

Tags associated with Crohn's disease are usually thicker and have a purplish indurated appearance. Biopsy and histology may then be diagnostic as they commonly contain granulomas.

Anal warts

Anal warts are usually, but not always sexually transmitted. Their presence should therefore alert the clinician to the possible presence of other sexually transmitted disease.

Anal warts need to be distinguished from the much rarer mucosal lesions of secondary syphylis (condylomata lata). The latter are flatter and moister.

Management

Warts are usually treated with a topical application of 25% podophyllin or trichloracetic acid, but are commonly resistant to treatment. Intralesional injection of interferon has been tried with promising results. If all else fails surgical excision under general anaesthetic may be required and carries about a 75% chance of cure.

Anal tumours

Epidermoid carcinomas of the anus are most commonly squamous, but may also be basal cell tumours. They are commoner in homosexuals and may complicate or be mistaken for anal warts.

Management

Small lesions may be locally excised, but radiotherapy is the mainstay of treatment for epidermoid carcinoma. Trials are still being performed to assess the benefit of chemotherapy in addition, but radical surgery is no longer thought to be necessary.

Wide excision is necessary however for some of the rare anal tumours including malignant melanoma, mucinous adenocarcinoma occurring in anal canal glands (this causes recurrent anorectal fistulas), Bowen's disease and Paget's disease.

Bowen's disease is squamous carcinoma *in situ*. It often presents with chronic pruritus and may be treated by laser photocoagulation. Paget's disease, quite unlike Paget's disease of the nipple, is an intraepithelial mucinous carcinoma, which probably arises in the subepidermal apocrine glands.

▶ **Treatment of epidermoid anal cancer**

Radiotherapy is the preferred treament for epidermoid cancer of the anus

Skin conditions affecting perianal skin

Conditions affecting the anal skin are often difficult to diagnose from appearance alone and are likely to need referral for a dermatological opinion and biopsy if chronic. Differential diagnoses include simple lichenification associated with chronic pruritus ani, the premalignant condition lichen sclerosus et atrophicus, leukoplakia, fungal infection, lichen planus or lesions of more generalised diseases such as eczema or psoriasis.

Prolapse and solitary rectal ulcer syndrome

Prolapse (**Fig. 5.13**) may involve either the full thickness of the rectal wall (procidentia) or prolapse just of the mucosa, which may be either external or internal. Mucosal prolapse usually affects the anterior rectal wall. It is commonly internal (i.e. not presented through the anus), and is as a result often misdiagnosed. It results in a feeling of incomplete defaecation and tenesmus, which may be associated with rectal bleeding. Trauma to the mucosa may result in ulceration 6–10 cm above the anal verge, usually a single ulcer, hence 'solitary rectal ulcer', but not infrequently there may be more than one ulcer.

Patients with solitary rectal ulcer are often accused of self-digitating or unusual sexual activities, but usually there is no evidence for either and the ulcer is probably the result of a combination of local ischaemia and trauma directly related to the mucosal prolapse.

Management

The ulcer should be biopsied and the histological appearances are characteristic. There is obliteration of the lamina propria by fibromuscular hyperplasia, which streams up at right angles to the muscularis mucosae (**Fig. 5.2**). Glands may be seen in the submucosa ('colitis cystica profunda').

The perineum should be observed with the patient bearing down, but if the prolapse is internal a defaecating proctogram will be necessary to demonstrate the prolapse. Surgical fixation of the posterior rectal wall is usually effective at preventing this prolapse and allowing the ulcer to heal. Medical therapies are usually ineffective although it may be worth a preliminary trial of bulking agents.

Complete prolapse (procidentia) in an adult requires surgical correction as soon as the diagnosis is made. The procedure is usually posterior fixation to the sacrum using some form of synthetic mesh, but in frail or very elderly patients the sphincters may be encircled by a strip of synthetic mesh (Thiersch procedure), a procedure that only requires two very small perineal incisions. These operations are usually effective, preventing further prolapse in more than 90% of patients, but the sphincters are always weak and incontinence remains a problem in up to 50%.

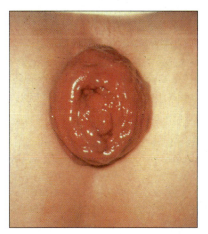

Fig. 5.13 Rectal prolapse in an infant with diarrhoea.

Faecal incontinence

If the faeces are liquid then the first aim should be to establish the cause and treat the diarrhoea, remembering that spurious diarrhoea due to severe constipation is common in the elderly. Incontinence of formed faeces is a distressing condition, which is often mismanaged.

Management

The obstetric history should be noted since damage to the sphincters is often the result of traumatic childbirth. The cutaneous anal reflex should be tested to exclude a neurological lesion, and the anal sphincters should be checked carefully on digital examination, noting the tone, the presence of any obvious defects and the ability to contract. Sigmoidoscopy should be performed to exclude rectal carcinoma and solitary rectal ulcer. If these tests reveal no obvious abnormality the patient should be referred to a centre specialising in anorectal problems and equipped to perform anorectal manometry and myography. Transanal ultrasound scanning may also be helpful in demonstrating defects in the external sphincter.

Traumatic sphincter disruption usually needs surgical repair. Other cases may respond to biofeedback, but surgical treatment (postanal repair) may be effective for those with structurally intact sphincters.

Pruritus ani

In the absence of either local disease of the anal canal or generalised pruritus, pruritus ani is nearly always the result of imperfect local hygiene.

Frequent bathing or showering supplemented by the use of impregnated tissues after evacuation will usually allow the condition to settle. Local allergic reactions to topical local anaesthetic preparations may compound the problem.

Proctalgia (rectal pain)

This is a frustrating condition for both patient and doctor. Seldom is a cause or an effective treatment found. Solitary rectal ulcer sydrome and associated mucosal prolapse should be excluded, but are usually associated with symptoms of incomplete evacuation or tenesmus. The pain is thought usually to result from spasm of the levator ani muscle.

Warm baths, simple analgesia and reassurance are usually all that can be offered, but there have been reports of good results with electrogalvanic stimulation of the levator ani.

Coccygodynia

Coccygodynia (pain in the coccyx) is equally perplexing. The diagnosis is confirmed by pain on movement of the coccyx.

Treatment is usually by injection of local anaesthetic, though occasionally resection of the coccyx is resorted to with rather mixed results.

Anorectal abscess

Underlying Crohn's disease, haematological conditions such as leukaemia and immune deficiency states may all be predisposing factors although most patients are otherwise healthy, but develop infection in an anal crypt, which then tracks along the anal ducts through the anal sphincter and then spreads. Abscesses may be:

- Perianal.
- Ischiorectal.
- Intersphincteric.
- Supralevator.
- Pelvirectal (Fig. 5.14)

Intersphincteric or supralevator abscesses are diagnosed by digital rectal examination, which reveals a tender mass.

Management

It is a general rule that all tender masses in the anorectal anatomical spaces contain pus and require drainage whether or not they are fluctuant. Delayed drainage may lead to further extension of the sepsis. It is no longer thought necessary to carry out extensive `deroofing' and 'saucerisation' so patients are usually able to return to work with little delay.

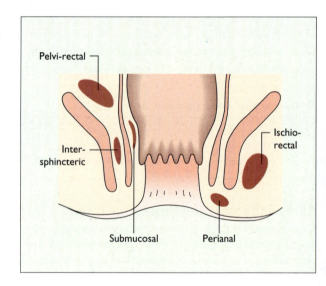

Fig. 5.14 Anatomy of perineal abscesses.

▶ **Drainage of anorectal abscesses**

Tender masses in the anorectal spaces contain pus and require drainage whether or not they are fluctuant

Anorectal fistula

Fistula formation is a common complication of anorectal abscess. Anal crypt infection spreads internally along a track, forming an abscess as described above, and when this abscess drains to the exterior a fistula is inevitable unless the original track from the anal crypt to the abscess has sealed.

Management

The treatment is usually surgical, but depends on two factors:

• The site of the proximal opening.
• The presence or absence of Crohn's disease.

An examination under anaesthetic will often be necessary to determine the site of the proximal opening although a low track will usually be palpable as a thick cord running towards the anal canal from the internal opening.

High fistulas require surgical correction by a specialist anorectal surgeon as repair of the sphincter (and covering colostomy) may be necessary. An alternative approach to a high fistula is to use a seton suture. The lower part of the track is first laid open and a suture tied around the remaining sphincter. This then slowly migrates through the sphincter and healing takes place by fibrosis so that the track is opened without impairing sphincter function.

In Crohn's disease (Figs 5.15–5.17) the standard surgical approach to fistulas can be disastrous, resulting in extensive perianal infection without granulation or healing. In Crohn's disease treatment should be as conservative as possible. Oral metronidazole, 400 mg three times daily, taken for up to three months may help reduce local sepsis and allow healing. If this fails then a period of enteral feeding with an amino acid-based feed (e.g. EO28) or a whole protein low residue feed (e.g. Triosorbon) may result in the fistula closing.

However, Crohn's fistulas often open up again when the patient returns to a normal diet. Conservative surgery using a loose seton suture may be successful and is increasingly used. If this fails diversion, either by a temporary (split ileostomy) or permanent ileostomy may be necessary for disabling symptoms due to perineal Crohn's disease.

▶ **Conservative approach to perianal Crohn's disease**

> Extensive surgery to perianal Crohn's disease is likely to lead to disaster with poor healing and fistulation, particularly if there is active rectal disease.

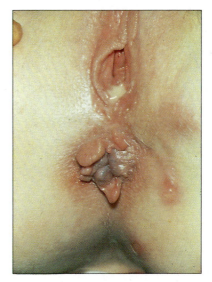

Fig. 5.15 Perianal Crohn's disease with fistulae.

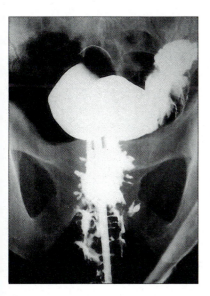

Fig. 5.16 Barium enema showing multiple fistulae and sinuses due to Crohn's disease. Enteral feeding with bowel rest and prolonged therapy with metronidazole for up to three months may be helpful in this situation to allow local sepsis to resolve, but a defunctioning stoma is likely to be required because of its severity.

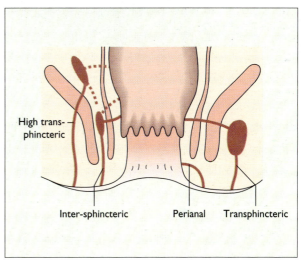

High trans-phincteric

Inter-sphincteric   Perianal   Transphincteric

Fig. 5.17 Anatomy of perineal fistulae.

FURTHER READING

Haemorrhoids

Cocchiara JL. Hemorrhoids. A practical approach to an aggravating problem. *Postgrad Med* 1991; **89**(1): 149–52.

Hancock BD. ABC of colorectal diseases. Haemorrhoids. *Br Med J* 1992; **304**(6833): 1042–4.

Anal fissure

Penninck F, Lestar B, Kerremans R. The internal anal sphincter: mechanisms of control and its role in maintaining anal continence. *Baillière's Clin Gastroenterol* 1992; **6**(1): 193–214.

Faecal incontinence

Bartolo DC. Gastroenterological options in faecal incontinence. *Ann Chir* 1991; **45**(7): 590–8.

Christiansen J. Advances in the surgical management of anal incontinence. *Baillière's Clin Gastroenterol* 1992; **6**(1): 43–57.

Kiff ES. ABC of colorectal diseases. Faecal incontinence. *Br Med J* 1992; **305**(6855): 702–4.

Pinho M, Keighley MR. Results of surgery in idiopathic faecal incontinence. *Ann Med* 1990; **22**(6): 425–33.

Speakman CT, Kamm MA. The internal and sphincter—new insights into faecal incontinence. *Gut* 1991; **32**(4): 345–6.

Anorectal fistula

Levien DH, Surrell J, Mazier WP. Surgical treatment of anorectal fistula in patients with Crohn's disease. *Surg Gynecol Obstet* 1989; **169**(2): 133–6.

Solitary rectal ulcer syndrome

Lam TC, Lubowski DZ, King DW. Solitary rectal ulcer syndrome. *Baillière's Clin Gastroenterol* 1992; **6**(1): 129–43.

Mackle EJ, Parks TG. Solitary rectal ulcer syndrome: aetiology, investigation and management. *Dig Dis* 1990; **8**(5): 294–304.

6
GASTROINTESTINAL BLEEDING

REACHING A DIAGNOSIS AND MANAGEMENT

The treatment of a patient with gastrointestinal bleeding usually has to be started before a clear diagnosis has been reached so the general principles of management will be considered together with the approach to diagnosis.

Is there significant gastrointestinal bleeding?

The patient may present with:

- Haematemesis (vomiting either bright red blood or altered blood described as 'coffee grounds').
- Melaena (passage of tarry black 'sticky' or liquid stools).
- Haematochezia (the passage of bright blood per rectum).
- Hypotensive shock without external evidence of bleeding, when rectal examination is particularly important and will usually reveal fresh or altered blood.

If it is clear that there has been a significant bleed the patient must be admitted to hospital even if the bleeding appears to have stopped and the patient is haemo-dynamically stable. For several reasons it may not be clear whether a significant gastrointestinal bleed has occurred:

- Haemoptysis may be confused with haematemesis, but a patient with haemoptysis can often cough up a further sputum sample on demand, which frequently resolves the question.
- Swallowed blood from nose bleeding may cause confusion and conversely patients with profuse bleeding from oesophageal varices may have blood running from the nose.
- Patients who are vomiting from any cause may have small amounts of altered blood ('coffee grounds') in the vomitus.
- Recent ingestion of oral iron or bismuth preparations, liquorice, spinach or dark beers (stout or Guinness) may all cause very dark motions that mimic melaena.

If in doubt the stool should be tested for occult blood using a guaiac test. Oral iron preparations do not interfere with this test at normal faecal pH.

Stabilisation

The first priority is to ensure that the patient's haemodynamic status is stabilised. An intravenous line should be set up and blood cross-matched as the first priority. The haemoglobin concentration, platelet count and prothrombin time should be checked. If there is hypotension (systolic pressure < 100 mmHg) or other evidence of continued bleeding, a central venous line should be inserted into a subclavian or internal jugular vein to allow early detection of hypovolaemia.

The commonest and most serious error in the management of gastrointestinal bleeding is underestimation of the extent of bleeding with consequent under transfusion and late intervention. The hospital mortality for gastrointestinal bleeding had remained depressingly constant at around 10% for many years. More recent surveys are at last reporting lower mortalities around 3%. The increasing age of patients presenting with gastrointestinal bleeding may also have obscured further improvement.

Further reduction in mortality is likely to come mainly from better monitoring of the bleeding patient rather than from any dramatic developments in therapy. Pulse and blood pressure should be monitored every half hour for the first four hours and if there has been significant hypotension the central venous pressure should also be monitored.

The threat to the patient from further bleeding is greatly increased if the patient is anaemic. If the haemoglobin concentration is less than 10.0 g/dl the patient should receive a blood transfusion even if haemodynamically stable. A reasonable approach is to transfuse one unit (500 ml) of blood for every gram that the haemoglobin is below 10 g. If the patient is not hypovolaemic and particularly if the patient is also elderly it may be necessary to transfuse plasma-reduced blood and administer intravenous frusemide to prevent fluid overload.

History and examination

When the intravenous line has been set up and the cross match requested, a more detailed history should be taken from the patient with particular attention to drug therapy, alcohol intake, previous episodes of gastrointestinal bleeding and previous intra-abdominal surgery.

The patient should be examined carefully, particularly for the following signs, which may help point to a diagnosis:

- Signs of liver disease or portal hypertension (the presence of oesophageal varices is the only factor that will significantly alter the initial management).
- Vasculitic skin lesions.
- Haemangiomas.
- Telangiectasia.
- Previous aortic surgery.

Where is the bleeding?

Haemetemesis is nearly always due to a lesion proximal to the ligament of Treitz, but in melaena the lesion will be distal to that point in up to 35% of patients and may even be in the colon. Conversely the passage of bright red blood per rectum may result from brisk bleeding in the upper gastrointestinal tract. Aspiration via a nasogastric tube may help to resolve the question, but carries a slight risk of provoking further bleeding by dislodging blood clot particularly if the lesion is in the oesophagus.

Since the practice of gastric lavage with ice-cooled water has been shown to have no therapeutic value the use of nasogastric tubes can now be restricted to occasional diagnostic use in patients with persistent melaena of obscure cause.

Fibreoptic endoscopy

Fibreoptic endoscopy has much the highest diagnostic yield of any investigation for upper gastrointestinal bleeding and has superceded barium meal examination. A diagnosis will be made in up to 90% of patients with haematemesis (**Figs 6.1** and **6.2**).

The diagnostic yield falls sharply if the endoscopy is delayed for more than 24 hours and in the early days of endoscopy it used to be common to endoscope all bleeding patients within a few hours of admission. Although this

▶ **Management of gastrointestinal bleeding**

- Set up intravenous line
- Check haemoglobin, platelets, prothrombin time, partial thromboplastin time
- Cross match blood
- Central venous line if systolic blood pressure < 100 mmHg
- Transfuse if haemoglobin < 10 g/dl or if low central venous pressure and/or systolic blood pressure < 100 mmHg
- Endoscopy

sounds ideal it often resulted in inadequately resuscitated patients being endoscoped in the middle of the night by relatively inexperienced endoscopists, sometimes with inadequate nursing support. A blocked endoscope and an unclear diagnosis were then a common consequence. Most centres have therefore adopted a policy of endoscoping patients on the next available routine list.

Selected patients will still need out-of-hours emergency endoscopy. These will include:

- Patients who are thought likely to have oesophageal varices who would benefit from early injection sclerotherapy.
- Patients who have rebled or have massive bleeding (more than four units in the first 12 hours).
- Elderly patients in whom there is a considerable mortality if rebleeding occurs.

The endoscopy should usually be performed with cautious intravenous sedation and it is vital to have adequate nursing assistance to ensure patency of the airway and adequate oxygenation throughout.

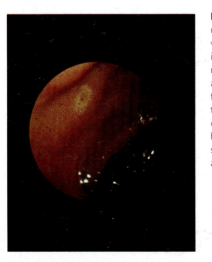

Fig. 6.1 Duodenal ulcer with central visible vessel. This indicates an increased risk for rebleeding and is an indication for endoscopic therapy (bicap diathermy, laser, heater probe, sclerotherapy or adrenaline injection).

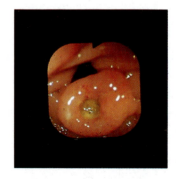

Fig. 6.2 Secondary carcinoma in the gastric antrum. The 'volcano' appearance of a mound of normal mucosa with central ulceration is similar to that seen in leiomyoma.

► **Endoscopy in gastrointestinal bleeding**

> **Next routine list for most patients but emergency endoscopy for patients with:**
>
> - Evidence of liver disease
> - Known varices
> - Rebleeding
> - Massive bleeding (more than four units in the first 12 hours)
> - Over 70 years of age

► **Therapeutic endoscopy for bleeding**

> - Injection of adrenaline +/- sclerosant
> - Bicap diathermy
> - Heater probe
> - Laser therapy
>
> These techniques have all been shown to reduce rebleeding. It is not clear which is superior, but one of these techniques should be used if there is a visible vessel at endoscopy.

Normal endoscopy: what next?

Fibreoptic endoscopy fails to give a diagnosis for about 10% of patients with haemetemesis and a higher proportion of patients with melaena.

Many of these patients will have had a small bleed from a Mallory–Weiss tear. If a history can be obtained of a blood-free vomitus preceding the haemetemesis and particularly if there was recent consumption of alcohol it is reasonable to assume that there has been a Mallory–Weiss tear and not investigate further unless bleeding recurs. The tears are often small and heal rapidly so are easily missed if the endoscopy is done 24 hours after the bleed.

If bleeding persists there is a wide range of tests that can be used to establish the site of bleeding. These include enteroscopy, angiography, isotope scanning, computerised tomography (CT) and colonoscopy. The large number of tests reflects their inadequacy, but if properly used in appropriate circumstances and in an adequately prepared patient an accurate diagnosis can nearly always be established. The choice of test will depend on the circumstances.

^{99m} Technetium pertechnetate scanning for Meckel's diverticulum

In a child or young adult with melaena, a Meckel's diverticulum containing ectopic gastric mucosa should be suspected. Gastric mucosa concentrates the isotope ^{99m}Tc pertechnetate (not technetium colloid) following its intravenous injection so scanning with this agent should be an early investigation in the younger patient (**Fig. 6.3**). Bleeding from a Meckel's diverticulum is extremely rare in people over 40 years of age.

Colonoscopy

In the older patient, lesions in the caecum and ascending colon such as carcinoma or angiodysplasia (**Fig. 6.4**) are relatively common so colonoscopy should usually be the next investigation after upper gastrointestinal endoscopy.

Bowel preparation is difficult. It is usually worth performing the procedure initially after simple rectal washouts with phosphate enemas have been performed until the enema is returned reasonably clear. This will usually allow the site of colonic bleeding to be determined, but if angiodysplasia is suspected it may be necessary to repeat the procedure after a more vigorous bowel preparation as the lesions are easily missed unless there is good visibility.

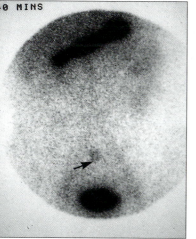

Fig. 6.3 Technetium pertechnetate scan showing uptake in normal stomach and in gastric-type mucosa in a Meckel's diverticulum (arrowed) Courtesy of Dr M Critchley.

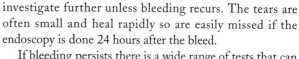

Fig. 6.4 Angiodysplasia in the caecum. Lesions of this size can be effectively treated by diathermy, but larger lesions may need resection.

Colonoscopy is the initial investigation of choice in the patient with fresh rectal bleeding.

Angiography

Angiography should be considered if both upper gastrointestinal endoscopy and colonoscopy have proved negative. Extravasation of contrast media is only likely to be seen if bleeding is occurring at the rate of 0.5 ml/minute or greater. Vascular lesions such as angiodysplasia (**Fig. 6.5**) and tumours of the small intestine may be demonstrated in the absence of bleeding, but colonoscopy is more accurate for the diagnosis of colonic angiodysplasia.

^{99m}Technetium colloid scanning or labelled red cell scanning

Extravasation of isotope may be detected by abdominal gamma scanning following an intravenous injection of ^{99m}technetium sulphur colloid or chromium-labelled red cells. The results of this test are sometimes more intriguing than useful as at best the bleeding site is localised to one quadrant of the abdomen and this is of limited value if it is not known whether it is in the colon or small intestine.

▶ **Investigating endoscopy-negative bleeding**

- Meckel's scan if under 40 years of age
- Colonoscopy
- Angiography (will only detect bleeding site if blood loss > 0.5 ml/minute)
- Enteroscopy
- Combined enteroscopy and laparotomy
- On-table angiography (at laparotomy)

The above steps are followed sequentially with increasing desperation if bleeding persists without diagnosis. Laparotomy should only prove necessary to establish the diagnosis in well under 0.5% of gastrointestinal bleeds.

Enteroscopy

Fibreoptic enteroscopy of the small intestine should be the most logical approach to the diagnosis of obscure gastrointestinal bleeding, but endoscopy of the small intestine is very difficult and manageable instruments are only just becoming available. It is however relatively easy to pass a long endoscope (e.g. colonoscope) via the mouth into the proximal jejunum and this can be very useful since the distal duodenum and jejunum are the commonest sites for small intestinal tumours and aorto-enteric fistulae (**Figs 6.6 and 6.7**). This is an underused technique.

Combined enteroscopy and laparotomy

If all other diagnostic tests have failed the final and probably most rigorous test is fibreoptic inspection of the whole small intestine performed at laparotomy. The endoscope (a full-length colonoscope) can be inserted either by mouth or through an enterostomy and the intestine can be gently telescoped over the instrument by the surgeon while the mucosa is inspected by the endoscopist. Interpretation may be difficult as trauma to the mucosa may result in petechial haemorrhages, which can mimic angiodysplasia.

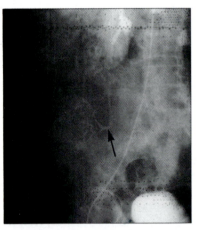

Fig. 6.5
Angiographic demonstration of caecal angiodysplasia. There is a vascular blush associated with a characteristically prominent draining vein (arrowed).

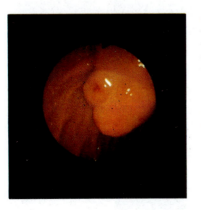

Fig. 6.6 Carcinoma of the ampulla of Vater viewed with a side-viewing duodenoscope. These lesions usually cause iron-deficiency anaemia or jaundice rather than frank haemorrhage.

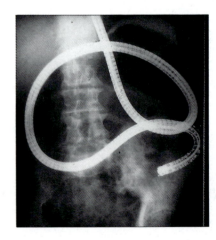

Fig. 6.7 Enterosopy to visualise the distal duodenum, a common site for gastroscopy-negative, colonoscopy-negative bleeding. In this case a standard colonoscope has been passed via the mouth into the proximal jejunum. Push-enteroscopes are now available for this purpose.

Investigating anaemia

The first step in the investigation of anaemia should always be an assessment of the blood film and full blood count including mean corpuscular volume.

If there is evidence of macrocytosis then serum and red cell folate, serum vitamin B_{12} and direct and indirect Coombs' test should be performed and if no clear conclusion is reached then a referral to a haematologist should be made. A low serum B_{12} should be followed by a Schilling test to differentiate between intrinsic factor deficiency and malabsorption. A combination of low B_{12} and raised serum folate is highly suggestive of small bowel bacterial overgrowth (folate is synthesized by bacteria).

If the anaemia is normocytic, haematinics should also be checked, together with erythrocyte sedimentation rate, serum immunoglobulins and renal function. This should be followed by haematological referral if no clear explanation is found.

Microcytic anaemia should always be considered to be due to chronic blood loss in a patient of Northern European extraction. In races with a high incidence of thalassaemia, haemoglobin electrophoresis should be checked. Faecal occult blood testing is not helpful in most cases since a negative result may merely indicate that bleeding is intermittent and should not be taken to exclude gastrointestinal blood loss.

The sequence of investigation is much as for acute gastrointestinal bleeding except angiography is much less likely to be helpful. Upper endoscopy is usually performed first because it does not require bowel preparation, but an efficient approach is to prepare the patient for colonoscopy and perform both upper and lower bowel endoscopy under sedation at the same appointment.

There are a number of important points to note in the interpretation of the significance of any abnormal findings.

- It is particularly important to note that duodenal ulcer, uncomplicated hiatus hernia and colonic diverticular disease are not causes of chronic iron-deficiency anaemia.
- Acceptable causes (if other lesions have been excluded) include chronic use of NSAIDs, peptic oesophagitis, inflammatory bowel disease, poor diet in adolescence, partial gastrectomy, achlorhydria, small bowel diverticulosis and even oesophageal varices, which do not always bleed massively.

Iron deficiency in patients with previous partial gastrectomy or achlorhydria often respond well to a combination of oral iron and vitamin C (100 mg taken at the same time as the iron) when oral iron alone has failed.

CONDITIONS CAUSING GASTROINTESTINAL BLEEDING: NATURAL HISTORY AND MANAGEMENT

Bleeding peptic ulcer and the effects of NSAIDs

Natural history

Duodenal and gastric ulcers account for about 65% of upper intestinal bleeds. Before the advent of effective medical anti-ulcer therapy it was estimated that the incidence of bleeding was about 5%/year in patients with peptic ulceration. Patients, particularly those with gastric ulcers, often give no history of previous indigestion. Blood is an effective buffer so patients are usually free from pain at the time of bleeding.

There has been a marked increase in admissions for intestinal bleeding in the elderly over the past 20 years, which parallels the increased ingestion of NSAIDs. Although the risk has been estimated at only one episode of clinically significant bleeding for every 6000 NSAID prescriptions, there were already 22 million such prescriptions in the UK in 1983 and at that time it was suggested that there might be as many as 4000 deaths/year in the UK from NSAID-related ulcers.

▶ **Iron-deficiency anaemia**

Caused by:

- Carcinoma or lymphoma of the oesophagus, stomach, ampulla, duodenum, jejunum, ileum or colon
- Chronic NSAID use
- Peptic oesophagitis
- Oesophageal varices
- Achlorhydria +/- pernicious anaemia
- Partial gastrectomy
- Coeliac disease
- Inflammatory bowel disease
- Small bowel diverticulosis
- Intestinal telangiectasia
- Angiodysplasia
- Inadequate diet in an adolescent

Is not caused by:

- Benign peptic ulceration
- Uncomplicated hiatus hernia
- Dietary deficiency in an otherwise healthy adult (except exceptionally)
- Diverticular disease of the colon

▶ **Bleeding duodenal ulcers**

- Bleeding duodenal ulcers are often pain free at the time of bleeding

▶ **NSAID-related gastrointestinal bleeding**

> One significant bleed/6000 NSAID prescriptions

Management

PREVENTING REBLEEDING

No form of medical treatment other than good supportive management has been shown to affect the mortality in patients with bleeding peptic ulcers. The prescription of histamine H_2 antagonists is logical since they are so effective at healing the ulcers, but there is little evidence that the early use of intravenous H_2 antagonists reduces the risk of rebleeding. Antifibrinolytic therapies such as tranexamic acid have also been tried without convincing success, but further studies are still needed. If the bleeding settles with medical treatment, therapy with H_2 antagonists should usually be continued indefinitely as an early study suggested that the risk of further episodes of bleeding from untreated duodenal ulcer disease is as high as 75%. Patients who are positive for *H. pylori* should probably have eradication therapy, although the association between *H. pylori* and complicated ulcer disease is not as strong as for uncomplicated disease.

A wide range of local therapies directed against the bleeding vessel have been tried. These include laser coagulation, bicap electrocoagulation and heater probe coagulation all of which are applied using a fibreoptic-endoscope. None of these techniques has yet been shown to have a convincing impact on mortality, but this may well simply be due to the very large numbers of patients needed for any study to show this. For each of these techniques there is some evidence of reduced morbidity, for example reduced transfusion requirements.

A simpler technique, which is producing equally impressive results is the endoscopic injection of adrenaline (with or without sclerosants such as ethanolamine oleate or absolute alcohol) into or around the bleeding vessel. There are numerous variations to this approach, but a reasonable protocol is to place four injections up to a maximum of 10ml of 1:10 000 adrenaline around the visible vessel or site of active bleeding. Subsequent injections of sclerosant (e.g. 5% ethanolamine 0.5–2 ml) may then be placed into and around the bleeding vessel although current evidence suggests this may not be necessary. Initial injections of adrenaline should be around rather than directly into the vessel so as to avoid precipitation of rebleeding.

IF THERE IS REBLEEDING

Rebleeding occurs during the same hospital admission in about 50% of patients with gastric ulcers and about 25% of those with duodenal ulcers. It is the major cause of mortality. In one study of 89 patients, endoscopic demonstration of continued bleeding, adherent blood clot or a

▶ **Endoscopic stigmata and rebleeding**

> **Risk of bleeding is higher than 50% if any of the following stigmata are present, and 6% if they are absent**
> - Active bleeding
> - Adherent blood clot
> - Visible vessel

visible vessel in the ulcer crater carried a risk of rebleeding of 51% compared with 6% for those without these findings, with mortalities of 21% and 0% respectively in each group. Elderly patients are particularly at risk of dying from rebleeding, and some centres therefore advocate a policy of early surgery in patients over 70 years of age if these endoscopic stigmata are present.

SURGERY

The indications for surgery in patients with bleeding peptic ulcers are contentious. Age is an important factor since death from bleeding in patients under the age of 65 is fortunately extremely rare whether they are managed medically or surgically. There are however occasional young patients in whom bleeding is torrential and emergency surgery life-saving. There are no clearly established guidelines, but a reasonable empirical approach is to consider the presence of any of the following as an indication for surgery:

- The need to transfuse more than four pints of blood.
- The occurrence of rebleeding.
- The presence of adherent blood clot or visible vessels at endoscopy in a patient over 65 years of age (unless this can be treated endoscopically).

The operation will vary according to the nature of the lesion and the preference of the surgeon, but for a duodenal ulcer will usually consist of oversewing of the ulcer and for a gastric ulcer will be partial gastrectomy. Some surgeons combine oversewing of a duodenal ulcer with truncal vagotomy and pyloroplasty, but this lengthens the operation time, has its own complication rate and is probably unnecessary in view of the potent ulcer healing properties of the H_2 antagonists. In most centres patients with ulcers with visible vessels are treated initially by endoscopic therapy.

▶ **Indications for surgery for actively bleeding ulcers**

> - Transfusion requirement higher than four pints
> - Rebleeding despite endoscopic therapy

Gastric erosions

Causes of gastric erosions include generalised sepsis, extensive burns (Curling's ulcer), central nervous system injury (Cushing's ulcer) and NSAID medication.

Management

Prevention by use of H_2 antagonist or proton pump inhibitor prophylaxis in high-risk patients is easier than treatment of established lesions. Bleeding due to extensive erosive gastritis can be very difficult to manage.

The only effective surgical treatment is total gastrectomy, which carries an appreciable mortality and high morbidity. No medical treatments are of unequivocal benefit. Embolisation is usually ineffective for gastric bleeding because of extensive anastomoses and may result in dangerous infarction. Local endoscopic therapy with diathermy coagulation or laser is occasionally helpful.

If the patient has been taking NSAIDs it is reasonable to give a prostaglandin derivative such as misoprostil, and for patients with associated portal hypertension, the beta blocker propranolol and/or somatostatin infusion may be beneficial.

Oesophageal varices

Oesophageal varices account for 5–10% of admissions for intestinal bleeding, the size of the problem being proportional to the prevalence of alcoholism in the community.

Aetiology and pathogenesis of portal hypertension

The normal portal venous pressure is about 10 mm Hg, but rises to 20–40 mm Hg in portal hypertension. The causes of portal hypertension may be classified as:

- Pre-sinusoidal (i.e. on the portal venous side of the liver).
- Sinusoidal.
- Post-sinusoidal (on the hepatic venous side of the liver) (**Fig. 6.8**).

Distinction between these three groups can be made on the basis of hepatic venography with hepatic vein wedged pressure measurement.

PRE-SINUSOIDAL PORTAL HYPERTENSION

The hepatic vein wedge pressure is characteristically low or normal in presinusoidal portal hypertension since there is resistance to the flow of blood towards the liver. Common causes of presinusoidal portal hypertension include:

- Portal vein thrombosis.
- Schistosomiasis.
- Primary biliary cirrhosis (in which the portal tracts within the liver take the main brunt of the injury).

Portal vein thrombosis is most commonly caused by portal pyaemia due to intra-abdominal sepsis. This is often due to missed or delayed treatment of appendicitis or neonatal umbilical sepsis, which may be the result of umbilical vein catheterisation. Although the liver receives at least half its oxygen supply via the portal vein, thrombosis of this vein does not usually cause any significant derangement of hepatic function, ascites is rare unless there was pre-existing liver disease, and life expectancy is good providing the oesophageal varices can be dealt with. Portal vein occlusion may also occur as a consequence of tumour infiltration, usually in pancreatic cancer, in which case the prognosis is very poor.

Splenic vein thrombosis without thrombosis of the main portal vein may occur, usually as a consequence of pancreatic disease. It is important to recognise since, unlike other causes of portal hypertension, it may be effectively treated by splenectomy.

Diagnosis of portal vein thrombosis can usually be made at ultrasound examination. This usually shows an abnormal leash of collateral vessels around the hilum of the liver. Splenic vein thrombosis usually requires angiographic imaging for a definite diagnosis (usually the venous phase of a splenic arteriogram rather than by direct splenic venography, which requires direct splenic puncture), but new non-invasive imaging techniques such as Doppler ultrasound and magnetic resonance scanning are gradually reducing the need for invasive angiography.

Acute mesenteric vein thrombosis: Usually portal vein thrombosis causes few problems initially and the patient

▶ **Causes of portal hypertension**

Pre-sinusoidal causes

- Portal vein thrombosis
- Splenic vein thrombosis
- Primary biliary cirrhosis
- Schistosomiasis

Sinusoidal causes

- Cirrhosis

Post-sinusoidal causes

- Heart failure
- Constrictive pericarditis
- Vena cava web (Budd–Chiari syndrome)
- Hepatic vein thrombosis (Budd–Chiari syndrome)
- Veno-occlusive disease (Bush tea, chemotherapy)

may present years later with bleeding varices. Occasionally, however there is acute impairment of venous return from the intestine, particularly if the mesenteric veins themselves are thrombosed. The patient presents acutely with abdominal pain, shock, splenomegaly and intestinal bleeding. The bleeding usually results from a diffuse ooze from the congested intestinal mucosa and there is often haemoconcentration as well as hypovolaemia. There may be extensive infarction of the small intestine with a very high mortality.

SINUSOIDAL PORTAL HYPERTENSION

In sinusoidal portal hypertension, which is usually due to cirrhosis, the hepatic vein wedged pressure reflects the raised portal pressure.

POST-SINUSOIDAL PORTAL HYPERTENSION

In post-sinusoidal portal hypertension both the wedged and free hepatic vein pressures will be elevated if heart failure is the cause, but more commonly it will prove impossible to obtain a wedge pressure since hepatic vein thrombosis or occlusion is the major cause of this type of portal hypertension. Occlusion may be due to a surgically correctable web in the vena cava.

Hepatic vein thrombosis may occur as a result of a clotting disorder or in women receiving oral contraceptives. It gives rise to the Budd–Chiari syndrome. There is intense congestion of the liver with deranged liver function and tense ascites, which may have a high protein content. The caudate lobe escapes injury because it drains directly into the vena cava so becomes markedly hypertrophied. There are occasional long-term survivors, but the prognosis is generally poor with survival of only a few months without surgical therapy. Transplantation is now the main form of therapy, but good results have also been achieved by portocaval shunting, which decompresses the liver.

Veno-occlusive disease: Post-sinusoidal portal hypertension (Fig. 6.8) can also occur due to toxic injury to the hepatic veins caused by pyrrolizidine alkaloids in 'bush' teas drunk in the West Indies, India and Egypt or as a result of chemotherapy or hepatic irradiation given as treatment for leukaemia. It may also occur as part of the graft versus host reaction in patients who have received a bone marrow transplant.

Clinical features of portal hypertension

The main features of portal hypertension are oesophageal varices, splenomegaly, ascites and porto-systemic encephalopathy (Figs. 6.9–6.14). Ascites and encephalopathy are discussed in Chapter 15. Oesophageal varices do not always cause massive bleeding and may either cause low-grade blood loss with iron deficiency anaemia or be asymptomatic. As sclerotherapy may itself induce bleeding asymptomatic varices should be left untreated.

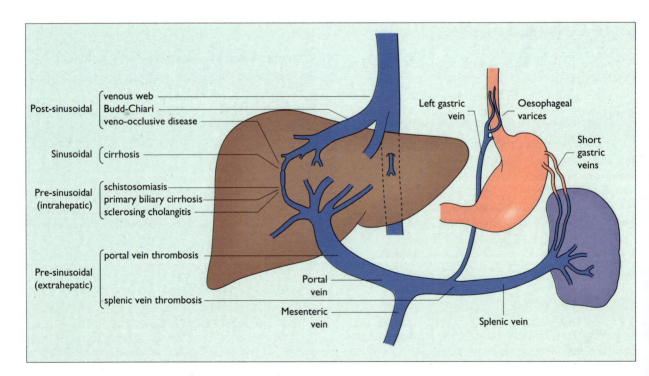

Fig. 6.8 Anatomy of portal hypertension.

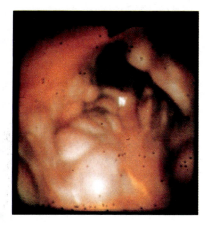

Fig. 6.9 Endoscopic view of large oesophageal varices.

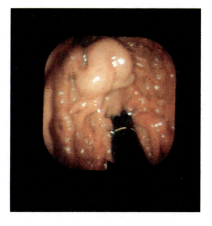

Fig. 6.10 Endoscopic view of varices in the gastric fundus. Treatment of varices in this site can be especially difficult. Conventional sclerotherapy often merely produces overlying ulceration, sometimes with disastrous results. Better results may be achievable with injection of acrylic resins, but some form of devascularisation or shunt procedure may be necessary.

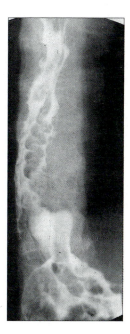

Fig. 6.11 Oesophageal varices seen on barium swallow. Despite their dramatic appearance they do not cause dysphagia.

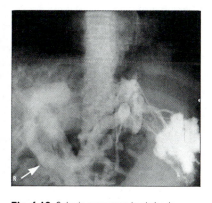

Fig. 6.12 Splenic venogram in cirrhosis. There is a hugely dilated umbilical vein (arrowed) coming off the left intrahepatic branch of the portal vein. The patient had a loud venous hum in the epigastrium (Cruveilhier–Baumgarten syndrome). Courtesy of Prof S Sherlock.

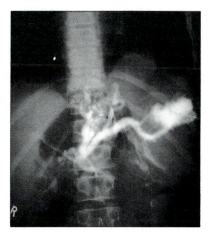

Fig. 6.13 Splenic venogram in portal vein thrombosis. The splenic vein is patent, but ends abruptly in a mesh of disorganised vessels at the hepatic hilum.

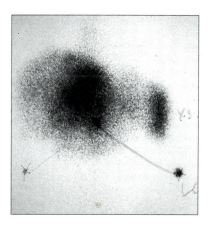

Fig. 6.14 Technetium colloid isotope scan in Budd–Chiari syndrome (hepatic vein thrombosis). There is increased uptake by a hypertrophied caudate lobe in the epigastrium with markedly diminished uptake throughout the rest of the liver. This appearance is highly specific for Budd–Chiari, but is only seen in approximately 50% of patients with the syndrome.

The patient may have distended abdominal veins. The classic caput medusae in which distended veins radiate from the umbilicus is rare and the veins more commonly run longitudinally. The direction of blood flow is the same as normal (i.e. away from the umbilicus) unless there is obstruction to the inferior vena cava in which case the blood flows upwards in the veins of the lower abdomen. There may be an audible venous hum (Cruveilhier–Baumgarten syndrome) between the umbilicus and the xiphisternum due to collateral flow from the portal system via the umbilical vein. This is a useful sign as it implies patency of the portal vein.

Management of variceal bleeding

GENERAL PRINCIPLES

The general principles for managing variceal bleeding include the following:

- At least four pints of blood should be cross matched if the diagnosis is suspected because bleeding may be massive.
- Prothrombin time should be checked and fresh frozen plasma given if it is prolonged by more than three seconds. Disordered coagulation is common due to underlying liver disease.
- Infusion of intravenous saline must be avoided as it will quickly lead to accumulation of ascites in a cirrhotic patient.
- The platelet count should be checked and platelets transfused if available if the count is less than 60,000/dl.
- Blood and melaena should be cleared from the intestine as quickly as possible to reduce the risk of encephalopathy. This should be achieved by frequent magnesium sulphate enemas and oral lactulose syrup, 20 ml 8-hourly. Oral neomycin, 1 g 6-hourly, may also be given if the patient is known to have cirrhosis.
- Early endoscopy should be performed as soon as the patient is haemodynamically stable.

ENDOSCOPIC THERAPY

Endoscopic sclerotherapy is the mainstay of treatment. Controlled trials have shown a reduction in rebleeding rates in the first three months from about 41% to 29%, and mortality at two years from 52% to 25%. Repeated sclerotherapy will usually lead to eradication of the varices after about six or seven courses of treatment, although occasional patients will have varices that are more resistant.

Techniques vary, but the procedure is usually performed using a fibreoptic endoscope under intravenous sedation. Ethanolamine oleate and hydroxypolyethoxydodecane have both been used successfully as sclerosants. The sclerosant is injected either directly into the varix or submucosally into the surrounding tissue. Submucosal injections should be of small volume (e.g. 0.5–1 ml) or extensive ulceration will result. A maximum volume of 20 ml sclerosant is injected during each session. The technique is surprisingly safe, but oesophageal ulceration is common and may lead to stricturing and chemical mediastinitis may result in chest pain and fever, which may last for 2–3 weeks. Oesophageal perforation is rare.

Sclerotherapy probably has some effect at stopping the acute bleed, but its main effect is the reduction of rebleeding. Most units perform weekly injections for the first month and then monthly until the varices have been eradicated. There is some evidence that a policy of repeating sclerotherapy only when rebleeding occurs may be as

effective and requires fewer endoscopies/patient. Mortality is to a large extent related to the degree of impairment of liver function. Patients with ascites and hypoalbuminaemia have a very high mortality while patients with portal vein thrombosis usually have near normal hepatic function and have a very low mortality from bleeding.

Endoscopic therapy should not be used prophylactically in patients with varices who have not bled as studies have shown that the risk of bleeding as a result of the injection therapy outweighs the prophylactic benefit. Endoscopic banding of varices is increasing in popularity, but further studies are needed to assess its relative efficacy in comparison with sclerotherapy.

DRUG THERAPY

Drug therapy has an established role in the therapy of bleeding oesophageal varices.

- **Vasopressin**, 20 units in 100 ml 5% dextrose given intravenously over 15 minutes, reduces splanchnic blood flow, but causes coronary artery spasm, which can be dangerous in patients with coronary atheroma and controlled data demonstrating its efficacy is scanty. Glyceryl trinitrate, 0.4 mg subcutaneously, may be given at the same time to reduce the coronary vasospasm. The longer acting Glypressin, 2 mg 6-hourly by continuous infusion, is less well tried, but there is evidence that it might be more effective.
- **Intravenous somatostatin**, 250 µg/hour as a continuous intravenous infusion given after a bolus of 5µg, and its synthetic analogue, octreotide, 100 µg subcutaneously twice daily, are probably more effective than vasopressin and have the considerable advantage that they do not cause coronary spasm. They are particularly useful for controlling bleeding before sclerotherapy.
- **Propranolol** lowers portal pressure and was shown in a large French study to reduce rebleeding considerably. Other studies have produced less impressive results, but it probably has some prophylactic effect and seems very safe. If patients bleed while receiving beta blocker therapy resuscitation may be made slightly more difficult by the lack of appropriate haemodynamic response to blood loss. Because of this beta-blocked patients who are hypotensive as a result of bleeding should probably be given intravenous glucagon (1 mg in adults) to reverse myocardial depression.

BALLOON TAMPONADE

If bleeding persists despite endoscopic sclerotherapy and vasopressin or somatostatin, control can usually be achieved temporarily by direct compression of the varices using a Sengstaken balloon.

There are a number of variations on this technique. Control can usually be achieved by the use of a single gastric balloon, which is inflated with 300 ml of air (instillation of radiographic contrast, particularly barium, may necessitate a laparotomy for removal of the balloon!). The balloon is then pulled up into the fundus of the stomach under firm traction. This can be achieved by tying a 500 ml bag of dextrose to the aspiration tube of the balloon using a long string and suspending the bag over the end of the bed. This is more comfortable for the patient if the balloon has been passed through the nose with the help of local anaesthetic gel. This should control bleeding in about 90% of cases, but if it fails the oesophageal balloon can be inflated to 40 mm Hg. The balloon should be deflated after 12 hours and should not be left *in situ* for more than 24 hours otherwise severe oesophagitis will result with inevitable rebleeding when the balloon is removed (**Fig. 6.15**).

SURGERY AND TRANSHEPATIC PORTAL-SYSTEMIC SHUNTING
Surgical options include:

- Decompression of the portal system via a porto-caval shunt.
- Obliteration of the varices by high gastric or oesophageal transection.
- Devascularisation of the stomach.

Until the development of transhepatic shunting, oeso-phageal transection was the least invasive of these procedures and since the advent of stapling guns, which allow simultaneous transection and reanastomosis to be performed relatively quickly can be performed with what is a reasonably low mortality (10–30%) for such a life-threatening condition. It may be particularly difficult to perform in patients who have had previous variceal sclerosis. Varices tend to reform so the incidence of rebleeding after one year is high.

Devascularisation procedures are more difficult, but are particularly useful in the minority of patients who are bleeding from gastric varices. Porto-caval shunting is very effective at lowering portal pressure and preventing re-bleeding from varices, but it has a high mortality when performed as an emergency (up to 50%) and carries an unacceptable and unpredictable risk of long-term encephalopathy, which can be very disabling and distressing for patient and relatives.

It is now possible to perform a shunt transhepatically. A catheter is inserted via the internal jugular vein into the hepatic vein, a fine needle is then passed through this catheter and passed via the hepatic vein to puncture a branch of the portal vein. This allows the passage of a guide wire over which a dilating ballon is passed, followed by an expanding metal stent to maintain the patency of the portal-hepatic venous connection (**Figs. 6.16–6.19**). This technique is increasing in use and carries the considerable advantage that it does not entail any disruption of the liver or surrounding tissues that might make subsequent transplantation more difficult. It does, however, carry an appreciable risk of inducing encephalopathy.

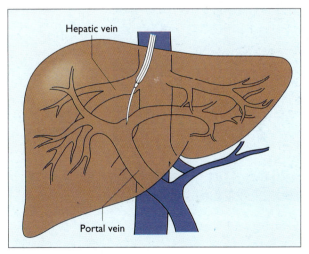

Hepatic vein

Portal vein

Fig. 6.16 Diagram showing the first stage in the procedure of transhepatic porta-systemic shunting. A needle is being advanced from the hepatic vein to puncture the portal vein. Courtesy of Dr R Edwards.

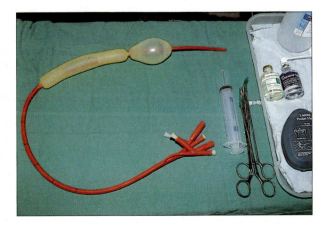

Fig. 6.15 A 'Minnesota' version of the Sengstaken balloon. The gastric balloon is inflated with approximately 300 ml of air and put on gentle traction (e.g. using a 500 ml bag of saline attached by string and suspended over the end of the bed). The oesophageal balloon is only rarely necessary to control bleeding, but can be inflated for up to 12 hours at 40 mm Hg pressure. Courtesy of Dr Y Yiannakou.

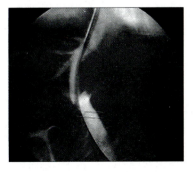

Fig. 6.17 A wire followed by a catheter have been passed to connect the hepatic and portal veins. Courtesy of Dr R Edwards.

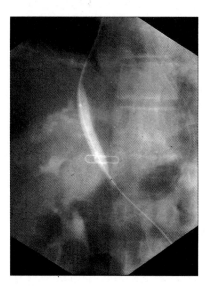

Fig. 6.18 The track between the hepatic and portal veins is being dilated using a balloon catheter. Courtesy of Dr R Edwards.

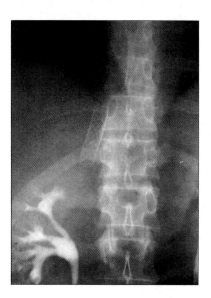

Fig. 6.19 An expanding metal 'stent' has been inserted to form a permanent bridge between the hepatic and portal veins. The false passage then becomes endothelialised. Courtesy of Dr R Edwards.

VARICES IN OTHER SITES

Varices in the gastric fundus are common in patients with portal hypertension, but fortunately bleed relatively infrequently. They are not amenable to endoscopic sclerotherapy, which usually results in severe ulceration of the overlying mucosa with disastrous results. If they are the site of major bleeding some form of surgical therapy is usually required. This could be transhepatic shunting, high gastric transection or a devascularisation procedure.

Varices may rarely cause problems in the small intestine or colon. They may cause particular problems around the stoma in patients who have had a previous ileostomy.

Portal hypertensive gastropathy

In some patients with portal hypertension bleeding occurs as a generalised ooze from the stomach rather than from oesophageal varices although these often coexist. The endoscopist sees a speckled dusky appearance to the gastric mucosa. The frequency with which this condition is diagnosed varies considerably from unit to unit reflecting the difficulty of determining whether oesophageal varices have contributed to the bleeding. Treatment should usually be medical with somatostatin analogue (octreotide) for short-term therapy and propranolol prophylaxis.

Mallory–Weiss tear

Haemorrhage induced by vomiting was recognised by Avicenna, but was more recently redescribed by Mallory and Weiss, who noted its frequent association with alcohol ingestion. One or more longitudinal tears occur at the gastric cardia at or just below the squamo-columnar mucosal junction. There is often an associated small hiatus hernia, and tearing occurs when the cardia has been forced into the thorax. Bleeding is usually minor and transient, but may occasionally be massive requiring surgical repair.

Dieulafoy's syndrome

In this syndrome there is an unusually prominent submucosal artery in the fundus of the stomach, which erodes through the mucosa causing a single small ulcer. Bleeding may be marked, but the ulcer is easily missed so all the endoscopist may find is a collection of blood in the gastric fundus. The condition is almost certainly underdiagnosed. Surgery is usually required although endoscopic sclerotherapy is occasionally successful.

Leiomyoma

Benign tumours of smooth muscle and connective tissue (leiomyomas) are not uncommon in the stomach, oesophagus and small intestine. Gastric leiomyomas have a characteristic endoscopic appearance. They are covered by normal gastric mucosa except for a central ('volcano crater') ulcer, which may bleed. Biopsy may be difficult to obtain since most of the lesion is submucosal and may require prior diathermy snaring to denude the overlying normal mucosa. This should not be performed if the patient has recently bled.

Management

Although the entire lesion may look tempting to snare this should not be done since the tumours typically have a 'dumbbell' shape and require full thickness excision. The tumours are often multiple and small bowel barium examination should be performed. Malignancy may be difficult to exclude on histology, but malignant potential is closely related to size, being commoner in lesions larger than 4 cm diameter.

Leiomyosarcomas are associated with a 25–30% five-year survival after resection. Benign leiomyomas are fortunately much commoner and are often asymptomatic.

Meckel's diverticulum

Meckel's diverticulum results from incomplete closure of the ileal end of the vitelline duct. It is sited within 100 cm (usually 85 cm) of the ileocaecal valve and occurs in 1–3% of the population. Gastric mucosa is present in about 40% and haemorrhage is then common. This usually presents as rectal bleeding in children under two years of age and accounts for about 50% of cases of lower intestinal bleeding in children.

Bleeding may occur at any time up to early adult life, but is rare over 40 years of age, presumably because ulceration and bleeding have usually occurred by then if ectopic gastric mucosa is present.

Diagnosis is by ^{99m}technetium scanning, which is positive in about 75% of patients, or by angiography. Barium studies are seldom helpful. Surgical resection is required if the diagnosis is confirmed.

▶ **Meckel's diverticulum**

- Found within 100 cm of the ileo-caecal valve
- Occurs in 1–3% of the population
- Gastric mucosa present in 40%
- Accounts for 50% of lower gastrointestinal bleeding in children
- Bleeding rare in people over 40 years of age

Aorto-enteric fistulae

Bleeding into the small intestine from an abdominal aortic aneurysm may occasionally occur without previous surgery, but is more commonly a complication of previous aortic aneurysm repair. There may be back pain from the expanding aneurysm, but it is more commonly painless. Bleeding is often massive, but may surprisingly be self-limiting. If a patient with a known aortic aneurysm has upper gastrointestinal haemorrhage and a normal gastroscopy it should be assumed that the bleeding is coming from the aneurysm. Fibreoptic endoscopy of the distal duodenum may reveal blood, but is unlikely to show the actual bleeding site. Angiography may be hazardous and is often unhelpful unless the patient is actively bleeding. CT scanning may occasionally show gas within the wall of the aortic graft indicating infection by gas-forming organisms, which is the usual cause of graft failure.

Management

None of these investigations has a high yield and it is usually better to proceed to laparotomy as soon as the diagnosis is suspected providing endoscopy has shown no alternative source of bleeding. Surgical correction is however a major undertaking and carries a mortality of approximately 50%.

RARER CAUSES OF SMALL INTESTINAL BLEEDING

Carcinoma of the small intestine

Carcinoma of the small intestine is rare, but presents with bleeding in 15%. It usually affects the distal duodenum so can often be detected if a suitable endoscope (e.g. colonoscope or enteroscope) is passed down to the third and fourth parts of the duodenum. Lymphoma of the small intestine can also present with bleeding. It may be very difficult to diagnose, small bowel enema (enteroclysis) probably having the best diagnostic yield. Crohn's disease of the small intestine, small bowel diverticulosis and ulcerative jejunoileitis may rarely present with intestinal bleeding.

Peutz–Jeghers syndrome

Peutz–Jeghers syndrome is an autosomal dominant condition characterised by hamartomatous polyps of the stomach, small and large intestine together with spotty melanin pigmentation around the mouth, hands, feet and genital areas. By adult life all the pigmented lesions except those on the buccal mucosa have usually faded. The polyps are most prominent in the small intestine where they may cause obstruction, intussusception or bleeding. They have a slight, but definite malignant potential, the overall frequency of cancer of the intestine being 3%. Ovarian and testicular tumours also occur in 5–10% of patients.

Bleeding from the biliary and pancreatic ducts via the ampulla of Vater

Bleeding from the biliary and pancreatic ducts via the ampulla of Vater occurs occasionally and is particularly difficult to diagnose. Haematobilia is rare unless there has been a previous liver biopsy, but may occasionally occur spontaneously in patients with vascular liver tumours. Bleeding from the pancreatic duct is probably commoner and is usually the result of chronic pancreatitis complicated by a pancreatic cyst eroding an aneurysmal splenic artery. The patients typically have intermittent quite large bleeds yet gastroduodenoscopy done shortly after may be normal or simply show a small amount of blood in the second part of the duodenum. Endoscopic pancreatography is sometimes diagnostic, with filling defects seen in the pancreatic duct followed by direct visualisation of clot passing through the papilla when the catheter is withdrawn.

Haemorrhagic telangiectasia

Haemorrhagic telangiectasia may be either inherited or acquired. Lesions may occur at any site in the intestine or stomach and may present either with chronic iron deficiency anaemia or acute bleeding. Acquired telangiectasia occurs in association with collagen disorders such as scleroderma and the CREST syndrome.

Hereditary telangiectasia most commonly presents with recurrent nose bleeds in childhood and affected individuals may have telangiectasia on the hands and particularly under the tongue (Fig 6.20). In severe forms of the disease there may be massive shunting through pulmonary arteriovenous fistulae and cirrhosis may develop.

Management

Treatment is frustrating because of the multiple lesions, which are often inaccessible to the endoscope even with modern enteroscopes. Lesions that can be reached can be treated by laser or diathermy coagulation. Treatment with oestradiol has been shown to reduce the frequency of rebleeding.

COLONIC BLEEDING

Diverticulosis

Diverticulosis is probably the commonest cause of colonic bleeding in the adult although it has been overdiagnosed in the past because of failure to recognise angiodysplasia. Bleeding is usually acute and severe and chronic low-grade blood loss with iron deficiency anaemia does not occur. It is thought that a faecolith erodes an arteriole at the base of the diverticulum. The bleeding diverticulum is on the right side of the colon in 65% of the patients.

Management

Colonoscopy is essential to determine the site of bleeding and exclude angiodysplasia otherwise an inappropriate operation may be performed.

Colorectal cancer and polyps

Approximately 30% of patients with colonic cancer present with bleeding (Fig. 6.21); in most of these the tumour is in the rectum and easily diagnosed. More proximal tumours usually cause chronic blood loss rather than sudden massive bleeding.

Bleeding is usually only a problem with large polyps 2 cm or more in diameter. The commonest are adenomas, but bleeding also occurs with the much rarer hamartomas that occur not only in Peutz–Jeghers syndrome, but also in other familial hamartoma syndromes such as juvenile polyposis and in the acquired Cronkhite–Canada syndrome.

Angiodysplasia

Angiodysplastic lesions may affect any part of the intestine, but are commonest in the terminal ileum, caecum and ascending colon. They are probably always acquired and usually affect elderly patients approximately 50% of whom have some form, of cardiac disease, (aortic stenosis in 25%). The aetiology is unclear, but it has been suggested that the lesions arise as a result of chronic intermittent obstruction of submucosal veins and dilatation of the veins draining the lesion is a characteristic feature on angiography. In approximately 15% of patients bleeding is massive, while 15% of patients present with iron-deficiency anaemia.

Diagnosis of colonic lesions is made by colonoscopy, but angiography may be used to show more proximal lesions.

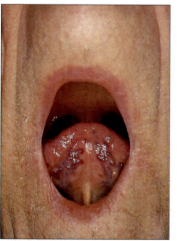

Fig. 6.20 Hereditary haemorrhagic telangiectasia. It is always worth checking under the tongue for telangiectasia in any patient with unexplained iron deficiency.

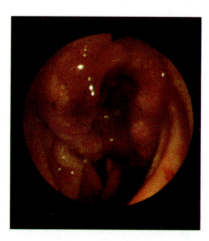

Fig. 6.21 Bleeding from a carcinoma in the descending colon.

Management
Small lesions can be treated by colonoscopic diathermy, but extensive lesions require surgical resection.

Colonic ulceration
Inflammatory bowel disease, either Crohn's disease or ulcerative colitis may present with rectal bleeding although there is more commonly diarrhoea in addition.

Solitary ulcers of the colon may present with bleeding. The three main sites for solitary ulcers are the rectum, sigmoid and the caecum.

- In the rectum, they are nearly always associated with rectal mucosal prolapse so treatment usually entails surgical correction of the prolapse.
- In the sigmoid, ulcers usually occur as stercoral ulcers in association with severe constipation.
- Caecal ulcers often have no obvious explanation, but have been reported in leukaemic or immunosuppressed patients in association with cytomegalovirus infection.

Pneumatosis coli (cystoides intestinalis)
Pneumatosis coli is a curious condition characterised by extensive gas-filled cysts, which may involve the small and large intestine. There is an extensive range of conditions with which it may be associated, in particular pyloric stenosis and chronic lung disease. Cysts vary in size from a few millimetres to several centimeters in diameter and may be either subserosal or submucosal. They are often asymptomatic, but may give rise to lower abdominal cramping pain, rectal bleeding or diarrhoea. (See page 94.)

Management
If the patient has chronic lung disease the cysts may resolve with administration of oxygen. Resolution has also been described following treatment with metronidazole.

Marathon runner's colon
Long-distance runners occasionally develop rectal bleeding and diarrhoea within hours of a long run (usually of marathon proportions). This is a self-limiting condition, but presumably indicates mucosal ischaemia.

Vasculitis of the intestine
Vasculitis of the intestine may occur as part of a number of systemic diseases including:

- Polyarteritis nodosa.
- Behçet's syndrome.
- Systemic lupus erythematosus.
- Rheumatoid arthritis.
- Dermatomyositis.

Abdominal pain is the commonest symptom due to ischaemia or even infarction of the bowel, but there may be bleeding from ischaemic ulcers.

In all these conditions the radiological appearances may mimic Crohn's disease. Indeed the similarities between Behçet's syndrome and Crohn's disease are so great it has even been suggested that they are forms of the same disease. Both conditions are associated with arthritis, uveitis, mouth ulcers and ulceration of the colon or ileum moreover resin injected blood vessel casts of resected Crohn's disease intestine show evidence of microvascular damage. In Behçet's syndrome genital ulcers are typically present, but are uncommon in Crohn's disease and cerebral vascular lesions and venous thrombosis are also commoner in Behçet's disease.

Diagnosis of mesenteric vasculitis usually requires vascular angiography, but evidence of vasculitis elsewhere, particularly on renal biopsy if nephritis is present makes the diagnosis easier. Polyarteritis nodosa may be associated with detectable serum antineutrophil antibodies (pANCA and cANCA, 'p' for perinuclear staining; 'c' for cytoplasmic staining). This pANCA is mainly directed against myeloperoxidase in contrast to the pANCA found in about 60% of cases of ulcerative colitis, which is thought to be directed mainly against other neutrophil granule contents such as lactoferrin.

Management
Systemic vasculitis is a grave condition, but may respond to immunosuppression, usually with a combination of corticosteroids and either azathioprine or cyclophosphamide.

Degos' disease
Degos' disease is a rare disease which usually affects young men and is characterised by the presence of necrotic skin lesions and vasculitis of the gut, often resulting in infarction.

Henoch–Schönlein purpura
Henoch–Schönlein purpura often occurs in association with streptococcal A infection of the oropharynx and consists of a triad of purpura, arthritis and abdominal pain. Intestinal bleeding occurs in up to 50% and there may occasionally be intussusception or even infarction. Purpura are typically present in rows on the, buttocks and lower abdomen. There may also be glomerulonephritis, which can result in acute renal failure. The disease is almost always self-limiting and has a good prognosis. (See chapter 18.)

Ehlers–Danlos syndrome
Ehlers–Danlos is probably a group of several different syndromes with varying patterns of inheritance, either autosomal dominant, recessive or X-linked. Collagen is abnormal and this results in joint laxity, poor wound healing and intermittent gastrointestinal bleeding.

BLEEDING AND COAGULATION DISORDERS

Haematological disorders may result in intestinal bleeding as a direct consequence of the coagulopathy or as a result of bleeding into the bowel wall with subsequent infarction.

- Haemophiliacs rarely bleed from the intestine unless there is a lesion such as peptic ulceration or oesophageal varices (in association with hepatitis C-related cirrhosis).
- In von Willebrand's disease there is also a platelet defect and spontaneous intestinal haemorrhage is commoner. Moreover there is a recognised association between von Willebrand's disease and intestinal angiodysplasia.
- Prolongation of the prothrombin time to more than five times control due to warfarin therapy may cause spontaneous bleeding.
- Intestinal bleeding is common in the presence of disseminated intravascular coagulation (DIC).
- Severe thrombocytopenia may be associated with gastrointestinal bleeding, but this usually only occurs in the presence of some other lesion such as the intestinal ulcers that may affect any part of the intestine in the leukaemic patient.

A coagulopathy or bleeding disorder should be considered in any patient with unexplained intestinal bleeding. Screening should initially consist of prothrombin and partial thromboplastin (or kaolin–cephalin) times and platelet count and haematological advice should be sought if these are abnormal.

Colon cancer and colonic polyps

Clinical features

Right-sided lesions typically present late with microcytic anaemia, weight loss, abdominal pain and possibly a palpable mass in the right iliac fossa whereas left sided lesions tend either to cause obstructive symptoms earlier or present with frank rectal bleeding. Overall approximately 50% of patients present with altered bowel habit, constipation or more commonly diarrhoea, and about 30% with bleeding. About 25% present as an acute emergency due to obstruction, bleeding, pericolic abscess, perforation or jaundice due to secondary deposits.

Epidemiology

The average incidence (number of new cases/year) worldwide for colon cancer is 17/100,000 males and 15/100,000 females, and for rectal cancer is 12/100,000 males and 8/100,000 females. Incidence is about 60 times higher in developed countries (ranging from 30/100,000 in parts of the USA to less than 1/100,000 in parts of Africa). The risk of colon cancer rises rapidly in populations migrating from low-risk to high-risk areas (e.g. Japanese emigrants to the USA). This suggests that environmental factors are more important than genetic factors in determining the marked geographical variation in incidence.

DIFFERENCES BETWEEN RIGHT AND LEFT COLON CANCER AND RECTAL CANCER

Colon cancer has been increasing in incidence since 1950 whereas rectal cancer is becoming less frequent. Currently the distribution of cancers around the colon is approximately:

- Caecum and ascending colon, 25%.
- Transverse colon, 13%.
- Descending colon, 6%.
- Sigmoid, 36%.
- Rectum, 20%.

There is a 5% higher proportion of rectal cancer in men and 5% higher proportion of caecal cancer in women.

Aetiology

Many large studies have shown associations between colorectal cancer and diet. The most impressive associations are with high fat consumption and low dietary fibre intake. Some studies have analysed their data separately for proximal and distal lesions and have shown that high fat consumption tends to correlate with proximal tumours and

▶ **Risk factors for colorectal cancer**

- High animal fat intake
- Low fruit and vegetable fibre intake
- High beer intake
- Cholesterol-lowering diets and drugs (proximal colon cancer)
- Cholecystectomy (proximal colon cancer)
- Familial adenomatous polyposis coli
- Inflammatory bowel disease
- [a] Hereditary non-polyposis colon cancer

▶ **Relationship between polyps and cancer**

- Distal colon cancers usually arise from polyps
- Average lag time from polyp to cancer is 10 years
- 50% of people over 65 years of age have one or more adenomatous polyps
- Proximal colon cancers usually arise from flat lesions

low fibre with distal. Animal fat seems more important than vegetable fat and there is some evidence that it is fruit and vegetable fibre rather than cereal fibre that is protective.

Cholesterol-lowering drugs and even low cholesterol diets have also been associated with an increased risk for colon cancer and there is some contentious evidence that cholecystectomy predisposes to an increased risk for proximal cancer.

High consumption of beer, but probably not other alcohols, and a low intake of calcium and vitamin D are also linked with a high risk for colon cancer.

RELATIONSHIP TO ADENOMATOUS POLYPS

Adenomatous polyps are uncommon in the caecum and ascending colon and in this site most colon cancers probably start as flat dysplastic lesions. In the distal colon however it is thought that almost all cancers develop from malignant change within adenomatous polyps.

All adenomatous polyps by definition show some degree of dysplasia, but this increases in severity in association with increasing size of the polyp so that less than 1% of polyps less than 1 cm diameter are cancerous, whereas about 15% of those larger than 2 cm diameter are cancerous.

Tubular polyps (about 75% of the total) are less likely to be malignant (2% overall) than tubulovillous (23% of the total, 6% malignant) or villous (5% of the total, 18% malignant). In the rectum and caecum tubular adenomas on stalks are rare, whereas flat (sessile) villous adenomas are relatively common (Figs 6.22, 6.23; see also 6.30–6.32).

▶ **Familial polyposis coli**

- Familial polyposis coli accounts for 1% of colorectal cancer
- Familial non-polyposis colon cancer (Lynch syndromes) accounts for at least 10% of colorectal cancer

Adenomatous polyps are remarkably common in developed countries. Their frequency increases with age and it is reported that the prevalence rises to 50% in the over-60s.

The annual conversion rate from adenoma to cancer has been estimated in a Norwegian study to be 3% for polyps over 1 cm diameter, rising to 17% in the presence of villous components and to 37% in the presence of severe dysplasia. It should be pointed out that severe dysplasia may well occur in one part of a polyp that already shows frank malignant change in another part so that cancer can not be excluded until the whole polyp has been removed.

RELATIONSHIP TO INFLAMMATORY BOWEL DISEASE

Idiopathic ulcerative colitis and colonic Crohn's disease are both associated with increased risk for colon cancer. The overall relative risk compared with age-matched controls is approximately an 11-fold increase.

- In patients with extensive ulcerative colitis the cumulative risk for colon cancer is 1% at 10 years and about 7% at 20 years.
- The risk for patients with colonic Crohn's disease is less well documented, but recent studies suggest that it is probably similar.

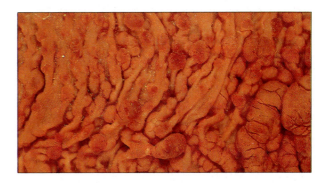

Fig 6.22 Familial adenomatous polyposis. Hundreds of adenomatous polyps are present. The incidence of colon cancer is virtually 100% unless prophylactic colectomy is performed.

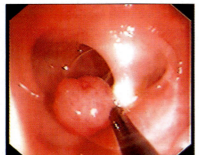

Fig. 6.23 Snare diathermy of an adenomatous colonic polyp.

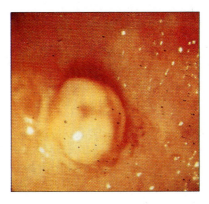

Fig. 6.24 A pseudopolyp associated with ulcerative colitis. It is an island of hyperplasia that has been surrounded by ulceration at some time in the past. These polyps are not pre-malignant; cancer in the colitic colon usually arises as a flat lesion.

Several factors suggest that the increased risk for cancer is not simply a reflection of the chronicity of inflammation:

- There is no increased risk, even for rectal cancer, in patients whose disease is confined to the rectum.
- The anatomical distribution of cancers in colitis bears no relation to the typical distribution of inflammation, caecal cancers in some studies have been commoner than rectal.
- The relative risk for colon cancer, compared with age-matched controls probably remains constant with time.
- Age at onset of colitis is a more important determinant of the age-matched relative risk than duration of disease.

All these features suggest that patients with ulcerative colitis may be inheriting an increased risk for colon cancer that is not dependent on the presence of inflammation for its generation.

The tumours develop as flat lesions without passing through a macroscopic polyp stage and this makes screening particularly difficult. The inflammatory pseudopolyps, which are commonly seen in long-standing colitis have no malignant potentia (**Fig. 6.24**).

The cost-effectiveness of screening in long-standing colitis is debatable, but most authorities recommend screening patients with extensive colitis of more than seven years duration with toal colonoscopy and multiple biopsy every two years. High-grade dysplasia is an indication for repeat colonoscopy within six months and the presence of any raised dysplastic lesion is an indication for colectomy.

FAMILIAL ADENOMATOUS POLYPOSIS
Approximately 1% of patients with colon cancer have this autosomally dominant inherited condition, which has been shown to result from point mutations in a gene localised to chromosome 5q.21.

Patients start to develop multiple colonic adenomatous polyps in their teens and the colon becomes carpeted with 100–5000 adenomas. There is an average lag time of about ten years from polyp to cancer so that colon cancer is an inevitable consequence if the colon is not resected. Although most patients are easily identifiable when young, 10% present when over 50 years of age. Approximately 20% have a negative family history.

Some patients may have a range of lesions outside the colon. This used to be thought to be a separate syndrome (**Gardner's syndrome**), but has now been shown to be due to a defect at the same gene. These lesions may include:

- Other intestinal tumours, particularly adenomas or carcinomas of the ampulla of Vater, which is the main cancer-related cause of death in patients who have had total colectomy.

- Gastric polyps (adenomas, carcinoids and fundic gland hyperplasia).
- Osteomas of the skull, mandible and long bones.
- Benign soft tissue (desmoid) tumours.
- Papillary carcinoma of the thyroid.
- Adrenal adenomas and carcinoma.
- Brain tumours (Turcot syndrome).
- Hypertrophy of the retinal pigment epithelium.

Both the retinal and the mandible abnormalities are so common in familial polyposis (up to 90%) that they may be used as useful (but not sole) screeening tests.

Management
Total colectomy is mandatory and should be performed at some time in the teens (e.g. at 17–18 years of age) or on diagnosis if the patient presents later. Many patients are now having an ileal pouch procedure with ileo-anal anastomosis. Children sometimes tolerate direct ileo-anal anastomosis surprisingly well without pouch construction.

There is controversy about the advisability of leaving the rectum and performing ileo-rectal anastomosis. More than 50% will develop cancer in the rectum within 20 years although this risk may be lowered to about 10% by six-monthly proctoscopy and fulguration of large adenomas.

First-degree relatives should be screened from 13 years of age by flexible sigmoidoscopy or colonoscopy, repeated every 2–3 years until 40 years of age.

Polyp growth may be slowed by taking NSAIDs or high-dose vitamin C, but neither of these measures are sufficently powerful to affect the need for colectomy.

NON-POLYPOSIS FAMILY CANCER SYNDROMES
Whereas familial polyposis only accounts for about 1% of colon cancer at least 10% of colon cancers are the result of inherited non-polyposis syndromes (**Lynch syndromes**). Two syndromes are recognised:

- **Cancer family syndrome** in which there is an inherited tendency to develop cancer at multiple sites including colon, ovary, endometrium, stomach, brain and lung.
- **Hereditary site-specific colon cancer** in which there is a tendency to develop cancers of the proximal colon, which may be multiple and are often mucinous. These typically occur in 40–50-year-olds (i.e. 20 years earlier than the peak incidence for non-inherited colon cancer). They are typically right-sided colon cancers, which usually arise from flat rather than polypoidal lesions.

First-degree relatives should be screened by total colonoscopy at three year intervals from 20 years of age.

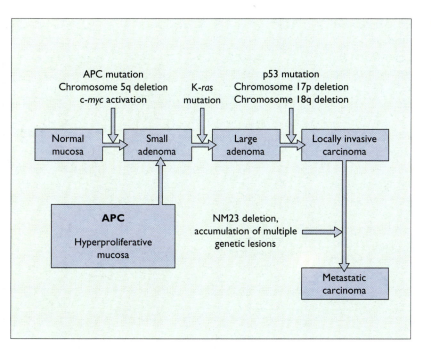

Fig. 6.25 Vogelstein's hypothesis for the multi-step evolution of colon cancer. Adenomatous polyposis coli (APC) mutations may occur either in all cells of the body (familial polyposis coli) or only in adenomatous or carcinomatous cells (sporadic colon cancer).

Pathogenesis

A widely accepted hypothesis put forward by Vogelstein is that there is a sequence from hyperplasia to dysplasia to malignancy and finally invasion and metastasis and that several (up to six or seven) mutations affecting oncogenes or tumour suppressor genes occur during this process (**Fig. 6.25**). The commonest of these are mutations in the p53 tumour suppressor gene, which can be detected in 60–70%. These mutations result in overexpression of the p53 protein, which is a membrane transport protein. Other mutations detectable within the tumour include the oncogenes c-*myc* and c-Ki-*ras*, the latter also coding for a membrane protein whereas c-myc encodes a nuclear phosphoprotein involved in cell proliferation. The familial polyposis gene (APC) is mutated within the tumour cells of about 50% of non polyposis cancers and is thought to be another tumour suppressor gene.

Although hyperplasia is thought to be a general precursor of cancer, by the time the cancer is established proliferation slows down and is less than the surrounding tissue. The doubling time for colon cancers has been estimated in one radiological study to be 620 days. It is therefore probably common for colon cancers to take up to five years to become symptomatic.

Pathology

Carcinomas of the caecum and ascending colon, despite starting as flat lesions, typically become bulky and polypoid, similar to those in the rectum, whereas tumours of the distal colon usually involve most of the circumference producing an 'apple core' stricturing lesion. Annular growth is probably accounted for by the circular arrangement of lymphatics. The tumours are adenocarcinomas and secrete variable amounts of mucin, a high molecular weight (approximately 10×10^6 Dalton) glycoprotein, which can be identified by histochemical stains for carbohydrate such as periodic acid–Schiff or alcian blue. In poorly differentiated tumours gland formation and mucus synthesis are less marked.

Cygnet ring cells may be seen. These are cells in which the nucleus is shifted to one side by intracytoplasmic mucus. Approximately 15% of tumours contain large extracellular lakes of mucus. These are termed **mucinous** or **colloid** cancers and are commoner in patients with inherited non-polyposis cancer or cancer complicating ulcerative colitis. The rarer **scirrhous** tumours contain sparse glands and dense fibrosis.

STAGING

The first stage in spread of the tumour is usually penetration through the muscularis mucosae although occasional poorly differentiated tumours may metastasise to distant sites beforte the muscularis is breached. Subsequent spread is then either by direct invasion (particularly in the rectum, which lacks a serosal covering) followed by spread along lymphatics to draining nodes or blood borne, usually to liver, but also portal-vertebral communications (Batson's vertebral venous plexuses) to lumbar and thoracic vertebrae. Lung deposits are usually thought to have spread from the liver.

Prognosis correlates well with the degree of invasion and metastasis. The staging system used is usually based on that described by Dukes in 1929 and modified by Astler and Coller (Fig. 6.26). The scheme is as follows:

- A: limited to the mucosa.
- B1: extending into, but not through the muscularis mucosa.
- B2: through the muscularis, but without lymph node involvement.
- C1: 1-4 lymph nodes involved.
- C2: five or more nodes involved.
- D: distant metastases (modification by Turnbull).

Five-year survivals are approximately:

- Stage A: 80%.
- B1: 65%.
- B2: 45%.
- C1: 45%.
- C2: 15%.
- D: <1%.

Poorly-differentiated tumours or tumours of mucinous, scirrhous or signet ring types all have a worse prognosis. Tumours in which a high proportion of the cells have an abnormal DNA content, (aneuploidy) as assessed by flow cytometry, also have a worse prognosis.

Management

Surgical resection is the only effective treatment for colon cancer. The overall prognosis has improved disappointingly little: over the past 40 years the five-year survival has probably improved slightly from 50% to about 65%. It seems likely that much of this improvement is due to earlier diagnosis.

Adjuvant chemotherapy or chemotherapy as sole therapy for advanced disease have been disappointing although 5-fluorouracil plus levamisole or folinic acid has shown a modest benefit in controlled studies.

Adjuvant pre-operative radiotherapy has not been shown to improve survival and results in delayed surgery and difficulties in accurate staging. Postoperative radiotherapy for patients with lymph node metastases shows some promise, but there is no convincing evidence from controlled trials for increased survival.

Surgical resection is aimed at removing the tumour, at least 5 cm of healthy bowel either side plus the regional lymph nodes and mesentery. There is no evidence that more radical lymph node resection improves survival. For rectal tumours a distal margin of 2 cm of normal bowel beyond the lesion is acceptable. With the use of new stapling devices it

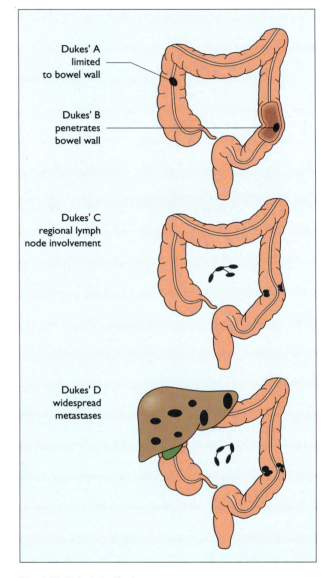

Fig. 6.26 Dukes' classification.

may thefore be feasible in some patients to perform a sphincter saving resection of tumours within three to four centimetres of the anorectal junction providing that there is no local invasion. Rectal ultrasonography may well help to evaluate this.

Hepatic metastases are present at initial presentation in up to 25% of patients, and the primary tumour should still be resected conventionally unless the patient is thought too unfit to tolerate the procedure. This is partly to prevent subsequent bowel obstruction, which is extremely unpleasant for the patient and partly because promising results are being obtained in some patients by partial hepatic resection. This is still experimental and the indications are still unclear.

Some surgeons advocate waiting approximately three months after the bowel resection and then rescanning. This is to allow micrometastases to grow (in the hope that no further hepatic metastases will form after the primary tumour has been removed).

If repeat scanning then shows only one or two metastases in a resectable segment of liver partial hepatectomy is performed. This is a technique in which there have been considerable surgical advances recently, partly as a result of ultrasonic and water jet dissectors combined with the use of intraoperative ultrasound to delineate the anatomy and identify the position of major vessels. Operative mortality as a result is about 2% in some specialist centres. Five-year survivals in these selected patients of 20–34% have been reported. Although controlled trials have not yet been reported these results are considerably better than would otherwise be expected for this group of patients.

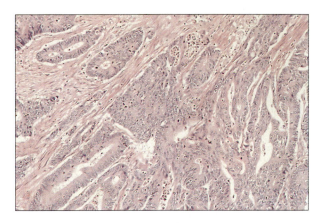

Fig. 6.27 Histological appearances of colon cancer. Disorganised glands are seen containing dysplastic cells with large, darkly staining nuclei.

FOLLOW-UP AFTER COLONIC RESECTION
Up to 5% of patients have a second synchronous cancer at presentation and about 35% have one or more adenomatous polyps elsewhere in the colon. There is therefore a good justification for performing colonoscopy within a few months of surgery if it has not been performed before surgery. Subsequent risk for the development of new (metachronous) tumours is about 5% and about 50% of these will arise within the first five years after the initial resection. Some surgeons therefore advocate regular colonoscopic screening every two years thereafter. The benefit from this is likely to be rather slight and these patients should have a lower priority than patients screened because of a strong family history of cancer. This is an important point when resources are limited since there is a natural tendency to offer screening or surveillance more readily to patients who are already known to the hospital (partly reflecting medico-legal awareness) rather than actively seeking new 'high-risk' patients for surveillance, yet it is the latter group who are far more likely to benefit.

Carcinoembryonic antigen *(CEA)* is a glycoprotein present in low concentrations in normal tissues and tends to rise in concentration in blood in a range of epithelial malignancies. Its sensitivity (36% for Dukes' A and B) and specificity are too low for use in diagnosis or screening, but a rising CEA after resection will detect about 60% of recurrences. The sensitivity may be improved by combining this with another serological test such as CA19.9. This is only of use if the surgeon is then going to act on this information by performing a second look laparotomy. It has been suggested that this may be indicated in about 5% of patients overall, but there is as yet no clear evidence that it improves survival. CEA needs to be measured at least three-monthly to allow a reasonable chance of resecting any detectable recurrence.

SCREENING AND PREVENTION
In view of the depressing lack of evidence for benefit from chemotherapy or radiotherapy it is likely that most progress in the foreseeable future is likely to result from earlier diagnosis or prevention.

Earlier diagnosis is aimed at increasing the proportion of cases diagnosed as Dukes' stage A. A modest improvement may result from better patient awareness so that they consult early for altered bowel habit or rectal bleeding however more substantial improvement requires diagnosis of asymptomatic cases. This is at present mainly being achieved by screening for occult blood loss.

The daily faecal blood loss in the normal individual is usually about 1 ml, but the upper end of the normal range (2 ml/day) is just sufficient to produce a positive occult blood test by Hemoccult. Tumours of the sigmoid colon and rectum result in average faecal occult blood loss of 1.8–1.9 ml, tumours of the transverse colon and rectum average 1.5 ml loss, and tumours of the ascending colon and caecum average 9.3 ml blood loss. The way the test is performed is critically important. The sensitivity is improved by adding a drop of water to the slide before development of the colour reaction. This improves the overall sensitivity from 81% to 92% when two samples of each of three consecutive daily stools are tested. Improving the sensitivity of the test in this way also increases the false-positive rate to about 7%, but this can be improved by avoiding red meat, peroxidase-containing foods (brassicas, turnips, radish) and NSAIDs for three days before the test. The test depends on the pseudoperoxidase activity of haemoglobin, which reacts with guaiac and hydrogen peroxide to give a green colour. About 20–30% of the positive patients will then be found to have adenomas and 2–5% to have cancer. It can be seen from the average blood loss that distal colon and rectal tumours are much less likely to be picked up than caecal or ascending

▶ **Colon cancer**

- 65% five-year survival
- Hepatic metastases at presentation in 25% of patients
- 5% of patients have a second (synchronous) colon cancer at presentation (35% have a second (synchronous) cancer at presentation if the primary lesion is in the rectum)
- 5% of patients develop subsequent (metachronous) colon cancer

colon. It has therefore been suggested that occult blood screening should be combined with flexible sigmoidoscopy. This however raises the cost considerably and this is rapidly becoming the limiting factor.

A large study in Minnesota, USA, has shown a 33% reduction in colon cancer mortality as a result of annual occult blood screening using Hemoccult with hydration (three faecal samples each studied twice) with colonoscopy for positive results. Screening every two years however produced only a 6% fall in mortality.

The consensus at present is that the best available approach would be to screen all asymptomatic people over 50 years of age who have an average risk for colon cancer by:

- Annual Hemoccult on three consecutive faecal samples (with rehydration and dietary restriction).
- Colonoscopy if positive Hemoccult.
- Flexible sigmoidoscopy in all patients every three years.

The cost for each life saved has been estimated to be at least 30,000 US dollars.

Screening of patients with a strong family history for colon cancer is very important and should be performed by twice yearly colonoscopy from 20 years of age because these patients tend to develop proximal colon cancers at an early age.

There is a strong suspicion that diet is strongly related to the risk for colon cancer although a causal relationship is difficult to demonstrate. It seems likely that a diet low in animal fat and high in fruit and vegetable fibre will reduce the risk and effect. Recent coronary prevention trials have also shown the surprising result that once daily low-dose aspirin significantly lowers the risk for colon cancer, possibly by a similar mechanism to the inhibition of polyp formation by NSAIDs.

OTHER COLONIC MALIGNANCIES

Lymphoma

Primary lymphoma of the colon is rare, accounting for only 0.5% of colonic malignancies and 10–20% of primary gastrointestinal lymphomas. Lesions may be infiltrative, polypoid or massive and stricturing may occur. Predisposing conditions include ulcerative colitis, long-term immuno-suppression, radiation therapy, or ureterosigmoidostomy. Increased risk of rectal lymphoma has been reported in homosexual men.

Management

Treatment is usually by a combination of surgery and chemotherapy, sometimes combined with radiotherapy. Cases are too rare for therapeutic trials so the optimal regimen is unclear. Five-year survival is about 35%.

Carcinoid

Rectal carcinoid accounts for about 10% of carcinoid tumours and for 1% of rectal malignancies. There is a high rate of synchronous rectal carcinoma. About 15% metastasize, but carcinoid syndrome is very rare.

Carcinoid tumours elsewhere in the colon acount for less than 10% of colonic tumours, but behave aggressively with a high rate of metastasis. Treatment should be excision and five-year survival is about 80%.

OTHER COLONIC POLYPS

Hyperplastic (metaplastic) polyps

Hyperplastic polyps are the commonest polyps found in the colon. Crypts are elongated and the epithelium has a papillary appearance (**Figs. 6.28** and **6.29**). It has been suggested that they result more from a failure of mature epithelial cells to drop off rather than from an increased rate of proliferation.

Hyperplastic polyps are statistically associated with cancer, 90% of patients with rectal cancer have these polyps elsewhere in the rectum for example, but it is generally accepted that the polyps themselves have no pre-malignant potential. They are nearly always small (< 5 mm) sessile polyps, but cannot be reliably distinguished from adenomas on macroscopic appearance.

Juvenile (hamartomatous) polyps

Juvenile polyps are commonest in early childhood (**Fig. 6.33**) and are often familial. They consist of dilated cystic glands and a widened, oedematous lamina propria. They are commonest in the rectum. These polyps carry a slightly increased risk for malignancy because they may contain adenomatous components and should in any case be removed because of the high risk of bleeding.

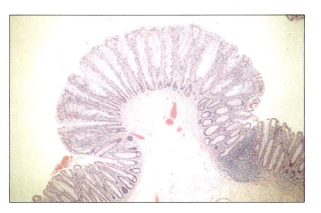

Fig. 6.28 Metaplastic colon polyp (low power). These polyps are very common and are not themselves pre-malignant except when rarely they contain areas of adenomatous change.

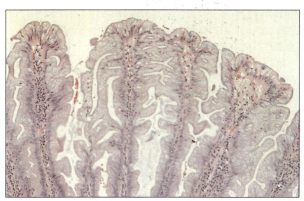

Fig. 6.29 Metaplastic polyp (high power). Hypertrophied mucus-filled crypts are seen.

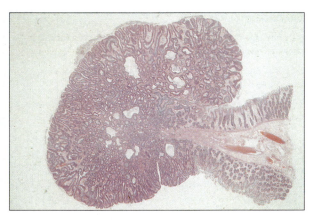

Fig. 6.30 Tubular adenoma. This is typically attached (as here) to a stalk covered by normal mucosa. This allows complete cure by snare diathermy even if there are carcinomatous changes confined within the adenoma.

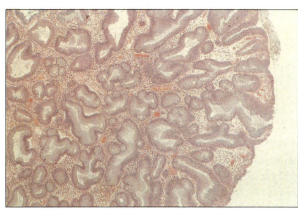

Fig. 6.31 Tubular adenoma (high power) showing dysplastic glands.

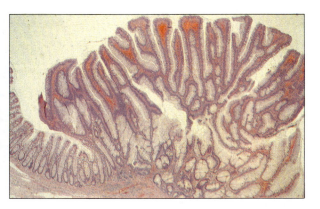

Fig. 6.32 Villous adenoma with typical frond-like appearance. These adenomas are usually larger than tubular adenomas (i.e. larger than 2 cm diameter), have a higher rate of malignant change and may cause marked secretory diarrhoea with hypokalaemia.

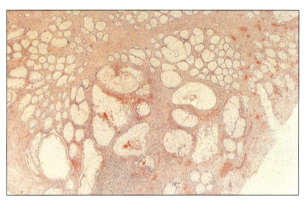

Fig. 6.33 Juvenile polyp showing the typical appearance of dilated, mucus-filled glands. When multiple they have a slight, but definite, premalignant potential.

Peutz–Jeghers (hamartomatous) polyps

Hamartomas are benign tumour-like proliferations of normal tissue arranged in an abnormal and disorganised fashion. Peutz–Jeghers polyps differ from juvenile hamartomas in that the lamina propria is normal and the polyp consists of marked smooth muscle hyperplasia. The polyps:

- Are always multiple.
- Are commoner in the small intestine.
- Carry a low, but definite risk of malignant change.
- Occur as part of an autosomal dominant syndrome that is also characterised by mucocutaneous pigmentation of the face, perianal area, hands, feet and genitals. Ovarian, breast or testicular (Sertoli cell) tumours may occasionally occur.

Cronkhite–Canada syndrome

Cronkhite–Canada syndrome is an acquired syndrome that consists of multiple gastrointestinal polyps from the stomach to the rectum, dystrophic nails, hair loss, pigmentation, abdominal pain and malabsorption. The polyps are hamartomas with cystic retention similar to that seen in juvenile polps. The aetiology is uncertain and the outlook poor, but occasional patients respond to enteral feeding suggesting that there may be an underlying nutritional deficiency.

FURTHER READING

Upper gastrointestinal bleeding: general

Dudnick R, Martin P, Friedman LS. Management of bleeding ulcers. *Med Clin North Am* 1991; **75**(4): 947–65.

Fleischer D. Endoscopic hemostasis in non-variceal bleeding. *Endoscopy* 1992; **24**(12): 58–63.

Jones SC, Axon AT. Bleeding peptic ulcer endoscopic and pharmacological management. *Postgrad Med J* 1991; **67**(789): 606–12.

Johnston JH. Endoscopic risk factors for bleeding peptic ulcer. *Gastrointest Endosc* 1990; **36**(5 Suppl): S16–20.

Laine L. Rolling review: upper gastrointestinal bleeding. *Aliment Pharmacol Ther* 1993; **7**(2): 207–32.

Qureshi WA, Netchvolodoff CV. Acute bleeding from peptic ulcers. How to restore hemostasis and prevent recurrence. *Postgrad Med* 1993; **93**(4): 167–70, 175–8.

Reilly HF, al Kawas FH. Dieulafoy's lesion. Diagnosis and management. *Dig Dis Sci* 1991; **36**(12): 1702–7.

Rooney PJ, Hunt RH. The risk of upper gastrointestinal haemorrhage during steroidal and non steroidal anti inflammatory therapy. *Baillière's Clin Rheumatol* 1991; **4**(2): 207–17.

Steffes C, Fromm D. The current diagnosis and management of upper gastrointestinal bleeding. *Adv Surg* 1992; **25**: 331–61.

Sugawa C, Joseph AL. Endoscopic interventional management of bleeding duodenal and gastric ulcers. *Surg Clin North Am* 1992; **72**(2): 317–34.

Waye JD. Small bowel endoscopy. *Endoscopy* 1992; **24**(12): 68–72.

Lower gastrointestinal bleeding (general)

JFoutch PG. Angiodysplasia of the gastrointestinal tract. *Am J Gastroenterol* 1993; **88**(6): 807–18.

ones DJ. ABC of colorectal diseases. Lower gastrointestinal haemorrhage. *Br Med J* 1992; **305**(6845): 107–10.

Oesophageal varices

Binmoeller KF, Vadeyar HJ, Soehendra N. Treatment of oesophageal varices. *Endoscopy* 1994; **26**: 42–7.

Burroughs AK, McCormick PA. Prevention of variceal rebleeding. *Gastroenterol Clin North Am* 1992; **21**(1): 119–47.

Burroughs AK. Acute management of bleeding oesophageal varices. *Drugs* 1992; **44** Suppl. 2: 14–23.

Conn HO. Transjugular intrahepatic Portal-systemic shunts: The state of the art. *Hepatology* 1993; **17**: 148–155.

Garden OJ, Carter DC. Balloon tamponade and vasoactive drugs in the control of acute variceal haemorrhage. *Baillière's Clin Gastroenterol* 1992; **6**(3): 451–63.

Garden OJ, Carter DC. Natural history and prognosis of variceal bleeding. *Baillière's Clin Gastroenterol* 1992; **6**(3): 437–50.

Grose RD, Hayes PC. Review article: the pathophysiology and pharmacological treatment of portal hypertension. *Aliment Pharmacol Ther* 1992t; **6**(5): 521–40.

Idezuki Y. Transection and devascularization procedures for bleeding from oesophagogastric varices. *Baillière's Clin Gastroenterol* 1992; **6**(3): 549–61.

Kleber G, Ansari H, Sauerbruch T. Prophylaxis of first variceal bleeding. *Baillière's Clin Gastroenterol* 1992; **6**(3): 563–80.

Matloff DS. Treatment of acute variceal bleeding. *Gastroenterol Clin North Am* 1992; **21**(1): 103–18.

Richter GM, Roeren T, Roessle M, Palmaz JC. Transjugular intrahepatic portosystemic stent shunt. *Baillière's Clin Gastroenterol* 1992; **6**(2): 403–19.

Rodriguez Perez F, Groszmann RJ. Pharmacologic treatment of portal hypertension. *Gastroenterol Clin North Am* 1992; **21**(1): 15–40.

Sarin SK, Lahoti D. Management of gastric varices. *Baillière's Clin Gastroenterol* 1992; **6**(3): 527–48.

Terblanche J, Steigman GV, Krige JE, Bornman PC. Long-term management of variceal bleeding: the place of varix injection and ligation. *World J Surg* 1994; **18**: 185–92.

Westaby D. The management of active variceal bleeding. *J Hepatol* 1993; **17** Suppl. 2: S34–7.

Westaby D, Williams R. Status of sclerotherapy for variceal bleeding in 1990. *Am J Surg* 1990; **160**(1): 32–6.

Williams SG, Westaby D. Management of variceal haemorrhage. *Br Med J* 1994; **308**: 1213–17.

Portal hypertensive gastropathy

Rodriguez Perez F, Groszmann RJ. Clinical features, pathophysiology and relevance of portal hypertensive gastropathy. *Endoscopy* 1991l; **23**(4): 224–8.

Triger DR. Portal hypertensive gastropathy. *Baillière's Clin Gastroenterol* 1992; **6**(3): 481–95.

Colon cancer

Greenwald P. Colon cancer overview. *Cancer* 1992; **70** (5 Suppl.): 1206–15.

Colon cancer: molecular and genetic aspects

Burt RW, Bishop DT, Cannon Albright L, Samowitz WS, Lee RL, DiSario JA, Skolnick MH. Hereditary aspects of colorectal adenomas. *Cancer* 1992; **70** (5 Suppl.): 1296–9.

Cho KR, Vogelstein B. Suppressor gene alterations in the colorectal adenoma carcinoma sequence. *J Cell Biochem* Suppl. 1992; **16G**: 137–41.

Lynch HT, Watson P, Smyrk TC,*et al.* Colon cancer genetics. *Cancer* 1992; **70**(5 Suppl.): 1300–12.

Miller WH Jr, Dmitrovsky E. Oncogenes and clinical oncology. *Curr Opin Oncol* 1991; **3**(1): 65–9.

Potter JD. Colon cancer: do the nutritional epidemiology, the gut physiology and the molecular biology tell the same story? *J Nutr* 1993; **123**(2 Suppl.): 418–23.

Rustgi AK, Podolsky DK. The molecular basis of colon cancer. *Annu Rev Med* 1992; **43**: 61–8.

Colon cancer: screening

Lieberman DA. Targeted colon cancer screening: a concept whose time has almost come. *Am J Gastroenterol* 1992; **87**(9): 1085–93.

Mandel JS, Bond JH, Church TR, *et al.* Reducing mortality from colorectal cancer by screening for fecal occult blood. Minnesota Colon Cancer Control Study. *N Engl J Med* 1993; **328**(19): 1365–71.

Mandel JS, Bond JH, Bradley M, *et al.*. Sensitivity, specificity, and positive predictivity of the Hemoccult test in screening for colorectal cancers. The University of Minnesota's Colon Cancer Control Study. *Gastroenterology* 1989; **97**(3): 597–600.

Schatzkin A,. Freedman LS, Dawsey SM, Lanza E. Interpreting precursor studies: what polyp trials tell us about large bowel cancer. *J Natl Cancer Inst* 1994; **86**: 1053–7.

Colon cancer: treatment

Beatty JD. Immunotherapy of colorectal cancer. *Cancer* 1992 Sep 1; **70** (5 Suppl.): 1425–33.

Block GE. Colon cancer: diagnosis and prognosis in the elderly. *Geriatrics* 1989; **44**(5): 45–7, 52–3.

DeCosse JJ, Cennerazzo W. Treatment options for the patient with colorectal cancer. *Cancer* 1992 Sep 1; **70**(5 Suppl.): 1342–5.

Grem JL. Current treatment approaches in colorectal cancer. *Semin Oncol* 1991; **18**(1 Suppl. 1): 17–26.

Moertel CG. Accomplishments in surgical adjuvant therapy for large bowel cancer. *Cancer* 1992; **70**(5 Suppl.): 136471.

Steup WH. Surgery for cancer of the colon and rectum. *Ann Oncol* 1994; **5** (3): 91–5.

7
NAUSEA AND VOMITING

NEUROPHYSIOLOGY OF NAUSEA

The neurological pathways that mediate the sensation of nausea are poorly understood. It is assumed that they are probably the same as those which mediate vomiting, but there is also evidence that they overlap with the pathway that mediates the sensation of fullness or satiety. It follows from this that anorexia is a universal accompaniment.

Vomiting can be induced experimentally by electrical stimulation of the dorsal portion of the fasciculus solitarius in the medulla. The vomiting centre is close to the centres that control respiration and salivation and the process of nausea and retching usually involves activation of both these centres. When retching or 'dry heaves' occurs there is repeated herniation of the abdominal oesophagus and cardia into the thorax as a result of a sudden fall in intrathoracic pressure due to inspiratory effort against a closed glottis. This is associated with reflux of gastric contents into the oesophagus. The natural anti-reflux mechanisms of the oesophagogastric junction having thus been overcome, vomiting may then follow and is associated with a rise in intrathoracic pressure.

Close to the vomiting centre there is a chemoreceptor trigger zone in the floor of the fourth ventricle. Morphine, digoxin, many other drugs and also motion sickness act via stimulation of this centre. In addition sympathetic afferent fibres conduct signals back from the stomach to the vomiting centre and are probably responsible for the nausea associated with gastritis and staphylococcal food poisoning (Fig. 7.1).

REACHING A DIAGNOSIS AND MANAGEMENT

Abdominal pain is often associated with nausea or vomiting, but the diagnosis and management of conditions that cause this combination of symptoms have already been discussed in the section on abdominal pain so will not be dealt with again here in detail. Patients with duodenal ulcer may vomit even in the absence of pyloric stenosis and will often notice relief of the pain after vomiting. Pain associated with biliary colic or pancreatitis will not however be relieved by vomiting. Vomiting is common in acute pancreatitis but uncommon in patients with a perforated viscus and this may be a useful diagnostic clue.

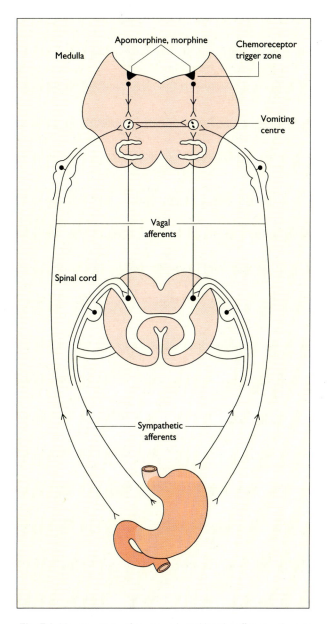

Fig. 7.1 Neuroanatomy of nausea and vomiting: the afferent pathways. The efferent pathways are via somatic motor nerves innervating the muscles of the pharynx, chest wall, diaphragm, and abdominal muscles, as well as vagal innervation of reverse peristalsis of the oesophagus.

CAUSES OF NAUSEA AND VOMITING

Pregnancy?

In a young woman with persistent vomiting this should be the first diagnosis to exclude. The vomiting may start shortly after the first missed period, so it is not uncommon for patients to be referred up to gastroenterology clinics for investigation of vomiting due to undiagnosed pregnancy.

Vomiting in pregnancy usually needs no specific treatment and resolves towards the end of the first trimester. Severe vomiting resulting in electrolyte or fluid depletion (hyperemesis gravidarum) affects about 3.5/1000 deliveries and requires hospital admission for fluid and electrolyte replacement and investigation for underlying causes such as twin pregnancy or hydatidiform mole. Oral pyridoxine is sometimes prescribed, but its efficacy (and mechanism) are not established.

Is there excessive alcohol intake?

Patients who habitually drink heavily often seem surprised when they develop alcohol-related gastritis and commonly fail to make any connection between the resulting vomiting and their alcohol intake. Alcoholic gastritis typically causes early morning retching or vomiting, usually of small volumes, the morning after heavy drinking. The vomit often contains flecks of blood.

Could drugs be responsible?

Many drugs will provoke nausea or vomiting by direct stimulation of the chemoreceptor trigger zone. Classical examples include morphine, dopamine agonists and digoxin, but it is also a common side-effect occurring in a minority of patients with most other drugs.

Is it hepatitis or liver failure?

Vomiting is a common feature of severe hepatic damage and may be the presenting symptom of fulminant viral hepatitis, hepatic failure due to poisoning (e.g. paracetamol or solvents), fatty liver of pregnancy, Reye's syndrome, idiosyncratic reaction to drugs or acute presentation of Wilson's disease. Blood should be checked for hepatic enzymes and if these are abnormal or there is a strong suspicion of liver failure, the prothrombin time should be checked.

Is there a metabolic cause?

Addison's disease is a particularly important condition to consider. Postural hypotension and mucosal pigmentation should be looked for. A high normal or raised plasma potassium is highly suggestive since vomiting will usually result in a fall in plasma potassium.

A short Synacthen test should be performed (plasma cortisol measurements before and one hour after intravenous injection of adrenocorticotrophic hormone). Hypercalcaemia and hyperthyroidism should also be considered.

Does the patient have diabetes?

It has been reported that up to 30% of diabetic patients experience intermittent nausea or vomiting. Often this is due to vagal autonomic neuropathy resulting in 'diabetic gastroparesis.' Patients with this condition typically have long-standing insulin-dependent diabetes and frequently have peripheral neuropathy and other signs of autonomic neuropathy such as postural hypotension, impotence, sweating and bladder dysfunction. There is marked delay in gastric emptying, which may be seen on barium meal, but is best demonstrated by gastric scanning after ingestion of a radiolabelled meal.

Vomiting often, but not always settles when diabetic control is improved. The prokinetic drug cisapride may then be helpful as may erythromycin, which has been shown to have a powerful prokinetic effect.

▶ **Causes of painless nausea and vomiting**

- Alcoholic gastritis
- Viral gastritis
- Food poisoning
- Gastric carcinoma
- Pyloric stenosis (Fig. 7.2)
- Duodenal obstruction (Figs 7.3)
- Biliary reflux following previous gastric surgery
- Diabetic gastroparesis
- Acute hepatitis
- Pregnancy
- Drugs
- Uraemia
- Hypercalcaemia
- Adrenal insufficiency
- Thyrotoxicosis
- Labyrinthitis
- Menière's disease
- Psychogenic

▶ **Causes of vomiting without nausea**

- Intracranial tumours
- Raised intracranial pressure
- Encephalitis
- Meningitis
- Migraine
- Cyclical vomiting

Is there a neurological cause?

The absence of nausea is not invariable in neurological vomiting and a neurological cause can easily be missed when vomiting is the only symptom. A careful neurological examination is required checking particularly for nystagmus, hearing loss, normality of gait, incoordination, and signs of raised intracranial pressure including papilloedema.

Is there a gastric cause?

Not all gastric lesions that cause vomiting are associated with pain so it is important to exclude gastric pathology. Possible gastric causes include carcinoma, which commonly presents with vague symptoms of bloating, belching and nausea without definite pain; other possibilities include gastritis (including rare conditions such as Ménétrier's hypertrophic gastritis or gastric Crohn's disease) and benign gastric ulceration. The management of these conditions is discussed in Chapter 1, pages 17–24. It has been difficult to prove whether *Helicobacter pylori*-associated superficial gastritis can itself cause symptoms. There seem to be some patients in whom eradication of *H. pylori* by appropriate therapy (e.g. bismuth plus two antibiotics) results in a resolution of symptoms.

A hair 'bezoar' may be an unexpected finding on endoscopy. It can often be broken up endoscopically thus preventing the need for laparotomy.

Is there intestinal obstruction?

If vomiting is persistent, intestinal obstrcution should be considered and a plain abdominal X-ray performed without delay (**Fig. 7.4**) providing pregnancy has been excluded. Vomiting due to obstruction will usually be accompanied by colicky abdominal pain and abdominal distension. This condition is discussed in detail on pages 39, 53–57.

Is there bile reflux gastritis?

Bile reflux gastritis is common in patients who have had a previous gastroenterostomy or partial gastrectomy. Endoscopically the mucosa is diffusely reddened, but there may be diagnostic changes of foveolar hyperplasia seen on histology.

Treatment is often unsatisfactory. Bile acid binding agents such as aluminium hydroxide and cholestyramine are worth trying. If these fail and the condition is severe then a surgical biliary diversion procedure may be the only option.

Is it cyclical vomiting?

Cyclical vomiting, usually occurring approximately in two-month cycles, most commonly presents in childhood, but may present in teenagers or young adults. It often seems to be a variant of migraine and may be associated with headache or abdominal pain. The condition may respond to propranolol. Care must be taken to exclude alternative gastrointestinal or neurological causes.

Is it the superior mesenteric artery syndrome?

Sometimes a barium meal examination performed in a patient with vomiting will show a dilated proximal duodenum with an apparent obstruction just to the right of the

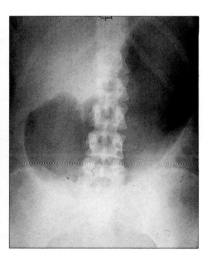

Fig. 7.2 Plain abdominal radiograph of a patient with benign pyloric stenosis. The patient has been vomiting and air-swallowing and has a distended air-filled stomach. The stomach would usually be fluid-filled. Naso-gastric aspiration should then be performed before endoscopy to prevent aspiration.

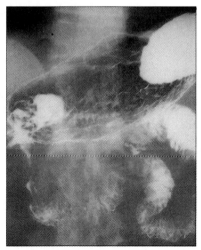

Fig. 7.3 Duodenal obstruction due to pancreatic cancer.

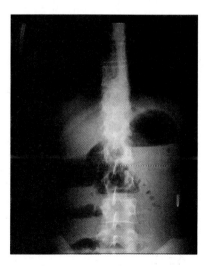

Fig. 7.4 Plain abdominal radiograph of a patient with small bowel obstruction.

midline. Angiography will show the superior mesenteric artery crossing over the duodenum at this point. The patients are usually thin, often female and have been reported to benefit from duodeno- or gastro-jejunostomy.

Many physicians are sceptical and believe that this is a functional syndrome and that the radiographic appearances are a normal variant. The rare possibility of a distal **duodenal carcinoma** should be considered in this situation.

Is it epidemic vomiting?

Epidemics of vomiting are quite common. The onset is usually sudden and vomiting may be severe and associated with headache, muscle aches and fever. Immune electron microscopy of faecal samples may confirm the presence of viruses such as Norwalk agent and human reovirus-like agent. Recovery occurs over 3–10 days.

Staphylococcus aureus food poisoning may cause a similar explosive onset of vomiting, but lasting usually for only 24 hours. It has an incubation period of 6–12 hours.

Is it psychogenic vomiting?

Patients with psychogenic vomiting are typically young women with stressful home situations. They usually freely admit to the vomiting, whereas patients with bulimia typically conceal the vomiting.

Treatment is generally very difficult. Response to conventional anti-emetics is usually poor. Resolution usually takes place slowly over one or two years, particularly if the patient is no longer in the situation that she finds stressful.

▶ **Features that suggest psychogenic vomiting**

- Vomiting during meals (organic causes usually result in vomiting after or between meals)
- Lack of preceding nausea
- The ability to delay vomiting until the toilet has been reached
- Apparent lack of concern

Is it rumination?

Rumination rarely occurs in adults. It is voluntarily induced regurgitation followed by reswallowing. The regurgitation is thought generally to occur as a result of forced inspiration against a closed glottis. It indicates psychological disturbance and is commoner in the mentally subnormal.

DRUG THERAPY OF VOMITING

Drug therapy may not be necessary if the cause of the vomiting, for example intestinal obstruction or alcohol abuse, can be identified and removed. If vomiting is chronic and intermittent, it is important to be wary of the potential for some of the commoner anti-emetics to cause unpleasant neurological side-effects in prolonged usage.

Phenothiazines such as prochlorperazine and chlorpromazine are effective in vomiting due to many causes including gastroenteritis, disorders of the middle ear and chemotherapy-induced vomiting. Their main disadvantages are sedation and extrapyramidal reactions.

Dopaminergic antagonists, such as metoclopramide and domperidone, are effective in vomiting due to both central and intestinal causes. Metoclopramide is usually safe and well tolerated in short term use, but can cause severe orofacial dyskinesia when therapy is prolonged; it is not always reversible on stopping the drug. Domperidone causes extrapyramidal reactions less commonly but may cause troublesome hyperprolactinaemia with galactorrhoea and amenorrhoea.

▶ **Dangers of long-term metoclopramide therapy**

Metoclopramide therapy should not be used long term because of the risk of neurological side-effects (oro-facial dyskinesia)

Prokinetic agents such as cisapride, which facilitates acetylcholine release and rarely causes troublesome side-effects, and erythromycin, may be effective when vomiting is due to gastric dysmotility as in diabetic gastroparesis.

Serotonin antagonists such as ondansetron, granisetron or tropisetron, are particularly effective in centrally-induced vomiting (as seen in cancer chemotherapy) where they may be used in combination with dexamethasone.

FURTHER READING

Vomiting

Allan SG. Antiemetics. *Gastroenterol Clin North Am* 1992; **21**(3): 597–611.

Jones AL, Cunningham D. Management of vomiting associated with cytotoxic therapy. *Br J Hosp Med* 1991; **45**(2): 85–8.

Read NW, Houghton LA. Physiology of gastric emptying and pathophysiology of gastroparesis. *Gastroenterol Clin North Am* 1989; **18**(2): 359–73.

Talley NJ. Review article: 5-hydroxytryptamine agonists and antagonists in the modulation of gastrointestinal motility and sensation: clinical implications. *Aliment Pharmacol Ther* 1992; **6**(3): 273–89.

8
EATING DISORDERS AND WEIGHT LOSS

THE PHYSIOLOGY OF APPETITE

There is good evidence that appetite is controlled by the hypothalamus, but the exact mechanisms are poorly understood. It used to be thought, on the basis of experimental studies in animals, that there were two main centres with opposing effects, one controlling appetite and the other satiety. It is now thought that this is an oversimplification and that there is a complex network of neuroendocrine tracts that interact within the hypothalamus. Intraventricular injection of cholecystokinin, thyrotrophin releasing hormone, somatostatin and bombesin all produce satiety in experimental animals, whereas injection of opiates, neuropeptide Y, gamma-aminobutyric acid and diazepam all stimulate appetite.

Nausea, which is also mediated by the hypothalamus, is invariably accompanied by anorexia, but anorexia is not invariably accompanied by nausea.

REACHING A DIAGNOSIS AND MANAGEMENT

Anorexia and weight loss

Exclusion of malignant disease
Malignant disease can be difficult to exclude in the absence of any localising symptoms. Family history of cancer and the age of the patient are important considerations in assessing the likely risk. Direct questioning should be used to check for any change in bowel habit, any abdominal discomfort, any recent cough or haemoptysis, gynaecological or neurological symptoms. Alcohol consumption should be noted since many patients are unaware of the high calorific content of alcoholic drinks and are surprised when they lose weight if they cut their alcohol intake.

A careful clinical examination is extremely important with particular attention to lymph nodes. Rectal examination and faecal occult blood testing should be performed.

In the older patient (e.g. over 40 years of age) a reasonable programme of screening tests would then include full blood count and erythrocyte sedimentation rate, liver biochemistry, chest X-ray, ultrasound scan of liver, pancreas,

▶ **Anorexia**

> Nausea is invariably accompanied by anorexia, but anorexia is not necessarily accompanied by nausea

kidneys and pelvis. Because difficulty in visualising the whole pancreas is common, it is also reasonable to check for the presence of one of the available pancreas cancer serological markers such as CAM17.1 or CA19.9. An alternative to ultrasound scanning is CT scanning, but this ought to include the whole abdomen and pelvis so it is probably preferable to perform ultrasound scanning first in the hope that this may limit the area that needs to be examined by CT and thus allow more detailed CT scanning of the relevant area with smaller cuts and use of contrast. A gastroscopy should be performed since gastric cancer may present as anorexia without pain. Distal duodenal biopsy can be taken at the same time to exclude coeliac disease.

If all these tests prove negative a reasonable approach is to review the patient again after a period of about two months and reweigh when the patient will often be found to have regained weight. It is particularly important to re-examine the patient thoroughly on subsequent review to check for lymph nodes or other masses that may have become apparent since the first examination.

▶ **Causes of anorexia and weight loss**

- Malignant disease
- Hyperthyroidism
- Adrenal insufficiency
- Diabetes
- Hyperparathyroidism
- Hypercalcaemia
- Coeliac disease
- Crohn's disease
- Intestinal parasitosis
- Intracranial lesion, particularly hypothalamic
- Anorexia nervosa

Exclusion of metabolic disease

Tests should include serum calcium, creatinine, glucose, thyroid function tests and plasma electrophoresis. If postural hypertension is present, a short synacthen test should be performed to exclude Addison's disease.

▶ **Excluding organic disease as a cause of weight loss**

- Careful dietary history. Has there been a recent reduction in alcohol intake? Are there any neurological symptoms?
- Careful clinical examination: check lymph nodes
- Full blood count, erythrocyte sedimentation rate, biochemical profile, thyroid function, serum calcium
- Faecal occult blood and microscopy
- Chest X-ray
- Ultrasound scan of abdomen (liver, pancreas and pelvis)
- Endoscopy and duodenal biopsy
- Pancreatic tumour marker assay (CA19-9 or CAM17.1)
- Consider adrenal insufficiency

Anorexia nervosa

Anorexia nervosa has a male to female ratio of approximately 1:15, which presumably reflects the greater pressure on females to correspond to the socially imposed perception that slimness is desirable. Surveys have shown that it probably affects 4% of females at some time. It is increasingly realised that there are many patients who do not fit all of the previously required diagnostic criteria, but who nevertheless have a significant eating disorder.

Characteristic features therefore may include some, but not necessarily all of the following:

- Loss of 25% of original body weight.
- Onset before 25 years of age.
- Distorted body image.
- Hoarding of food.
- Amenorrhoea.
- Lanugo hair.
- Bradycardia (< 60 beats/min).
- Low luteinising hormone and follicle stimulating hormone.
- Low T_4 and normal thyroid stimulating hormone.
- Low temperature.

Other psychiatric illnesses such as depression or schizophrenia should be excluded.

MANAGEMENT

The patient is often defensive or manipulative. Secretive vomiting or hoarding of food is usual. Purgative and/or diuretic abuse are common. Any patient who has lost more than 40% of their ideal body weight or who has lost over 25% of their weight within three months should be admitted to hospital. A target weight should be agreed with the patient. Meals should be taken at regular times and the patient should be sat with during and for one hour after each meal.

If the patient does not cooperate with this approach management can be very difficult. A wide range of approaches has been tried reflecting not only the different training, but often the different philosophical approach to life of the health care personnel involved. Thus some will sedate the patient with large doses of phenothiazines in order to reduce the problems of non-cooperation and then commence enteral or intravenous feeding. Others will regard this as an intrusion with the liberties of the patient (particularly if the patient is adult) and will see psychotherapy and gentle encouragement as the only acceptable course. The mortality is at least 5% however and many health care professionals find it unacceptable to watch a patient starving to death without attempting some form of assisted feeding. Enteral feeding should be started slowly in these circumstances because of the risk of gastric dilatation, vomiting and inhalation and also a risk of pancreatitis. Caloric intake should be increased gradually up to 3000 calories/day over a two-week period.

If treatment is successful the patient may develop better insight into the problem as her weight approaches normal. At this time careful discussions should be held with the patient and family members to attempt to resolve the underlying conflicts or anxieties that are often present. About 35–50% of patients make a complete recovery, but persistence of some form of eating disorder (often intermittent bulimia) into later adult life is common and may even persist into old age.

Bulimia

Bulimia (bingeing and self-induced vomiting), often complicates anorexia nervosa, but in less severe cases may be the main feature. There is then often a greater insight and the prognosis is generally better. In the short term however

▶ **Anorexia nervosa**

- Female:male ratio of 15:1
- Affects 4% of females at some time
- Purgative and/or diuretic abuse common
- Overlaps with bulimia
- Rapid feeding may cause gastric dilatation, inhalation, acute pancreatitis
- Mortality 5%

severe electrolyte disturbances may occur and can even be fatal. The combination of dehydration and hypokalaemia may result in urinary calculi and life threatening renal failure.

Obesity

Obesity is defined as a body weight that is 120% or more of the ideal weight for an individual's height. Approximately 25% of adults in the USA are obese and a slightly lower proportion in most European countries.

Mortality rates compared with those of optimal weight are:

- 28% higher with a body weight 120–29% of ideal weight.
- 46% higher with a body weight 130–139% of ideal weight.
- 88% higher with a body weight over 140% of ideal weight.

Mortality is increased from coronary artery disease and diabetes and there is a considerable increase in relative risk for a range of intestinal cancers. Among patients with a body weight higher than 140% of ideal weight **relative risks** are:

- Colorectal cancer: 1.73 for men, 1.22 for women.
- Stomach cancer: 1.88 for men, 1.03 for women.
- Pancreatic cancer: 1.62 for men, 0.61 for women.

The risk of gallstones more than doubles in people with gross obesity.

Aetiology and pathogenesis

Underlying **genetic defects** are very rare and invariably present in childhood. They may be divided into four groups:

- Syndromes with primary hypogonadism and no polydactyly such as Prader–Willi (these children have hypotonia, mental retardation, short stature and hypogenitalism).
- Syndromes with secondary hypogonadism and polydactyly such as Laurence–Moon, in which there is also retinal degeneration and mental deficiency.
- Syndromes with secondary hypogonadism without polydactyly such as Bardet–Biedl, in which there is also retinal degeneration and mental deficiency.
- Obesity without hypogonadism such as triglyceride storage disease, which is extremely rare.

These syndromes have autosomal recessive inheritance and are usually readily recognised by the combination of short stature and mental retardation.

Hypothalamic damage due to trauma or neoplasia is a rare cause of obesity, which may also be associated with disordered temperature regulation.

There is considerable argument as to whether 'simple' obesity is inherited. Fat children usually have fat parents, but this might reflect environmental influence. However children adopted at a young age by overweight foster parents are often of normal weight suggesting that environmental factors may be less important than genetic factors. Children of obese parents have been shown to have lower basal metabolic rates than children of normal-sized parents.

Management

A common course of events is for the patient to go on a 'crash' diet that is devoid of carbohydrate. Muscle glycogen will start to be broken down and as this is stored with four times its own weight of water there will be rapid weight loss for the first 2–3 weeks. This process will then slow down and ingestion of a relatively small amount of carbohydrate will rapidly undo the weight loss, the patient will become disheartened and give up. Even more drastic diets such as protein-only diets are dangerous, probably because of their low potassium intake, and may be associated with sudden death. A reasonable course is to:

- Explain to the patient that a loss of one kilogram of fat requires a negative balance of 7700 kcal (32 MJ) and that the patient will be doing very well if he/she eats 1000 kcal/day less than is required to maintain equilibrium. Weight loss averaging 1 kg/week is therefore the most that can be maintained for any reasonable period.
- Explain that successful dieting can not be achieved without feeling hungry, at least for the first 2–3 weeks and that considerable will-power will be needed.
- Explain that fat provides about 7 kcal/gram and alcohol more, compared with carbohydrate, which provides 4 kcal/gram. Reduction in alcohol and fat intake may therefore have a much more dramatic effect than carbohydrate restriction and will also result in a much healthier diet.
- Ask the patient to keep a diary of what he/she eats. This may highlight indulgences that the patient may have thought were less frequent than they are and also allows the doctor or dietician to advise on which items have the highest calorific content.
- The basic aim is a **permanent reduction insugar, fat and alcohol intake with maintenance of starch and protein levels**.

Commercial slimming organisations may benefit some patients, but their success rates are generally only of the order of 15–20%.

Drastic **surgical measures** such as gastric plication or implantation of a gastric balloon usually only produce short term weight loss for the first few months. Jejuno-ileal bypass has been abandoned because of high rates of severe arthritis and liver failure, apparently related to the presence of bacteria in the bypassed loop. Jaw wiring seems to most to be unacceptably barbaric and carries a considerable risk of inhalation if vomiting occurs.

Drugs are of limited value. Thyroid supplements lead to protein loss and are generally considered too unsafe. There are a range of amphetamine derivatives, which have been tried with some success. The most commonly used is fenfluramine. The use of short acting tablets may allow the use of a single daily dose at the time when the patient finds that he/she experiences greatest hunger. The drug should be

► **Aims of treating obesity**

- Permanent reduction in intake of sugar, fat and alcohol
- Maintenance of starch and protein intake

withdrawn slowly since depression may occur during withdrawal. The drug should only be used when dietary treatment alone has failed and then only in combination with a controlled diet.

FURTHER READING

Neuroendocrine control of appetite

Billington CJ, Levine AS. Hypothalamic neuropeptide Y regulation of feeding and energy metabolism. *Curr Opin Neurobiol* 1992; **2**(6): 847–51.

Curzon G. Serotonin and appetite. *Ann N Y Acad Sci* 1990; **600**: 521–30.

Kissileff HR. Is there an eating disorder in the obese? *Ann N Y Acad Sci* 1989; **575**: 410–19.

McCoy JG, Avery DD. Bombesin: potential integrative peptide for feeding and satiety. *Peptides* 1990; **11**(3): 595–607.

Morley JE. Appetite regulation by gut peptides. *Annu Rev Nutr* 1990; **10**: 383–95.

Morley JE. Appetite regulation: the role of peptides and hormones. *J Endocrinol Invest* 1989; **12**(2): 135–47.

Anorexia nervosa and bulimia

Beumont PJ, Russell JD, Touyz SW. Treatment of anorexia nervosa. *Lancet* 1993; **341** (8861): 1635–40.

Kerr JK, Skok RL, McLaughlin TF. Characteristics common to females who exhibit anorexic or bulimic behavior: a review of current literature. *J Clin Psychol* 1991; **47**(6): 846–53.

Nagel KL, Jones KH. Predisposition factors in anorexia nervosa. *Adolescence* 1992; **27**(106): 381–6.

Stewart DE. Reproductive functions in eating disorders. *Ann Med* 1992, **24**(4): 287–91.

Walsh BT, Devlin MJ. The pharmacologic treatment of eating disorders. *Psychiatr Clin North Am* 1992; **15**(1): 149–60.

Weiner H. Psychoendocrinology of anorexia nervosa. *Psychiatr Clin North Am* 1989; **12**(1): 187–206.

Miscellaneous

Robison JI, Hoerr SL, Strandmark J, Mavis B. Obesity, weight loss, and health. *J Am Diet Assoc* 1993; **93**(4): 445–9.

Silverstone T, Goodall E. Centrally acting anorectic drugs: a clinical perspective. *Am J Clin Nutr* 1992; **55**(1 Suppl.): 211S–214S.

9
WIND

DIAGNOSIS AND MANAGEMENT

Belching

Belching, particularly in association with satiety and nausea, may occasionally be a symptom of significant gastric disease, either benign or malignant. Endoscopy is therefore indicated if it occurs as a new symptom in a patient over 40 years of age.

In most patients however there is no underlying gastric pathology and the repeated belching results from repeated air swallowing. The air often does not enter the stomach, being noisily regurgitated shortly after it has been swallowed. This usually occurs as a response to stress.

The patient is often unaware of the air swallowing, but if reassurance is combined with an explanation of the mechanism the problem is usually considerably improved.

▶ **Belching**

- May indicate significant gastric pathology
- Usually results from excessive air swallowing

Flatus

Much of what we know about flatus has been learnt as a result of meticulous studies by the American researchers, Bond and Levitt. They have shown that the composition of flatus varies widely:

- Nitrogen 11–92%.
- Oxygen 0–11%.
- Carbon dioxide 3–54%.
- Hydrogen 0–69%.
- Methane 0–56%.

Hydrogen production is the result of bacterial fermentation of unabsorbed carbohydrate. Methane production varies considerably between individuals due to the presence or absence of methane forming bacteria. The methane producing status of most individuals seems to remain fairly constant throughout life and it is presumed that these organisms are established in the colon early in life. The faeces of methane producers can be recognised by their tendency to float!

Although excessive air swallowing may result in air reaching the anus within 20 minutes of being swallowed, air swallowing is rarely the cause of excessive flatus. Ingenious experiments have shown that the normal range of flatus excretion varies between 200–2000 ml/day resulting in an average of about 40 separate passages of gas in young adult male controls. Excessive flatus (although rarely meticulously documented) is almost always due to increased production of hydrogen and carbon dioxide as a result of bacterial fermentation of carbohydrate. This usually results from either:

- The ingestion of high quantities of poorly absorbed dietary fibre (e.g. beans).
- Malabsorption of carbohydrate due either to hypolactasia or more generalised malabsorptive syndromes.

Hypolactasia should therefore be excluded by lactose hydrogen breath test and reassurance given combined with dietary advice.

▶ **Bloating**

- Usually reflects disordered motility rather than increased gas

Bloating

Bloating may occasionally be postprandial fullness resulting from important gastric pathology. More commonly it is used to describe the generalised abdominal distension that is commonly a symptom in patients who have other features of the irritable bowel sydrome such as alternating constipation with diarrhoea and colicky abdominal pain. Studies using intestinal gas washout techniques have shown that these patients do not have an increased intestinal gas content, but do have greater reflux of the gas into the stomach than controls and also experience increased abdominal pain. The complaint of bloating is therefore usually a reflection of altered intestinal motility rather than of increased intestinal gas content.

Smooth muscle relaxants such as mebeverine or peppermint oil preparations may be effective therapy.

▶ **Excessive flatus**

- **Not** usually due to air swallowing
- Results from increased fermentation of carbohydrate by colonic bacteria
- May be due to carbohydrate malabsorption or excessive intake of fibre

Halitosis

It is not usually possible for patients to smell their own breath and when patients complain that their breath is offensive it is important to check whether this is something they have noticed themself or whether someone else has commented on it. Anxious individuals often believe incorrectly that their breath is offensive whereas people with offensive breath are often blissfully unaware of the problem. Bad breath is most commonly due to fermentation of debris in the mouth by bacteria as a result of poor oral hygiene and dental cavities. Sepsis either in teeth, gums or tonsils may be a cause. Elongation of the filiform papillae 'hairy tongue' may be a contributory factor and can be improved by daily brushing of the tongue with a toothbrush. Occasionally sepsis in other sites such as bronchiectasis or lung abscesses may give rise to bad breath. Specific causes include hepatic failure, uraemia and diabetic ketoacidosis.

▶ **Halitosis**

- Most commonly due to poor oral hygiene

Hiccups

Hiccups are involuntary, abrupt inspiratory movements occurring against a closed glottis and they can affect both diaphragms. They result either from stimulation of the afferent limb of the glottis reflex arc, e.g. by gastric, diaphragmatic or mediastinal disease, or by stimulation of the efferent limb, e.g. by brain stem lesions or drugs. The afferent limb consists of the vagus and phrenic nerves and the thoracic sympathetic chain and the efferent limb is the phrenic nerve. Appropriate investigations for intractable hiccups may therefore include CT scan to exclude pathology such as tumour or abscess adjacent to the diaphragm, or in the mediastinum, and CT or preferably NMR to exclude intracranial and brain stem pathology. Endoscopy may be helpful to exclude gastric or oesophageal disease.

If hiccups persist despite simple measures such as drinking ice-cold water, pulling the tongue, or stimulation of the nasopharynx with a catheter, then drug treatment may be required. Therapies which may help include chlorpromazine (25–50 mgs intravenously every six hours), metaclopramide (10mgs intravenously every four hours), or phenytoin (100mgs four times daily).

Intractable hiccups can occasionally be very serious, resulting in weight loss, arythmias and oesophagitis. Phrenic nerve crush may have to be considered in very severe cases when drug therapy has failed, but it is not always effective.

FURTHER READING

Wind

Danzl DF. Flatology. *J Emerg* Med 1992; **10**(1): 79–88.

Grimble G. Fibre, fermentation, flora, and flatus. Gut 1989; **30**(1): 6–13.

Lewis JH. Hiccups: causes and cures. *J Clin Gastroenterol* 1985; **7**: 539–43.

Levitt MD, Bond JH. Volume, composition and source of intestinal gas. *Gastroenterology* 1970; **59**: 921.

10
PROBLEMS AFTER GASTRIC SURGERY

INTRODUCTION

Vagotomy and partial gastrectomy are fortunately rarely necessary now in the treatment of benign disease. Nevertheless there are many patients who have had these procedures performed in the past and a substantial proportion of these patients suffer one or more of the problems associated with these procedures.

REACHING A DIAGNOSIS AND MANAGEMENT

Pain

Possible causes of epigastric pain following previous gastric surgery or vagotomy include:

- Recurrent ulceration.
- Stomal ulceration.
- Afferent loop syndrome.
- Gastric carcinoma.
- An unrelated diagnosis(e.g. pancreatic disease, gallstones).

Recurrent or stomal ulceration?

Recurrent duodenal ulceration occurs after vagotomy in about 4–5% of patients in most series, although reported recurrence rates range as high as 25%. Many of these patients can be shown by means of the gastric acid response to insulin to have an incomplete vagotomy. There is nowadays little need to confirm this since treatment of recurrent ulcers should be medical whether the vagotomy is incomplete or not. Recurrence rates are convincingly lower after the combination of vagotomy and antrectomy (about 1%) so in the very occasional patient who refuses to take medical treatment antrectomy might be indicated.

Stomal ulceration (**Fig. 10.1**) was notoriously common when gastroenterostomy was performed without vagotomy for the treatment of duodenal ulceration when the stomal ulcer rate was 30–35%; stomal ulcer rates of about 5–10% occur following vagotomy and gastroenterostomy. About 60% of the stomal ulcers are asymptomatic and may present with bleeding without previous pain.

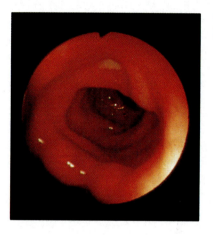

Fig. 10.1
Endoscopic view of stomal ulcer. Such ulcers are easily missed on barium meal.

Large stomal ulcers may occasionally perforate into the colon resulting in a gastrocolic fistula with severe malabsorption and diarrhoea.

Both duodenal ulcer recurrence and stomal ulceration are very difficult to diagnose with certainty by barium examination and symptomatic patients with previous gastric surgery should always be investigated by endoscopy.

▶ **Investigation of the operated stomach**

> Endoscopy is much better than barium meal for evaluating the operated stomach

Zollinger–Ellison or retained antrum syndrome?

In all patients with recurrent or stomal ulceration the fasting serum **gastrin** should be checked to exclude either an underlying Zollinger–Ellison syndrome or the retained antrum syndrome.

Interpretation of a raised serum gastrin may be difficult. A serum gastrin lower than 100 pg/ml virtually excludes a diagnosis of Zollinger–Ellison syndrome, while a gastrin higher than 1000 pg/ml is virtually diagnostic; however values are more commonly obtained between these two extremes. If the serum gastrin is between 100–1000 pg/ml the first steps should be to to exclude hypercalcaemia (which results in hypergastrinaemia and also predisposes to peptic ulceration) and assess basal and pentagastrin-stimulated gastric acid output. A basal acid output higher than 15 mM/hr that is more than 60% of peak stimulated acid output is strongly suggestive of Zollinger–Ellison syndrome, but false-negative results are common because of difficulty in ensuring a complete collection in the operated stomach.

A retained antrum should be excluded by technetium pertechnetate scanning. If confirmed then surgery is likely to be necessary to excise the cuff of retained antrum at the end of the afferent loop.

Afferent loop obstruction syndrome?

Afferent loop obstruction syndrome is a rare complication of Polya gastrectomy or gastroenterostomy. Partial obstruction of the afferent loop results in distension with bile, particularly when the gall bladder contracts after a meal. The patient complains of severe epigastric pain after meals, which is often followed by vomiting of bile and relief of pain. Objective confirmation may be difficult and is probably best made by HIDA scanning with late films to show bile stasis in the afferent loop.

Surgical revision is usually required either with re-fashioning of the stoma or conversion to a Billroth 1 partial gastrectomy.

Gastric carcinoma

There is about a two-fold increased relative risk for gastric cancer 20 years after partial gastrectomy. It has been presumed that the gastrectomy itself increases the risk, perhaps by causing bile reflux, but recent studies suggest that *H. pylori* may also have a role in the induction of gastric cancer, possibly by reducing gastric juice vitamin C content.

Epigastric pain developing many years after gastric surgery is therefore an indication for endoscopy. Because cancer may be multifocal and because early lesions may look macroscopically innocuous it is important that multiple biopsies are taken. Metaplasia of the gastric mucosa is commonly seen. Although statistically associated with malignancy, it is not directly pre-malignant; however, colonic-type metaplasia (containing sulphomucin) is associated with a particularly high risk for malignancy and indicates the need for careful endoscopic review (**Figs 10.2** and **10.3**).

▶ **In recurrent or stomal ulceration consider:**

- Zollinger–Ellison syndrome
- Retained antrum syndrome

▶ **Pain following gastric surgery may be due to:**

- Recurrent ulcer
- Stomal ulcer
- Afferent loop syndrome
- Rapid gastric emptying
- Delayed gastric emptying
- Gastric cancer
- An unrelated problem

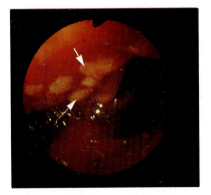

Fig. 10.2 Endoscopic appearance of intestinal metaplasia in the stomach following partial gastrectomy. The lesions (arrowed) are easier to see after spraying with methylene blue.

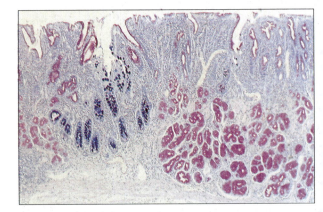

Fig. 10.3 Histological appearances of metaplasia in a biopsy from the gastric antrum. Intestinal-type goblet cells are stained blue (Alcian blue) with normal mucins staining magenta (Periodic Acid Schiff)

Vomiting

About 5–15% of patients have problems with vomiting after gastric surgery. Causes include biliary reflux gastritis (**Fig. 10.4**), stomal ulceration, afferent loop obstruction syndrome, post-vagotomy gastric stasis and the opposite: rapid gastric emptying with jejunal distension. The history should help distinguish some of these problems.

Symptoms of early dumping suggest rapid gastric emptying; afferent loop obstruction and biliary gastritis should be associated with vomiting of bile rather than postprandial vomiting of food and afferent loop obstruction and stomal ulceration are more likely to be associated with pain. In a difficult case satisfactory evaluation may require endoscopy, gastric emptying studies (performed by serial scanning after ingestion of a radiolabelled meal) and HIDA scan. Biliary reflux gastritis has a characteristic appearance of foveolar hyperplasia on gastric biopsy. It may respond to medical therapy with agents such as cholestyramine and aluminium hydroxide, which bind bile acids.

MANAGEMENT

Treatment of chronic vomiting after gastric surgery may be very difficult. Possible options include:

- Biliary gastritis: cholestyramine or aluminium hydroxide.
- Stomal ulcer: H_2 antagonist or proton pump inhibitor.
- Afferent loop syndrome: surgical revision.
- Rapid gastric emptying: small dry meals, guar, conversion to Billroth 1.
- Post-vagotomy stasis: small liquid meals, cisapride or other prokinetics.

Occasional patients have a diffficult combination of early dumping when they take liquids and early satiety with pain

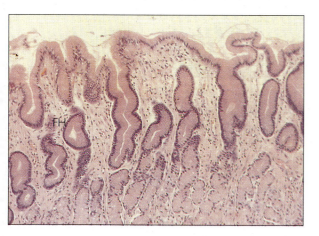

Fig. 10.4 Histological appearances of reflux gastritis showing the characteristic foveolar hyperplasia (FH) plus separation of crypts by oedema.

and vomiting if they take solids. In this situation the best that can usually be done is for the patient to modify the diet until a half-way compromise is reached.

▶ **Vomiting following gastric surgery may be due to:**

- Biliary reflux gastritis
- Stomal ulcer
- Rapid gastric emptying
- Delayed gastric emptying
- Afferent loop syndrome

Diarrhoea

Troublesome diarrhoea occurs in 5–10% of patients following vagotomy, but may affect up to 50% of those who have the common combination of vagotomy and cholecystectomy.

Possible mechanisms include bile salt diarrhoea, altered motility and small bowel bacterial overgrowth. Bile salt diarrhoea should be considered in any patient with post-vagotomy diarrhoea because about 50% will have a good response to oral cholestyramine. Bacterial overgrowth is particularly common following Polya gastrectomy and can be confirmed by lactulose hydrogen or ^{14}C glycocholate breath test.

Dumping

Dumping is probably the most devastating of the post-gastric surgery syndromes.

Early dumping

Early dumping is a combination of faintness and abdominal discomfort, which comes on within 10–20 minutes of eating, often while the meal is still in progress. It is useful to document the objective changes with a formal dumping provocation test. This can be performed by giving the patient a normal meal and then monitoring blood pressure and serum potassium every five minutes for the first 30 minutes. A typical response is a marked fall in both systolic and pulse pressure and a fall in serum potassium.

The mechanism for the haemodynamic changes is unclear. It is not simple hypovolaemia since intravenous infusion does not prevent either symptoms or hypotension. Similarly correction of the transient hypokalaemia also fails to improve symptoms. It seems likely that there is a complex release of vasoactive peptides and kinins.

MANAGEMENT

Treatment can be very difficult. The first step is to explain the likely mechanism to the patient and recommend frequent fairly dry meals in the hope that these will leave the stomach more slowly. If this fails, guar gum may be worth trying although results have generally been disappointing. Revision of the gastric surgery is often contemplated, but rarely successful. The somatostatin analogue, octreotide, given by twice daily subcutaneous injections is an expensive, but less invasive alternative, which sometimes produces good results in difficult cases.

Late dumping

Late dumping is faintness due to hypoglycaemia occurring 2–3 hours after a meal. The glucose tolerance test is characteristic with a rapid early rise to a high value at one hour, often associated with glycosuria, followed by a late fall. The mechanism of this is not fully understood. It is not a simple 'overshoot' in response to the rapid rise in blood glucose since late hypoglycaemia does not occur following large amounts of intravenous glucose. It probably reflects release of a peptide from the duodenum, possibly gastric inhibitory peptide, which sensitizes the pancreatic beta cells so that there is a greater release of insulin for any given rise in blood glucose.

MANAGEMENT

Treatment is much as for early dumping. A low carbohydrate intake may be helpful by inducing beta cell hypoplasia, but this probably has to be quite severe (less than 80–100 g/day) to be effective.

Weight loss

At least 50% of patients lose weight after partial gastrectomy. It is usually multifactorial. Early satiety is probably an important factor. Small bowel bacterial overgrowth with resulting fat malabsorption is probably an underestimated problem and should be sought if there is marked weight loss.

Anaemia

Anaemia is a common late complication of partial gastrectomy and often goes undetected for a long time because it develops insidiously long after the gastric surgery.

Iron deficiency is most common. It probably reflects the lack of:

• Acid, which helps solubilise dietary iron and allow its conversion from ferric to ferrous.
• Ascorbic acid, which is normally actively secreted in gastric juice and forms a complex with iron that is more soluble in the alkaline pH of the duodenum.

In the patient with iron-deficiency anaemia investigation will be required to exclude upper or lower gastrointestinal

malignancy, but if the investigations are normal it is reasonable to assume that the iron deficiency is secondary to the partial gastrectomy.

Management

A good therapeutic response is often achieved with a combination of oral iron and vitamin C when iron alone has previously failed.

If the anaemia is normocytic or macrocytic it is important to check serum vitamin B_{12}. Malabsorption of vitamin B_{12} following gastric surgery may be either due to lack of intrinsic factor or bacterial overgrowth. These can be distinguished by Schilling test (absorption of B_{12} with and wihout intrinsic factor) and breath testing for bacterial overgrowth. Whatever the cause of the low B_{12} the patient should be treated with regular three-monthly supplements (hydroxycobalamin, 1000 μg, intramuscularly) for life.

▶ **Treatment of iron deficiency after gastrectomy**

The response of a patient who has had a gastrectomy to treatment for iron deficiency is often considerably improved if the iron is taken with ascorbic acid (vitamin C, 100 mg)

Malabsorption

Some degree of malabsorption is usual following gastric surgery and is usually multifactorial. There may be inefficient mixing of food with bile and pancreatic juice, inadequate pancreatic and gallbladder responses to food and bacterial overgrowth. Malabsorption is occasionally clinically obvious with frank steatorrhoea, but much more commonly it is insidious, contributing to weight loss, anaemia and osteomalacia without any obvious bowel symptoms to suggest malabsorption.

Management

It is reasonable practice to prescribe prophylactic low-dose calcium and vitamin D supplementation to patients (particularly the elderly) with previous gastric surgery.

The usually mild malabsorption that occurs after gastric surgery may unmask a previously subclinical level of malabsorption due to some other condition such as coeliac disease. Endoscopic duodenal biopsies should be taken to exclude coeliac disease in any patient with clinical evidence of malabsorption.

FURTHER READING

Delcore R, Cheung LY. Surgical options in postgastrectomy syndromes. (Review). *Surg Clin North Am* 1991; **71**(1); 57–75.

Eagon JC, Miedema BW, Kelly KA. Postgastrectomy syndromes. *Clin North Am* 1992; **72**(2); 445–65.

Farthing MJ. Octreotide in dumping and short bowel syndromes. (Review.) *Digestion* 1993; **54** Suppl. 1; 47–52.

Harju E. Metabolic problems after gastric surgery. (Review.) *Int Surg* 1990; **75**(1); 27–35.

Lamers CB, Bijlstra AM, Harris AG. Octreotide, a long-acting somatostatin analog in the management of postoperative dumping syndrome. An update. (Review.) *Dig Dis Sci* 1993; **38**(2): 359–64.

Linehan IP, Weiman J, Hobsley M. The 15-minute dumping provocation test. *Br J Surg* 1986; **73**(10); 810–12.

Sawyers JL. Management of postgastrectomy syndromes. *Am J Surg* 1990; **159**(1); 8–14.

Tovey FI, Hall ML, Ell PJ, Hobsley M. A review of postgastrectomy bone disease. (Review.). *J Gastroent Hepat* 1992 **7**(6): 639–45.

Tovey FI, Godfrey JE, Lewin MR. A gastrectomy population: 25–30 years on. *Postgrad Med J* 1990; 66(776): 450–6.

11

OESOPHAGEAL PAIN AND DIFFICULTY WITH SWALLOWING

REACHING A DIAGNOSIS

Oesophageal pain

A carefully taken history is particularly important in the diagnosis of oesophageal pain. There are three main types of oesophageal pain:

- **Heartburn,** a retrosternal burning discomfort that is often made worse by bending or lying flat.
- **Oesophageal colic,** a severe retrosternal discomfort that is similar to and often indistinguishable from cardiac pain and which may radiate to the neck, jaw or arms.
- **Odynophagia,** a pain that occurs on swallowing.

Is it heartburn?

Heartburn is usually relieved by antacids and may occasionally be accompanied by reflux of bitter or sour fluid into the mouth. More commonly 'waterbrash' occurs. This is a reflex outpouring of saliva which is not specific for acid reflux and may occur in many other upper gastrointestinal disorders. Heartburn may be precipitated by relaxation of the lower oesophageal sphincter caused by alcohol or smoking. Most patients give a clear description of retrosternal burning, which is diagnostic of reflux.

The mechanism by which the normal oesophagogastric sphincter prevents acid reflux is poorly understood. The muscle tone of the lower oesophageal sphincter and the position of the sphincter with relation to the diaphragm are probably both of equal importance. Most patients with reflux symptoms have a hiatus hernia, but the converse does not apply and demonstration that a hiatus hernia is present is itself of little help in diagnosis or management.

INVESTIGATION

If heartburn responds well to symptomatic treatment with antacids there is no need for further investigation. If it cannot be readily controlled by antacids endoscopy should be performed to assess the degree of inflammation endoscopically and histologically.

There is little correlation between severity of heartburnand the extent of mucosal damage, but more vigorous therapies such as anti-reflux surgery should usually be avoided if endoscopy reveals minimal or no inflammation. Columnar epithelialisation of the lower oesophagus is also important to diagnose because of its associated increased risk for adenocarcinoma and is another justification for endoscopy in this group of patients.

A barium swallow examination will demonstrate the presence of a hiatus hernia or strictures, but is poor for assessing inflammation or columnar epithelialisation and is only helpful if the patient complains of dysphagia.

Quantification of acid reflux requires 24-hour pH monitoring and can therefore only be performed on selected patients, particularly any patient being considered for anti-reflux surgery. Interpretation of the results of pH monitoring is contentious. Some regard a fall of pH to 5 or below as significant, while others require a fall to below pH4, and it is still not clear whether duration or frequency of reflux episodes or a combination of the two is the best criterion. Documented evidence of acid reflux should be obtained before recommending anti-reflux surgery.

Is it oesophageal colic?

The distinction between oesophageal colic (spasm) and cardiac pain is one of the most difficult diagnostic problems that confronts the general physician. If the pain only occurs on exercise it is much more likely to be cardiac, but it has to be remembered that oesophageal reflux can also be precipitated by exercise and oesophageal colic is often precipitated by acid reflux.

Antacid therapy is not always effective at preventing oesophageal spasm and nitrates and calcium antagonists are effective in both conditions; therefore therapeutic trial does not help to clarify the diagnosis. The Bernstein acid perfusion test is the traditional way of resolving the problem. 0.1 N HCl is infused at a rate of 6-8 ml/minute via a tube sited in the middle third of the oesophagus. Acid is then

▶ **Endoscopic appearances in oesophagitis**

Symptoms of oesophagitis correlate poorly with endoscopic appearances exchanged for physiological saline without the patient's knowledge. Pain with acid, but not with saline is taken as a positive result. Many normal subjects experience discomfort with the acid infusion however and in any case the oesophageal pain that mimicks cardiac pain is due to spasm rather than acid reflux and the two are not always related.

A barium swallow examination may occasionally be helpful if it shows evidence of one of the more extreme forms of oesophageal dysmotility such as the 'corkscrew' oesophagus. The only logical solution at present seems to be to monitor intra-oesophageal pressure and electrocardiograph (ECG) for long enough for the patient to have experienced at least one spontaneous attack of pain, but this is often impractical. Pain that is associated with non-propagating muscular contraction in the oesophagus with no ECG change can then be assumed to be oesophageal. Such testing is clearly very laborious and is at present only carried out in a few centres and on a minority of patients. It is however more logical and less invasive than turning to coronary angiography early in the patient's diagnostic workup.

A reasonable practical approach is to assume that the pain is oesophageal in origin if the exercise ECG is normal, and treat accordingly with a combination of anti-reflux therapy and an antispasmodic, such as nifedipine.

Is it odynophagia?

Patients with reflux oesophagitis commonly experience some discomfort on swallowing, but intense pain on swallowing is a feature of oesophagitis due to infection with herpes simplex or cytomegalovirus. Endoscopy then reveals small circular or occasionally confluent ulcers and brush cytology shows characteristic inclusions. Treatment with acyclovir hastens a resolution of symptoms.

▶ **Odynophagia**

- Severe pain on swallowing is a feature of herpes or cytomegalovirus oesophagitis

Difficulty with swallowing

Is it globus hystericus?

It is usually possible to distinguish globus hystericus from dysphagia from the history. If a young patient gives a clear description of a constant feeling of a lump in the throat and careful inspection of the pharynx reveals no abnormality no further investigation is required and the patient can be reassured. Globus is a genuine symptom, albeit related to anxiety, and it is not appropriate to suggest that the patient is hysterical. In an older patient it may be more difficult to

distinguish this from cricopharyngeal spasm causing difficulty in initiating deglutition. Watching the patient attempt to drink a glass of water may help to make the diagnosis.

▶ **Globus versus true dysphagia**

- The feeling of a constant lump in the throat (globus) is almost always **functional**
- Difficulty with swallowing (dysphagia) is almost always due to an **organic** cause

Is it dysphagia?

Difficulty with swallowing must always be investigated as it is almost always due to organic disease. The patient's impression of the point where food sticks is a notoriously poor guide to the site of obstruction, but it is usually possible to assess whether the patient has difficulty in initiating deglutition or finds that the food sticks after it has been swallowed.

Is it due to cricopharyngeal dysfunction?

Difficulty in initiating deglutition occasionally occurs in severe anorexia, but usually indicates neuromuscular dysfunction affecting the cricopharyngeal muscle. This sometimes occurs in elderly frail patients without any obvious neurological disease elsewhere, but more commonly results from dysfunction of the bulbar muscles due to bulbar or pseudobulbar palsy or primary neuromuscular diseases such as motor neurone disease, myasthenia gravis or polymyositis.

Long-standing cricopharyngeal dysmotility is thought to be the major factor in the aetiology of pharyngeal pouch. This is a diverticulum arising between the upper border of the cricopharyngeus muscle and the inferior constrictor. If large it may cause dysphagia by compressing the adjacent oesophagus (**Figs 11.1** and **11.2**).

Is there an oesophageal stricture?

The history may give valuable clues to the nature of the obstruction. Dysphagia for solids in the absence of a previous history of heartburn is ominous and likely to be due to a malignant stricture whereas equal difficulty with liquids and solids, possibly associated with a lengthy history of regurgitation (but not heartburn), may suggest achalasia.

ENDOSCOPY OR BARIUM SWALLOW?

It is a very reasonable practice to perform a barium swallow as the initial investigation of dysphagia rather than endoscopy. There are two reasons for this:

- First, an upper oesophageal pouch may present with dysphagia and there is then a risk of perforation if endoscopy is performed particularly if the endoscope is not introduced under direct vision.
- Second, motility problems such as achalasia are very difficult to detect endoscopically as the increased tone at the lower oesophageal sphincter usually causes surprisingly little resistance to passage of the endoscope.

If there is any suggestion of an obstructing lesion on the barium swallow endoscopy should be performed. The endoscope should be introduced into the upper oesophagus under direct vision. Many experienced endoscopists however, perform endoscopy as the initial investigation, always taking care to introduce the endoscope into the upper oesophagus under direct vision.

Lesions that may be present include:

- An upper oesophageal web.
- A caustic stricture.
- A peptic stricture.
- A malignant stricture.
- A benign tumour.
- Achalasia.
- A Schatzki ring.

Upper oesophageal web

Webs are seen more often on barium swallow examination than by endoscopy and this discrepancy has not been adequately explained (Fig. 11.3). Localised spasm may account for some of the apparent webs seen on radiography. Endoscopically a web appears as a thin fibrous structure in the upper third of the oesophagus, and can easily be broken by the endoscope so is often missed if the endoscope is not passed under direct vision.

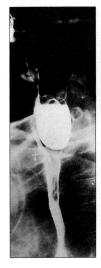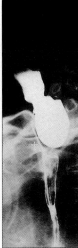

Fig. 11.1 Serial barium swallow in a patient with a pharyngeal pouch. This is usually associated with cricopharyngeal spasm.

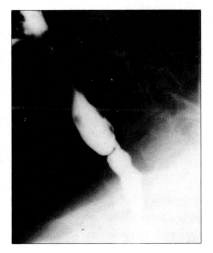

Fig. 11.3 Barium swallow showing oesophageal web in a patient with chronic iron deficiency.

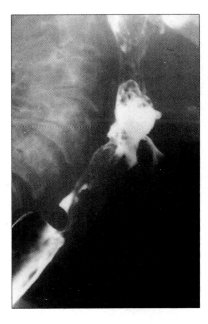

Fig. 11.2 Barium swallow demonstrating cricopharyngeal spasm.

Caustic stricture

Strictures resulting from accidental or deliberate ingestion of caustic substances are usually sited in the upper oesophagus and may be distinguished from peptic strictures by the presence of squamous mucosa below the stricture (**Figs 11.4** and **11.5**).

Peptic stricture

Peptic strictures can usually be recognised by the presence of circumferential slough. If they can be passed by the endoscope either with or without prior dilatation columnar epithelium (which has a deeper colour than squamous epithelium) can be recognised below the stricture, usually in association with a hiatus hernia (**Fig. 11.6**).

It must be emphasised though that benign and malignant strictures cannot be reliably distinguished by appearances alone. Biopsy samples should always be taken, but it may be difficult reliably to biopsy the relevant site because of the tangential approach. It is therefore particularly important to take multiple biopsies and brush cytology in addition. Cytology is more useful if performed before biopsy to avoid heavy contamination of smears by blood clot.

It is surprisingly uncommon to find a patient with peptic oesophageal stricturing who has intact incisor teeth. This presumably reflects either erosion of the teeth by long-standing acid reflux or possibly some as yet undiscovered defect in the saliva of patients with peptic stricturing.

Scleroderma

It is important to inspect the mouth for evidence of **scleroderma (systemic sclerosis)** or its milder variant the **CREST syndrome** where:

- C is dermal **C**alcinosis.
- R is **R**aynaud's sydrome.
- E is o**E**sophagitis.
- S is **S**clerodactyly.
- T is **T**elangiectasia.

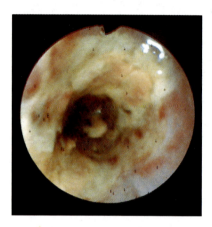

Fig. 11.4 Caustic oesophagitis resulting from inadvertent swallowing of denture-cleaning fluid

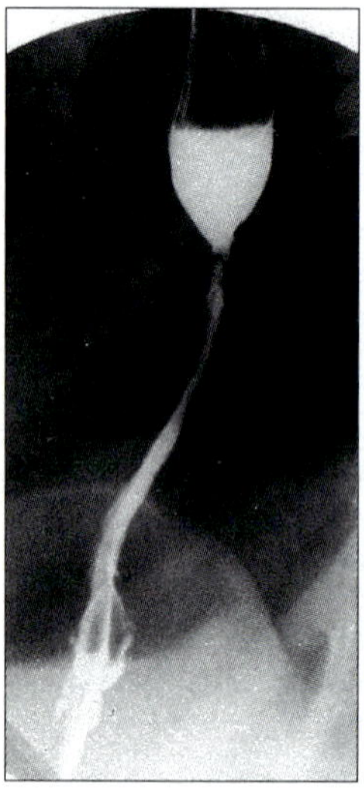

Fig. 11.5 Barium meal showing caustic oesophageal stricture (same patient as in Fig. 11.4).

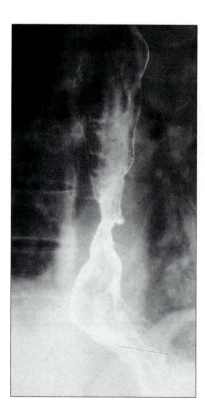

Fig. 11.6 Barium meal showing a benign stricture and an ulcer above a hiatus hernia.

It is very commonly associated with oesophageal dysmotility, oesophageal shortening with sliding hiatus hernia formation and severe oesophageal reflux.

Malignant stricture

Malignant strictures often have a fleshy irregular polypoid appearance with friable mucosa, but less slough than is seen in association with peptic strictures (**Fig. 11.7**).

Tumours may occur at any level in the oesophagus. The majority are squamous carcinomas. Although adenocarcinomas involving the lower oesophagus are not uncommon the majority of these arise from the gastric fundus. Because of this there are conflicting reports of the frequency of true adenocarcinoma of the oesophagus, some sources quoting figures as low as 5% for the proportion of true oesophageal carcinomas that are adenomatous. Invasion of the oesophagus by carcinoma of the left bronchus or from malignant mediastinal nodes is not uncommon.

Benign tumours

Benign tumours are rare and include leiomyomas, lipomas and lymphangiomas.

Achalasia

Achalasia produces subtle changes on endoscopy. There is usually only little or no resistance to passage of the endoscope through the cardia and greater difficulty in the absence of any mucosal abnormality should raise the suspicion of external compression by a low mediastinal tumour. Careful examination may show absence of peristalsis in achalasia. If the achalasia has been long-standing the oesophagus may be grossly dilated and contain a large residue of undigested food (**Fig. 11.8**).

Schatzki ring

A Schatzki ring appears similar to an upper oesophageal web, but is always sited in the lower oesophagus (**Fig. 11.9**). It is a fibromuscular ring occurring at the point where diaphragmatic fibres wrap around the oesophagus usually at the upper margin of a small hiatus hernia. It only extends about 2 mm into the lumen, but may cause bolus obstruction if the food is not well chewed.

Diagnosing oesophageal rupture

The sudden onset of epigastric pain and shock occurring shortly after vomiting suggest acute rupture of the oesophagus, first described by Boerhaave in 1724. The patient is usually a male who has just eaten a heavy meal. Profuse pallor, cyanosis, dyspnoea and sweating occur and signs of mediastinal air become apparent within a few hours (**Fig. 11.10**). These include crepitation over the chest wall and neck and there may be a systolic 'crunch' audible on auscultation over the heart. Rapid diagnosis is very important as mediastinitis with an associated high mortality inevitably follows.

A plain chest radiograph will show mediastinal air and a barium or gastrograffin swallow should be performed to determine the site of the perforation. A water-soluble

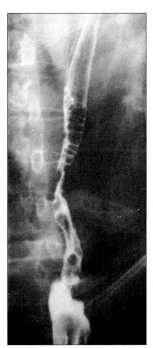

Fig. 11.7 A typically irregular stricture due to squamous carcinoma of the oesophagus.

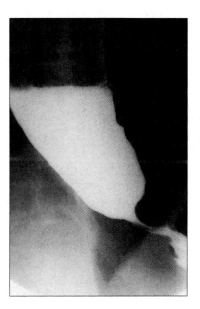

Fig. 11.8 Barium meal in a patient with achalasia showing the dilated oesophagus, the smooth beak-like stricture and absence of hiatus hernia.

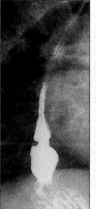
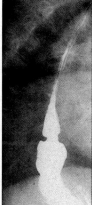

Fig. 11.9 Serial barium meal showing a Schatzki ring. This is a fibromuscular ring which is usually seen (as here) in association with a sliding hiatus hernia. Bolus obstruction may result if meat is not carefully chewed.

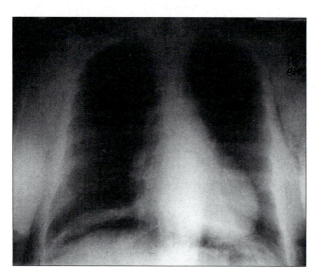

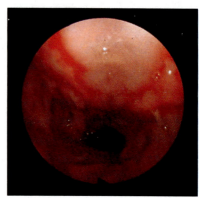

Fig. 11.11 Endoscopic appearances of severe reflux oesophagitis.

Fig. 11.10 Mediastinal emphysema and subdiaphragmatic gas following visceral perforation. It is most important to avoid feeding any patient with suspected oesophageal perforation until the diagnosis has been excluded as ingestion of food will almost always result in mediastinal sepsis with a high morbidity and mortality.

contrast agent such as gastrograffin is probably preferable as barium may cause an inflammatory reaction, but conversely, if the diagnosis is uncertain and inhalation of the contrast is a possibility water soluble contrast is less safe because it causes a vigorous pneumonitis if inhaled.

CONDITIONS CAUSING OESOPHAGEAL PAIN AND DIFFICULTY WITH SWALLOWING: NATURAL HISTORY AND MANAGEMENT

Oesophagitis

Aetiology and pathogenesis
Reflux oesophagitis is commonly termed 'peptic' although it is unclear what the major damaging factor is: acid, bile or pepsin being the main candidates (**Fig. 11.11**). Although antacids and sometimes even histamine H_2 receptor antagonists are relatively ineffective at treating reflux oesophagitis the proton pump inhibitors such as omeprazole and lansoprazole, which are extremely potent inhibitors of acid secretion, have been shown to be very effective therapy for oesophagitis. This suggests that acid is a major factor although its presence may just be ensuring an optimal pH (ie below pH 4.5) for peptic activity rather than having a directly damaging effect.

The reasons why some people suffer from excessive reflux are also unclear. Two factors which seem particularly important are a low pressure at the lower oesophageal sphincter and the presence of a hiatus hernia, but the relative importance of these is uncertain. Although almost all patients with endoscopic evidence of oesophagitis have a hiatus hernia, so do approximately 35% of asymptomatic people while there is only a poor correlation between randomly measured lower sphincter pressure and reflux symptoms.

A small minority of patients have a congenitally short oesophagus. This usually occurs in association with a hiatus hernia, but there may just be columnar epithelium extending up the lower oesophagus without a hiatus hernia. In either case severe reflux symptoms and even stricturing may occur in early childhood.

Reflux symptoms are extremely common in pregnancy possibly due either to raised intraabdominal pressure or hormonal effects on lower sphincter pressure. Oesophageal involvement by scleroderma causes particularly severe reflux combined with dysmotility resulting in oesophageal stricturing, dilatation and an increased risk for oesophageal cancer.

Many drugs reduce lower sphincter pressure and provoke reflux. These include alcohol, tobacco, and xanthine derivatives contained in coffee and chocolate as well as medicinal theophylline.

Management
Gravity is clearly a major factor in the cause of reflux and some benefit results from following a few simple guidelines. Much of the problem occurs at night and elevation of the head of the bed by 20 cm has been shown to have a beneficial effect. Overweight patients should try to lose weight and not wear tight clothing around the waist. Drugs such as alcohol, tobacco and coffee, which relax the lower oesophageal sphincter should be avoided. Although these methods bring some relief, in most patients some form of drug therapy is required (**Fig. 11.12**).

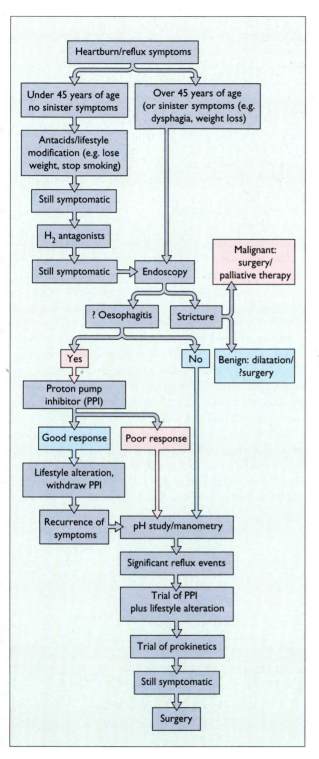

Fig. 11.12 Algorithm showing the management of heartburn.

DRUG THERAPY

Antacids

Most patients with intermittent heartburn can be adequately treated with antacids. It may be more convenient to take these in the form of chewable tablets that can be taken whenever symptoms occur. Some preparations combine antacid with the seaweed derivative sodium alginate. This helps to form a poorly soluble 'raft,' which floats on top of the gastric juice, the principle being that this will result in coating of the oesophagus whenever reflux occurs. These preparations are effective and easy to take although there is little evidence that they work better than antacids alone.

Histamine H$_2$ receptor antagonists

Although antacids are quite good at relieving heartburn they have little effect on oesophagitis. If patients still have unacceptably frequent symptoms despite antacid therapy endoscopy should be performed. The next step will be to prescribe histamine H$_2$ receptor antagonists, but because the course of therapy will probably have to be prolonged it is preferable to assess the extent of inflammation first. Histamine H$_2$ receptor antagonists are relatively much less effective in treating oesophagitis than in duodenal ulceration. Higher doses are often necessary (e.g ranitidine, 300 mg twice daily, or cimetidine, 800 mg twice or even four times daily). Once daily treatment is often inadequate.

Drugs that raise lower oesophageal sphincter pressure

Metoclopramide has been tried on the grounds that it raises lower oesophageal sphincter pressure, but it seems to have no additional therapeutic effect when prescribed with H$_2$ receptor antagonists and has a much poorer side-effect profile (particularly involuntary facial movements, which may not always reverse on stopping therapy).

Domperidone is another dopamine antagonist, which raises lower oesophageal sphincter pressure, stimulates peristalsis and speeds gastric emptying. It does not pass the blood brain barrier and the risk of extrapyramidal side-effects is low. Cisapride has similar effects, but works via a different mechanism, possibly facilitation of release of acetyl choline at nerve endings in the myenteric plexus. Cisapride seems to be at least as effective as metoclopramide, has fewer side-effects and may be a useful alternative or adjunct to histamine H$_2$ receptor antagonist therapy.

Proton pump inhibitors

Omeprazole, a substituted benzimidazole , acts as a proton pump inhibitor (i.e. by inhibiting the K$^+$/H$^+$ transporting adenosine triphosphatase in the parietal cells). It causes almost total suppression of acid output and this class of drug is without doubt the most effective drug for treating reflux oesophagitis (in doses of 20–40 mg daily). This may reflect the fact that it is necessary to raise the intragastric pH above 4.5 to inactivate pepsin. There was initially some anxiety about the long-term use of proton pump inhibitors because of reports that high doses cause carcinoid tumours in experimental animals as a result of stimulation by the elevated gastrin. They have, however, been used for many years now in patients with Zollinger–Ellison syndrome without any reported problems. There must remain some anxiety however about the wisdom of embarking on long-term therapy in young patients who may need treatment for decades. A reasonable compromise is to recommend that the patient has frequent drug 'holidays' (e.g. one month off in three) when less potent acid-suppressing medication is used.

Other medical therapies

Sucralfate, an aluminium hydroxide salt of sucrose-octasulphate, is designed to act by coating ulcerated mucosa thus providing an acid buffering layer. It has an efficacy roughly similar to H_2 receptor antagonists. Anxieties about aluminium accumulation preclude long term maintenance.

ANTI-REFLUX SURGERY

If medical therapy fails to produce satisfactory relief of symptoms or healing of ulceration then anti-reflux surgery should be considered. Unfortunately the wide range of surgical procedures reflects the fact that none of them is totally satisfactory. Some such as the Belsey procedure are performed via a thoracic approach, while others such as the Nissen procedure are performed via an abdominal approach.

The aim is generally to wrap (plicate) the fundus of the stomach around the lower oesophagus. Mortality is vey low (< 1%), but none of these procedures are minor and early complications, which affect about 10% include pleural effusions, wound infection and rarely gastric or oesophageal perforation. Dysphagia may result if the plication is too tight and occurs as a temporary feature in about 50%. Recurrence of reflux symptoms only affects about 10% in some series, but up to 50% in others followed over a 10-year period. In some centres anti-reflux procedures are being performed laparoscopically, but occasional major complications and even deaths have resulted and further studies are required before the overall success of this approach can be assessed.

It follows that the decision to undertake anti-reflux surgery should not be taken lightly. Suitable patients should be relatively young, have endoscopic evidence of significant mucosal damage, should usually have documented acid reflux and should have failed to respond to a trial of vigorous medical therapy, which should include at least three months treatment with high dose H_2 receptor antagonists or proton pump blockers. Patients with scleroderma or CREST syndrome should not be treated surgically because they have a generalised motility problem in addition to reflux and are likely to develop severe dysphagia after anti-reflux surgery.

Barrett's oesophagus

Columnar epithelialisation of the lower oesophagus was first described over 40 years ago by Barrett, but there is still considerable argument about its definition, aetiology and prognostic significance. The columnar epithelium normally extends up to 3 cm above the gastro-oesophageal sphincter, but extension above 3–5 cm is abnormal and is found in 10–16% of patients with reflux oesophagitis.

Argument about the precise limit of normal is of little clinical importance since the most worrying association with Barrett's oesophagus, the development of adenocarcinoma, is only significantly associated with extension of columnar epithelium 8 cm or more above the gastro-oesophageal junction (**Figs 11.13 and 11.14**).

Patients with extensive columnar epithelialisation of the lower oesophagus should probably be screened by annual endoscopy and multiple biopsies taken to exclude dysplasia or carcinoma although there is some anxiety about the effectiveness of this approach and studies have often failed to take into account the risk of commoner conditions such as colon cancer in this group of patients. Smokers and patients with intestinal-type rather than gastric-type metaplasia of the oesophagus are at particular risk of developing adenocarcinoma (**Figs 11.15 and 11.16**).

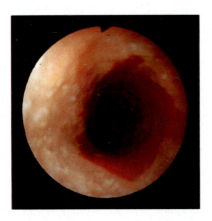

Fig. 11.13 Endoscopic appearances of Barrett's oesophagus in a patient with long-standing oesophageal reflux. Columnar epithelium (dark pink) is seen extending up the lower oesophagus.

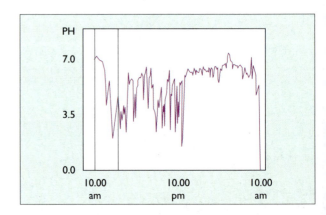

Fig. 11.14 24-hour oesophageal pH recording. Numerous episodes of acid reflux are seen in the first half of the recording (up until 10 p.m.).

Drug therapy usually has little or no effect on the degree of columnar epithelialisation although may possibly slow its rate of advance however the proton pump inhibitors have not been fully evaluated in this respect.

Peptic oesophageal stricture

Fibreoptic endoscopy has transformed the management of benign oesophageal stricturing. Dilatation can be carried out under intravenous sedation as a five-minute procedure.

A guide wire is passed under endoscopic control through the stricture, the endoscope is removed and a dilator passed over the guide wire. The dilator is usually either a metal olive shaped flexible rod or a tapering plastic rod and produces dilatation to a diameter of about 15 mm. The procedure is extremely safe and perforation is rare providing that care is taken to be certain that the guide wire is correctly sited. If there is any uncertainty about this the procedure should be done under X-ray control. Balloon dilators can also be used, but arguably have a higher rate of complications.

Most patients will eventually develop a recurrence of the stricture, but the timing of this is very variable being anything from a few weeks to years. The simplest approach to this is to ask the patient to contact directly when symptoms recur so that repeat dilatation can be organised without delay.

Caustic stricture

If a patient is seen shortly after accidental or deliberate ingestion of corrosives a poison centre should first be consulted if the nature of the swallowed fluid is known.

If the fluid is caustic, but not highly toxic systemically it may be better to avoid gastric lavage. A large bore nasogastric tube should be inserted to maintain oesophageal patency and a proton pump inhibitor should be administered. An urgent ENT opinion should be sought if there is any suspicion of laryngeal damage as emergency tracheostomy may be required.

If stricturing develops it is usually in the upper third of the oesophagus. It may be very severe with an intense fibrous reaction. Initial treatment when the inflammation has settled (usually after 2–3 weeks) should be endoscopic dilatation, but surgical resection and reconstruction may eventually be required.

Traumatic stricture

The commonest cause of a traumatic stricture is inappropriately prolonged use of a large bore nasogastric tube. Reflux occurs alongside the tube and severe damage may occur within 5–10 days.

The best policy is avoidance of this problem, but if stricturing has occurred it should be treated by endoscopic dilatation initially, although surgical excision and reconstruction may again be required if it is severe.

Stricturing also develops not infrequently following endoscopic sclerotherapy for oesophageal varices, but can usually be treated fairly easily by endoscopic dilatation.

Anastomotic stricture

Anastomotic strictures may be seen after total gastrectomy and oesophago-jejunostomy for gastric cancer or after oesophageal transection for emergency treatment of oesophageal varices. They can usually be safely dilated using a balloon dilator. Use of the bougie-type of dilator is usually unwise, partly because of the traction placed on the anastomosis and also because there is likely to be inadequate room beyond the stricture for safe passage of the bougie.

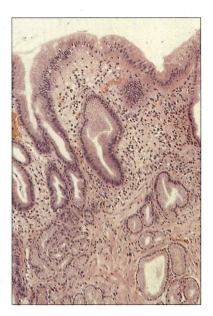

Fig. 11.15 Barrett's oesophagitis with gastric-type metaplasia. This carries very little increased risk for malignancy.

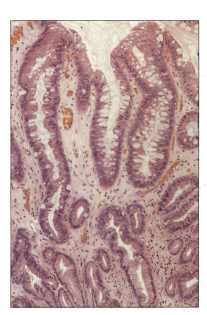

Fig. 11.16 Barrett's oesophagitis with intestinal-type metaplasia (note goblet cells). This carries a considerable risk for malignancy, particularly if the patient is a smoker.

Infective oesophagitis

Cytomegalovirus and herpes simplex may both cause oesophageal ulcers, either separate aphthoid ulcers or confluent ulceration. This may occur either as a result of primary infection or as a result of reactivation in an immunocompromised individual. Very severe pain on swallowing (odynophagia) may result and may prevent an adequate intake of fluids. A cause of immunodeficiency such as human immunodeficiency virus (HIV) infection should be sought and antiviral therapy commenced with intravenous acyclovir. This usually brings about impressive relief of symptoms within 24-48 hours.

Extensive oesophageal candidiasis can be very difficult to eradicate (**Fig. 11.17**). Oral nystatin or amphotericin should be tried initially. Inspection of the mouth is a poor guide to response as there is often a marked discrepancy between the degree of oral and oesophageal involvement. Systemic therapy may be needed particularly if there is evidence of *Candida* septicaemia; however, this will usually require intravenous amphotericin, which is highly nephrotoxic and should only be used when clearly indicated. Fluconazole may be used as a less toxic alternative, but is probably less effective in *Candida* septicaemia.

Achalasia

Natural history

Dysphagia for liquids and solids results and in some patients there may be episodes of severe pain due to spasm ('vigorous achalasia'). The oesophagus may gradually dilate to a very marked degree and regurgitation is a common feature and may result in recurrent inhalational pneumonia.

Aetiology and pathogenesis

Achalasia is a condition of unknown aetiology in which there is a marked reduction in the number of Auerbach's

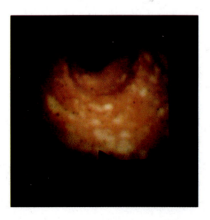

Fig. 11.17
Endoscopic appearances of *Candida* oesophagitis. Such appearance suggests the possible presence of human immunodeficiency virus (HIV) infection.

ganglion cells in the lower oesophagus. Heightened response to intravenous injection of synthetic acetylcholine (Mecholyl) is supportive evidence of denervation hypersensitivity. A similar end result is seen in **Chaga's disease**, a disease that occurs in Latin America as a result of infection with *Trypanosoma cruzi*. The two main consequences are:

- Disordered peristalsis.
- Lack of the normal relaxation of the lower oesophageal sphincter.

▶ **Features of achalasia**

- Dysphagia for solids and liquids
- Lack of heartburn
- Inability to belch
- Regurgitation common
- No mucosal abnormality
- Endoscope passes easily into the stomach
- Lack of organised peristalsis
- High lower oesophageal sphincter pressure

Management

Treatment is aimed at reducing lower oesophageal sphincter pressure. Drug therapy with calcium antagonists (e.g. sublingual nifedipine, 20 mg before meals) is sometimes effective in milder achalasia, but dilatation is usually required.

Dilatation is performed using a pneumatic balloon, which has a fixed maximum diameter of approximately 3 cm. The balloon is placed across the cardia under X-ray screening and inflated. A waist can be seen in the middle of the balloon when it is correctly sited and further inflation abolishes this waist. Full dilatation is maintained for about one minute and the balloon deflated. Reflation of the balloon then shows that the waist has been abolished. The treatment is successful in approximately 75% of patients and may be repeated if symptoms recur. Perforation is a serious complication that occurs in less than 2% of patients.

Surgical treatment should now be reserved for patients who have failed to respond to balloon dilatation and consists of longitudinal incision of the muscle coats around the lower oesophageal sphincter (Heller's procedure) This carries an appreciable risk of causing oesophageal reflux so most surgeons routinely perform an anti-reflux procedure at the same time.

▶ **Achalasia or 'pseudoachalasia': a diagnostic trap**

Radiological and manometric features of achalasia can be mimicked by carcinoma at the cardia

Oesophageal spasm

Painful oesophageal spasm may occur in association with generalised disorders of oesophageal motility such as achalasia, but is more often an intermittent event, the oesophageal motility returning to normal between attacks. Oesophageal reflux is a common aetiological factor (**Figs 11.18–11.21**).

Management

If reflux is present then treatment should initially be aimed at suppressing it. Various drug therapies have been tried for the spasm itself including anticholinergics, nitrates, hydralazine and nifedipine. Of these nifedipine, 20 mg sublingually before meals, is probably the most effective. Its effect lasts for approximately 60 minutes.

Cricopharyngeal spasm and oesophageal pouch

Cricopharyngeal spasm and oesophageal pouch are closely related. A pouch occurs as a pulsion diverticulum between the upper fibres of the cricopharyngeus and the lower fibres

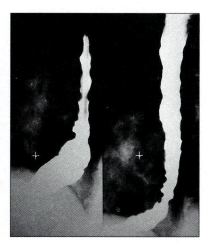

Fig. 11.18 Barium swallow in a patient with diffuse oesophageal spasm.

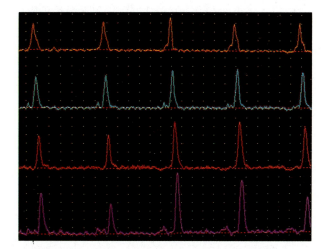

Fig. 11.19 Normal oesophageal motility. The four pressure recorders are sited at 5 cm intervals from orange (upper trace) down to purple (lower trace) in the body of the oesophagus. The horizontal gaps between the dots indicate five second intervals. Peristaltic waves are seen to progress normally down the oesophagus. Courtesy of T Norris.

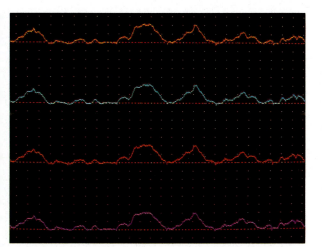

Fig. 11.20 Oesophageal motility in achalasia. Simultaneous (i.e. non-propagating) broad, low-amplitude contractions are seen without any normal peristalsis. Courtesy of T Norris.

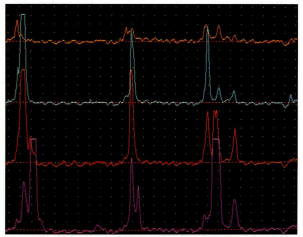

Fig. 11.21 Oesophageal motility in diffuse oesophageal spasm. Simultaneous prolonged contractions are seen that last up to 15 seconds (normal peristaltic waves last up to four seconds). Courtesy of T Norris.

of the inferior constrictor. As it fills dysphagia results from compression of the adjacent oesophagus. Regurgitation then produces relief of the dysphagia.

Management
Treatment is surgical and includes cricopharyngeal myotomy. The pouch is of secondary importance, but may be excised or invaginated. Cricopharyngeal myotomy is also beneficial in approximately 50% of patients with cricopharyngeal spasm due to neuromuscular disorders such as **motor neurone disease** and **Parkinsonism**, but selection of patients who are likely to benefit is very difficult. In many patients with neuromuscular disorders, dysphagia is due to incoordination of the tongue rather than cricopharyngeal spasm.

Other forms of oesophageal diverticula
Diverticula may also occur in the mid oesophagus as a result of traction by adjacent tuberculous mediastinal lymph nodes or as an epiphrenic diverticulum occurring as a pulsion diverticulum in the lower oesophagus in association with motility disorders. Rarely multiple tiny diverticula in the mid or lower oesophagus may also be seen in association with motility disorders (**Fig. 11.22**). These forms of diverticula do not usually require treatment.

Oesophageal web
Plummer–Vinson (Kelly–Patterson) syndrome has become extremely rare. It describes the association between longstanding iron deficiency and the development of atrophy and fibrous narrowing of the upper entry to the oesophagus with a high risk for later development of post cricoid carcinoma.

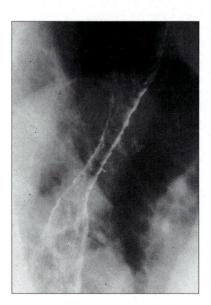

Fig. 11.22 Barium swallow showing intramural diverticulosis. The significance of this is unclear, but it is presumed to be the result of altered motility.

The appearance of a web is still seen quite commonly on barium swallow examinations, but endoscopy of these patients usually fails to show any mucosal abnormality and the appearances presumably result from spasm. When a web is present it may easily be missed unless the endoscope is passed under direct vision as it is easily broken down by passage of the endoscope.

Management
Biopsies should be taken and endoscopy repeated after a period of iron supplementation.

Schatzki ring
Schatzki's ring occurs in the lower oesophagus, probably always in association with a small hiatus hernia. They are thought to represent fibromuscular attachments running up from the diaphragm. They extend only about 2 mm into the lumen and are usually an incidental finding on barium swallow examination, but may cause bolus obstruction if unchewed meat is swallowed.

Management
A Schatzki ring can sometimes be split by endoscopic dilatation, but is often relatively resistant to dilatation and it may be necessary for the patient to continue to take care to chew well before swallowing.

Hiatus hernia
Hiatus hernia is notoriously overrated as a condition by the lay public and is often a cause of inappropriate chronic invalidity. Over 30% of asymptomatic people have a hiatus hernia. Hiatus hernias may be either sliding or rolling. Sliding hernias are commoner and are associated with symptomatic reflux in about 50%.

Treatment is aimed at the reflux and is not affected by the presence of or size of the hernia.

Rolling hiatus hernia and gastric volvulus
Rolling or paraoesophageal hernias cause dysphagia rather than reflux. If large they are invariably associated with some degree of gastric volvulus. This may be organo-axial, mesenteroaxial, or a combination of the two.

- In mesentero-axial volvulus the antrum rotates upwards to lie above and to the left of the fundus.
- In organo-axial volvulus the greater curve rotates upwards to lie above and to the right of the lesser curve (**Figs 11.23** and **11.24**).

▶ **Frequency of hiatus hernia**

Over 30% of asymptomatic adults have a hiatus hernia demonstrable on head-down tilt

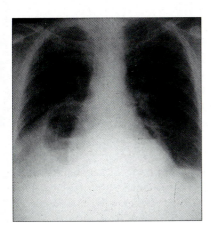

Fig. 11.23 Chest radiograph of a patient with a large diaphragmatic defect resulting in a rolling hiatus hernia. A rolling hernia of this size is usually associated with some degree of gastric volvulus, which should usually be surgically corrected and fixed providing the patient is sufficiently fit

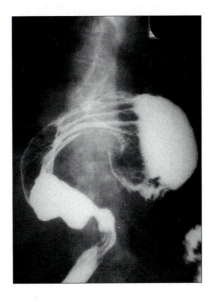

Fig. 11.24 Barium meal demonstrating organo-axial gastric volvulus within a rolling hiatus hernia.

Many patients are asymptomatic, but chronic discomfort, bloating, wind and embarrassingly loud borborygmi may occur. The most serious consequence is acute gastric strangulation. This presents as violent retching that tends to be unproductive, severe epigastric pain and shock. Mortality is about 50%.

MANAGEMENT

Surgery is often recommended whenever a large rolling hiatus hernia with associated gastric volvulus is diagnosed because of the high mortality associated with acute gastric strangulation, but many of the patients are elderly and it is unclear how high the risk of subsequent gastric strangulation is in patients with little or no symptoms.

▶ **Symptoms of rolling hiatus hernia**

Rolling hiatus hernias cause bloating and dysphagia, but not reflux

Oesophageal cancer

Natural history

Dysphagia is often very severe or total and not always easy to palliate. Even if the primary tumour can be successfully removed secondary spread occurs in at least 65% of patients.

The tumour may erode into other mediastinal structures resulting in oesophagobronchial fistulas with recurrent pneumonia or fistulation into the aorta with rapid exsanguination. Dysphagia, anorexia and weight loss are almost invariable, but severe pain usually indicates extension of tumour outside the wall of the oesophagus.

Non-metastatic manifestations include hypercalcaemia and ectopic ACTH production, but are uncommon.

Aetiology and pathogenesis

Oesophageal cancer is associated with smoking and heavy alcohol intake, particularly in combination. Epidemiological studies carried out in areas of high incidence in China have suggested the importance of dietary factors including a high intake of nitrates and vitamin C deficiency. Other factors include previous caustic stricturing, habitual ingestion of hot tea, exposure to ionising radiation and achalasia.

Management

Cancer of the oesophagus is a depressing disease. Five-year survival is about 3–5% and has been affected little by therapy.

CURATIVE THERAPY

Total cure can probably never be achieved by chemotherapy or radiotherapy alone although some centres have reported occasional cures (< 5%) with radiotherapy. Results for surgery are disappointing, but patients who survive clearance of macroscopic tumour have been reported as having five-year survivals of 6–35%.

Only about 30-50% of patients have resectable tumours and operative mortality averages approximately 10%. Careful preoperative screening is essential to define the patients who are likely to benefit from surgery. This should include liver ultrasound or CT scanning and chest radiography as a preliminary screen. Suspicious hepatic lesions should be biopsied. Histological proof of liver metastases is an obvious contraindication to resection. Tumours over 6 cm in length are also unlikely to be resectable.

Studies are still in progress to determine whether resectability can be better defined by using endoscopic ultrasound to assess depth of tumour invasion. In this technique an ultrasound probe is introduced endoscopically into the lumen of the tumour and gives a cross sectional view of the surrounding tissue, which allows an estimate of the depth of tumour invasion.

CT scanning has proved disappointing as a guide to assessing mediastinal involvement, but is useful to screen for lung or liver metastases. Lung function should be assessed by spirometry and blood gas analysis as severe chronic lung disease precludes transthoracic resection.

Low oesophageal adenocarcinomas, which are usually arising from the gastric fundus are often resectable via a trans-abdominal approach and have a relatively low operative mortality, however cure rates are if anything slightly worse than for mid oesophageal squamous tumours.

Surgical techniques vary considerably, but most surgeons are now bringing up the stomach for anastomosis rather than fashioning a new oesophagus from the left hemicolon.

PALLIATIVE THERAPY

If resection is not thought to be feasible or appropriate then palliation may be necessary to establish a lumen. It is now generally agreed that palliative oesophageal surgery should be avoided if at all possible as it has a mortality of about 30% and equally good palliation can be achieved non-surgically. Options include endoscopic intubation, radiotherapy and laser photocoagulation.

Endoscopic intubation

Endoscopic intubation requires a preliminary dilatation. This is more hazardous than dilatation of benign strictures and perforation rates of about 10% are reported. Providing the oesophageal tube is satisfactorily sited across the tear it usually seals off with conservative management. The same technique can also be used to cover a tracheo-oesophageal fistula, which may occur as a very unpleasant result of tumour erosion.

Endoprosthetic tubes come in a variety of lengths and diameters and are usually made from latex or silicone rubber. Tube placement is carried out under X-ray control and the tube is advanced over a guide wire, which has been sited endoscopically. The procedure can be carried out under heavy intravenous sedation.

The palliation achieved by a tube is variable. A satisfactory result is achieved in about 65% of patients. The patient should be instructed to chew food thoroughly or preferably to make sure that it has been minced. Intermittent draughts of a fizzy drink taken throughout meals help to ensure patency. Problems include slippage of the tube, overgrowth by tumour, obstruction by food and oesophageal reflux (particularly if the tube is placed across the cardia). Intubation is not suitable for high tumours as it results in constant discomfort due to awareness of the upper end of the tube (**Figs 11.25 and 11.26**). Promising results are being obtained with expanding metal stents, which achieve a wider lumen, at least initially.

Radiotherapy

Radiotherapy produces variable results. Initially oedema may result in worsening dysphagia and the patient should be intubated first if the lumen is already narrow. Oesophago-bronchial fistula is also more common after radiotherapy. Studies are currently being performed to assess intraluminal radiotherapy using [192]-iridium wire, which may allow better localisation of the therapy.

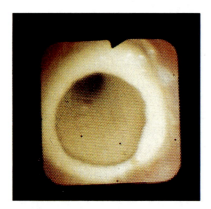

Fig. 11.25 Endoscopic view of a Celestin (Atkinson) tube in place through a malignant oesophageal stricture. Well-chewed food can usually be swallowed well, but frequent use of fizzy drinks during meals is advisable to prevent blockage.

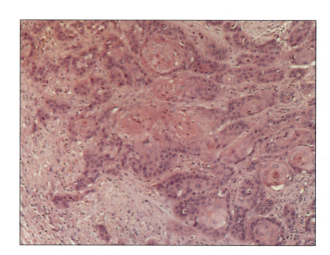

Fig. 11.26 Histological appearances of squamous cell carcinoma of the oesophagus. Nuclei are large and dark staining, and there is a high nucleus to cytoplasm ratio.

Laser therapy

Laser therapy is arguably the best form of palliative therapy currently available. The laser beam is used to burn a channel through the tumour after previous dilatation. The best results

are obtained with exophytic polypoid tumours rather than circumferential stricturing. Repeated therapy is required however and there is probably no prolongation of life.

FURTHER READING

Oesophageal diseases (general)

Dachman AH, Levine MS. Radiology of the esophagus. *Gastroenterol Clin North Am* 1991; **20** (4): 635–58.

Dancygier H. Endoscopic ultrasonography of the upper gastrointestinal tract. *Ballieres Clin Gastroenterol* 1991; **5** (1): 19–36.

Edwards LL, Quigley EM, Pfeiffer RF. Gastrointestinal dysfunction in Parkinson's disease: frequency and pathophysiology. *Neurology* 1992; **42** (4): 726–32.

Fulp SR, Castell DO. Scleroderma esophagus. *Dysphagia* 1990; **5** (4): 204–10.

Gorman RC, Morris JB, Kaiser LR. Esophageal disease in the elderly patient. *Surg Clin North Am* 1994; **74**: 93–112.

Richter JE. Investigation and management of non-cardiac chest pain. *Ballieres Clin Gastroenterol* 1991; **5** (2): 281–306.

Tytgat GN, Tio TL. Esophageal ultrasonography. *Gastroenterol Clin North Am* 1991: **20** (4): 659–71.

Barrett's oesophagus

Armstrong D. Reflux disease and Barrett's oesophagus. *Endoscopy* 1994; **26**: 9–19.

Bernstein IT, Kruse P, Andersen IB. Barrett's oesophagus. *Dig Dis Sci* 1994; **12**: 98–115.

Hassall E. Barrett's esophagus: congential or acquired? *Am J Gastroenterol* 1993; **88** (6): 819–24.

Phillips RW, Wong RK. Barrett's esophagus. Natural history, incidence, etiology and complications. *Gastroenterol Clin North Am* 1991; **20** (4): 791–816.

Gastroesophageal reflux

de Caestecker JS, Heading RC. Esophageal pH monitoring. *Gastroenterol Clin North Am* 1990; **19** (3): 645–69.

DeVault KR, Castell DO. Current diagnosis and treatment of gastroeesophageal reflux disease. *Mayo Clin Proc* 1994; **69**: 867–76.

Frierson HF Jr. Histology in the diagnosis of reflux esophagitis. *Gastroenterol Clin North Am* 1990; **19** (3): 631–44.

Goldstein JL, Schlesinger PK, Mozwecz HL, Layden TJ. Esophageal mucosal resistance. A factor in esophagitis. *Gastroenterol Clin North Am* 1990: **19** (3): 563–86.

Hill LD, Aye RW, Ramel S. Antireflux surgery. A surgeon's look. *Gastroenterol Clin North Am* 1990; **19** (3): 745–75.

Holloway RH, Dent J. Pathophysiology of gastroesophageal reflux. Lower esophageal sphincter dysfunction in gastroesophageal refllux disease. *Gastroenterol Clin North Am* 1990; **19** (3): 517–35.

Katz PO. Pathogenesis and management of gastroesophageal reflux disease. *J Clin Gastroenetrol* 1991; **13** (2): S6–15.

Orlando RC. Esophageal epithelial defence against acid injury. *J Clin Gastroenterol* 1991; **13** (2): S1–5.

Pope CE. Acid reflux disorders. *N Engl J Med* 1994; **331**: 656–60.

Ramirez B, Richter JE. Revies article: promotility drugs in the treatment of gastro-oesophageal reflux disease. *Aliment Pharmacol Ther* 1993; **7** (1): 5–20.

Stoker DL, Williams JG. Alkaline reflux oesophagitis. *Gut* 1991; **32** (10): 1090–2.

Traube M. The spectrum of the symptoms and presentations of gastroesophageal reflux disease. *Gastroenterol Clin North Am* 1990; **19** (3): 671–82.

Wu WC. Ancillary tests in the diagnosis of gastroesophageal reflux disease. *Gastroenterol Clin North Am* 1990; **19** (3): 671–82.

Achalasia and motility disorders

Atkinson M. Antecedents of achalasia. *Gut* 1994; **35**: 861–2.

Farr CM. Achalasia: new thoughts on an old disease [editorial]. *J Clin Gastroenterol Clin North Am* 1989; **18** (2): 195–222.

McCord GS, Staiano A, Clouse RE. Achalasia, diffuse spasm and non-specific motor disorders. *Ballieres Clin Gastroenterol* 1991; **5** (2): 307–35.

Nelson JB, Richter JE. Upper esophageal motility disorders. *Gastroenterol Clin North Am* 1989; **18** (2): 195–222.

Valori RM. Nutcracker, neurosis, or sampling bias? *Gut* 1990; **31** (7): 736–7.

Benign structures

Brady PG. Esophageal foreign bodies. *Gastroenterol Clin North Am* 1991; **20** (4): 691–701.

Grundy A. The radiological management of gastrointesinal strictures and other obstructive lesions. *Ballieres Clin Gastroenterol* 1992; **6** (2): 319–40.

Gumaste VV, Dave PB. Ingestion of corrosive substances by adults. *Am J Gastroenterol* 1992; **87** (1): 1–5.

Kikendall JW. Pill-induced esophageal injury. *Gastroenterol Clin North Am* 1991; **20** (4): 835–46.

Marks RD, Richter JE. Peptic strictures of the esophagus. *Am J Gastroenterol* 1993; **88**:1160–1173.

Oesophageal carcinoma

Becker HD. Esophageal cancer, early disease: diagnosis and currenmt treatment. *World J Surg* 1994; **18**:331–8.

Bremner RM, De Meester TR. Surgical treatment of esophageal carcinoma. *Gastroenterol Clin North Am* 1991; **20** (4): 743–63.

Ellis P, Cunningham D. Management of carcinomas of the upper gastrointestinal tract. *Brit Med J* 1994; **308**: 834–8.

Herrera JL. Benign and metastatic tumors of the esophagus. *Gastroenterol Clin North Am* 1991; **20** (4): 775–89.

Lerut TE, de Leyn P, Coosemans W, Van Raemdonek D, Cuypers P, Van Cleynenbreughel B. Advanced esophageal carcinoma. *World J Surg* 1994; **18**: 379–87.

Lightdale CJ. Endoscopic ultrasonography in the diagnosis, staging and follow-up of esophageal and gastric cancer. *Endoscopy* 1992; **24** (1): 297–303.

Moses FM. Sqaumous cell carcinoma of the esophagous. Natural history, incidence, etiology, and complications. *Gastroenterol Clin North Am* 1991; **20** (4): 703–16.

Nishihira T, Nakano T, Mori S. Adjuvant therapies for cancer of the thoracic esophagus. *World J Surg* 1994; **18**: 388–98.

Parker CH, Peura DA. Palliative treatment of esophageal carcinoma using esophageal dilatation and prosthesis. *Gastroenterol Clin North Am* 1991; **20** (4): 717–29.

Reilly HF, Fleischer DE. Palliative treatment of esophageal carcinoma using laser and tumor probe therapy. *Gastroenterol Clin North Am* 1991; **20** (4): 731–42.

Sagar PM. Aetiology of cancer of the oesophagus; geographical studies in the footsteps of Marco Polo and beyond [see comments]. *Gut* 1989; **30** (5): 561–4.

12
ORAL LESIONS

REACHING A DIAGNOSIS AND MANAGEMENT

Oral problems are frequently encountered by the physician and may reflect underlying gastrointestinal problems. The common problems affecting the oral mucosa are discussed here. Dental texts should be consulted for diseases of the teeth and gums. Oral problems of the patient with human immunodeficiency virus (HIV) are discussed in Chapter 17.

Non-ulcerative oral pain

The **sore tongue** is a common complaint.

Erythema migrans

The commonest finding is erythema migrans or benign migratory glossitis (**geographic tongue**). It affects children and adults and is associated with atopy. Map-like red areas are seen with intervening thickened filiform papillae. Sometimes they appear as scalloped red lesions with white margins. They change in pattern from day to day. It is usually asymptomatic, but may cause a sore tongue. No treatment is necessary. Geographic tongue occurs with increased frequency in association with Reiter's syndrome and psoriasis.

Glossitis

A **painful red tongue** is seen in glossitis caused by vitamin B_{12} or folate deficiency. Iron deficiency may also cause a painful red tongue, but a pale atrophic tongue is more usual. Deficiency glossitis may be accompanied by angular stomatitis and mouth ulcers. Other malabsorption states and chronic alcoholism (often associated with folate deficiency) may also cause a painful red tongue (**Fig. 12.1**).

▶ **Painful tongue**

> Vitamin B_{12}, folate and iron status should be checked even if the tongue looks normal

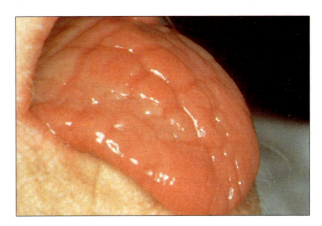

Fig. 12.1 Glossitis with generalised loss of the filiform papillae. Causes include deficiency of haematinics such as iron, vitamin B_{12} and folate, and acute candidal infection. Courtesy of Dr W Tyldesley.

Deficiency states may occasionally cause a painful, but normal looking tongue so assessment of blood ferritin, B_{12} and folate levels should be performed even in the absence of visible abnormality.

Oral dysaesthesia or glossodynia

Oral dysaesthesia or glossodynia is a burning sensation that usually affects the tongue, but patients may also complain of burning lips, gums and palate. The mucosa looks normal. It is often relieved by drinking or eating in contrast to inflammatory lesions in which these activities invariably provoke symptoms.

Evidence of candidiasis or type I herpes simplex infection should be sought. If no mucosal lesions are seen xerostomia and deficiency states should be excluded. If organic causes can be excluded the cause is probably psychogenic, possibly due to cancer phobia. Other unusual causes include diabetes mellitus and the ACE inhibitor captopril.

Painful mouth ulcers

Traumatic ulceration

Traumatic ulcers may result from accidental cheek biting, ill-fitting dentures or braces, burns and following dental anaesthetic. In children, ulcers associated with a torn labial fraenae may indicate child abuse.

Traumatic ulcers heal within a week if the cause has been removed. Patients should be reviewed after three weeks and if healing has not taken place, then the diagnosis should be reviewed, and a biopsy considered, especially if there is any possibility of malignancy.

Aphthous ulceration

Aphthous ulcers are common and easy to recognise. They affect at least 20% of the population at some time, but iron, folate or vitamin B_{12} deficiency are found in about 20% of patients and a blood count is essential. Associations with human leucocyte antigen A2, A11, B12 and DR2 have been recently been reported.

Aphthous ulcers are typically small, round or ovoid, with clearly circumscribed margins and tender, particularly when exposed to acidic drinks (**Fig. 12.2**). They last from 1-4 weeks before healing spontaneously and are often recurrent. Three varieties are described:

- **Minor aphthae** (MiRAS or Minor Recurrent Aphthous Stomatitis) are small, usually between 2–4 mm, number no more than five and occur mainly in the labial vestibule and floor of mouth. They are the most common and heal within ten days.
- **Major aphthae** (MaRAS) are large, exceeding 1 cm, may be multiple and heal in up to one month with scarring.
- **Herpetiform ulcers** are tiny, but may coalesce and appear as crops of ten or more. They are commonly found on the ventrum of the tongue and mainly affect females.

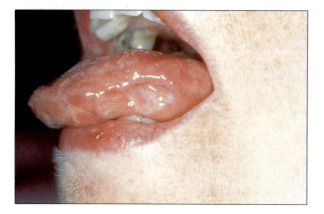

Fig. 12.2 Aphthous ulcers sited typically on the lateral border of the tongue. Coating is due to stasis resulting from the discomfort of the ulcers. Courtesy of Dr W Tyldesley.

▶ **Aphthous ulcers**

Iron, folate or vitamin B_{12} deficiency are present in 20% of patients

Aphthoid mouth ulcers may be associated with a wide range of **systemic diseases**. Gastrointestinal diseases associated with mouth ulcers include coeliac disease, Crohn's disease, ulcerative colitis and Behçet's syndrome. A persistent mouth ulcer in a patient with Crohn's disease should however

▶ **Conditions associated with mouth ulcers**

Infections

Herpes simplex
Herpes zoster
Infectious mononucleosis
Chickenpox
Tuberculosis
Syphilis
HIV

Gastrointestinal diseases

Coeliac disease
Crohn's disease
Ulcerative colitis

Skin diseases

Pemphigoid
Pemphigus
Erythema multiforme
Dermatitis herpetiformis
Epidermolysis bullosa

Haematological disorders

Anaemia
Neutropenia
Leukaemia

Rheumatological diseases

Systemic lupus erythematosus
Behçet's disease
Reiter's syndrome
Sweet's syndrome

Drugs

Cytotoxics

Radiotherapy

raise a suspicion of **oral Crohn's disease,** in which case biopsy is likely to reveal granulomas (**Fig. 12.3**). Any history of gastrointestinal disturbance in a patient with aphthoid ulcers should be taken as an indication for further investigation.

MANAGEMENT

Treatment with local measures such as antiseptic mouth-wash, good oral hygiene, or local corticosteroid preparations is all that is required for the vast majority of patients. If severe, systemic steroids may be necessary.

Thalidomide is sometimes an effective treatment in patients with giant orogenital ulceration with or without Behçet's disease, but because of teratogenicity, must be restricted to men and postmenopausal women. Moreover its use should be monitored carefully because of an appreciable risk of neuropathy.

Malignant ulceration

More than 90% of all malignant oral lesions are squamous cell carcinomas. They most commonly affect the lip (30%) and the tongue (25%).

The appearance of oral cancer is very variable. It may present as:

• A lump.
• A red or white patch.
• A fissure or an ulcer with rolled-up edges.

A high degree of clinical suspicion is necessary when chronic oral lesions are slow to heal. The presence of local lymphadenopathy must be sought. Many malignant ulcers arise from the premalignant conditions leucoplakia and erythroplasia. Pipe smoking (lip cancer), cigarette smoking, betel nut chewing (common among Southern Indians) or tobacco chewing all predispose to oral cancer. If there is any doubt the lesion should be biopsied.

MANAGEMENT

Treatment is by surgical excision (which may require extensive excision of regional lymph nodes) and radio-therapy. The prognosis of oral cancer is not good despite its easy accessibility to examination and biopsy and five-year survival is less than 50%.

Painless oral lesions

White lesions

White lesions are usually innocuous, caused by cheek biting or ill-fitting dentures. It is however important to differentiate these from the more clinically significant lesions including lichen planus, infections and premalignant leukoplakia. If in doubt biopsy is recommended.

LICHEN PLANUS

Lichen planus is a dermatosis, which may affect the oral mucosa alone or there may be other skin lesions as well. In the oral mucosa the lesions usually appear as white plaque-like lesions or reticular areas in the buccal and/or lingual mucosa (**Fig. 12.4**). The lesions usually only cause mild discomfort, but may be more painful. Lichenoid lesions are also found in systemic lupus erythematosus (SLE), in drug reactions, especially to non-steroidal anti-inflammatory drugs (NSAIDs) and in chronic renal failure.

Biopsy is generally recommended to exclude malignancy and lichen planus itself probably has a slight potential for malignant change hence should be regularly reviewed. Lichen planus may be controlled by topical corticosteroids.

LEUKOPLAKIA

Leukoplakia is recognised as a persistent adherent white patch (**Fig. 12.5**). It is important to recognise lesions that have a premalignant potential from innocuous ones. Uniform, flat, homogenous lesions are of low premalignant

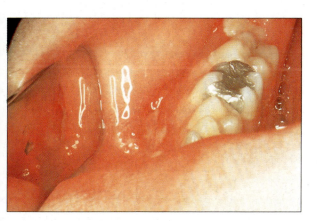

Fig. 12.3 Oral Crohn's disease. This shows similar 'cobblestoning' to that seen in the intestine. Biopsy characteristically shows non-caseating granulomas. Courtesy of Dr W Tyldesley.

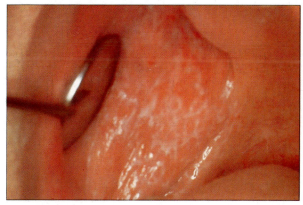

Fig. 12.4 Lichen planus. Erosions are formed by loss of atrophic areas of epithelium between the white reticulations. Courtesy of Dr W Tyldesley.

potential and may regress. However, speckled or nodular lesions with eroded areas are more sinister (**Fig. 12.6**). Most are associated with smoking, but occasionally syphylitic leukoplakia is still encountered.

Management of leukoplakia may be difficult, especially when extensive. Lesions should be biopsied, and if showing severe dysplasia, should be removed. Cessation of smoking (or treatment of syphilis if present) may lead to regression of symptoms. Patients with HIV infection are prone to develop the characteristic hairy leukoplakia (**Fig. 12.7**), which is discussed in Chapter 17.

ORAL CANDIDIASIS

White plaques, which resemble milk curds and are easily removed revealing a red mucosal surface are typical of oral candidiasis. They are common in infants, patients receiving inhaled steroids and patients immunosupressed by drugs (e.g. steroids, cyclosporin, cytotoxics) or HIV infection.

Occasionally the infection may be chronic and may lead to adherent plaques indistinguishable from leukoplakia and indeed may have a malignant potential too. The rare chronic mucocutaneous candidosis syndromes with associated hypoparathyroidism should then be considered.

Treatment of simple oral candidiasis is by topical nystatin or amphotericin, but in immunocompromised patients or those with chronic lesions, a systemic antifungal such as fluconazole is recommended.

Red lesions

ERYTHROPLASIA

The majority of red lesions are easy to recognise, but it is important to differentiate benign lesions from **erythroplasia**, which although rare, is premalignant. This presents as a red velvety lesion most often affecting the floor of the mouth and ventrum of the tongue or soft palate. It is often seen in

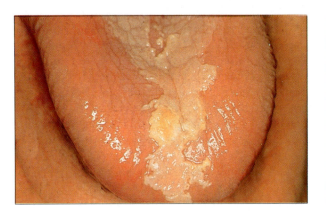

Fig. 12.5 Leucoplakia. Courtesy of Dr W Tyldesley.

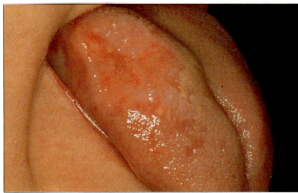

Fig. 12.6 Carcinoma of the lateral border of the tongue presenting as an erythematous patech.. Courtsey of Dr W Tyldesley.

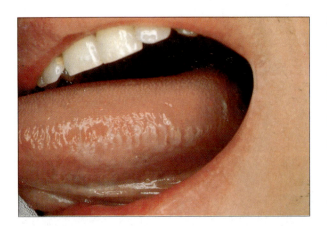

Fig. 12.7 Hairy leukoplakia in human immunodeficiency virus (HIV) infection. Courtesy of Dr W Tyldesley.

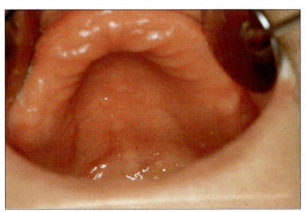

Fig. 12.8 Candidiasis (atrophic). This is the most painful form of oral candidiasis and is usually the result of corticosteroid or broad-spectrum antibiotic therapy. Courtesy of Dr W Tyldesley.

patients in their sixth and seventh decade. In 75–90% of patients it contains carcinoma *in situ*. Suspicious lesions must be biopsied and excised.

ORAL PETECHIAE

Oral petechiae, recognised as red pin-sized bleeding points, if asymmetrical may just be due to trauma, but are also seen in infectious mononucleosis, rubella and HIV infections.

ORAL TELANGIECTASIA

Oral telangiectasia are best seen under the tongue as part of hereditary haemorrhagic telangiectasia. They should be sought in patients with unexplained gastrointestinal bleeding or iron deficiency anaemia.

ORAL CANDIDIASIS

A painful red oral mucosa is most often caused by **oral candidiasis** and indeed oral candidiasis more often presents as red lesions rather than white plaques. It is associated with wearing of dentures, smoking, the use of steroid inhalers and immunosupression (**Fig. 12.8**).

Pigmented lesions

- Hyperpigmentation of the oral mucosa is seen in smokers and hypoadrenalism.
- In **Addison's disease**, the areas of pigmentation are usually in the traumatised sites of the buccal mucosa.
- Dark or purple lesions of **Kaposi's sarcoma** may be seen in patients with HIV infection (**Fig. 12.9**).
- A **brown-coated tongue** may be seen in smokers and those with xerostomia or poor oral hygiene.

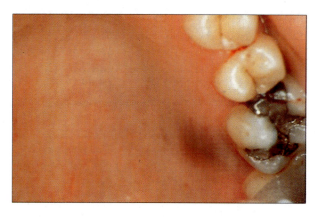

Fig. 12.9 Kaposi's sarcoma of the palate. This HIV-associated tumour is thought to arise from vascular endothelial cells and may affect any part of the gastrointestinal tract in acquired immune deficiency syndrome (AIDS). Courtesy of Dr W Tyldesley.

- The **furred, black hairy tongue** is caused by melanin-generating anaerobic bacteria and so may be found in patients receiving chronic antibiotic therapy (e.g. tetracycline) with poor oral hygiene or smokers.

Blisters

The blistering skin conditions **pemphigus** and **pemphigoid** can affect the oral mucosa, but the accompanying skin lesions usually make the diagnosis straightforward. **Mucus membrane pemphigoid**, which is not associated with more generalised lesions may be more difficult to diagnose. Drug reactions should always be included in the differential diagnosis. Other blistering skin lesions such as **epidermolysis bullosa** and **erythema multiforme** tend to cause oral ulcers rather than blisters.

FURTHER READING

Aphthoid ulcers

Vincent SD, Lilly GE. Clinical, historic, and therapeutic features of aphthous stomatitis. Literature review and open clinical trial employing steroids. *Oral Surg Oral Med Oral Pathol* 1992; **74**(1): 79–86.

Glossitis

Carter LC. Median rhomboid glossitis: review of a puzzling entity. *Compendium* 1990l; **11**(7): 446, 448–51.

Nally F. Diseases of the tongue. *Practitioner* 1991; **235**(1498): 65–71.

Zunt SL, Tomich CE. Erythema migrans—a psoriasiform lesion of the oral mucosa. *J Dermatol Surg Oncol* 1989; **15**(10): 1067–70.

Oral cancer

Lakshmi S, Nair SA, Pillai MR. Oral cancer and human papillomaviruses: is there a link? *J Surg Oncol* 1993; **52**(3): 193–6.

Nally F. Oral cancer—diagnosis and management. *Practitioner* 1992; **236**(1518): 812–7.

Pillai R, Balaram P, Reddiar KS. Pathogenesis of oral submucous fibrosis. Relationship to risk factors associated with oral cancer. *Cancer* 1992; **69**(8): 2011–20.

Sawyer DR, Wood NK. Oral cancer. Etiology, recognition, and management. *Dent Clin North Am* 1992; **36**(4): 919–44.

Silverman S Jr. Precancerous lesions and oral cancer in the elderly. *Clin Geriatr Med* 1992; **8**(3): 529–41.

Ward Booth P. Advances in the diagnosis and treatment of oral cancer. *Curr Opin Dent* 1991; **1**(3): 287–95.

Lichen planus

Eisen D. The therapy of oral lichen planus. *Crit Rev Oral Biol Med* 1993; **4**(2): 141–58.

Eisenberg E. Lichen planus and oral cancer: is there a connection between the two? *J Am Dent Assoc* 1992; **123**(5): 104–8.

Oliver GF, Winkelmann RK. Treatment of lichen planus. *Drugs* 1993; **45**(1): 56–65.

Shai A, Halevy S. Lichen planus and lichen planus-like eruptions: pathogenesis and associated diseases. *Int J Dermatol* 1992; **31**(6): 379–84.

Leukoplakia

Abbey LM. Precancerous lesions of the mouth. *Curr Opin Dent* 1991; **1**(6): 773–6.

Bouquot JE. Reviewing oral leukoplakia: clinical concepts for the 1990s. *J Am Dent Assoc* 1991; **122**(7): 80–2.

Greenspan D, Greenspan JS. Significance of oral hairy leukoplakia. *Oral Surg Oral Med Oral Pathol* 1992; **73**(2): 151–4.

Itin PH, Rufli T. Oral hairy leukoplakia. *Int J Dermatol* 1992; **31**(5): 301–6.

13
JAUNDICE

REACHING A DIAGNOSIS

Avoidable mistakes are still made in the diagnosis and management of patients with jaundice. Overinterpretation of serum biochemistry, inadequate radiological demonstration of the bile ducts, or failure to take a careful drug history are some of the commoner errors. The consequences of such mistakes can be serious, particularly if a patient with severe hepatitis is subjected to unnecessary laparotomy. Adhering to a logical series of steps should avoid these mistakes.

Is the hyperbilirubinaemia conjugated or unconjugated?

If an elevated serum bilirubin is the only biochemical abnormality there is a strong possibility that there is either excessive production of bilirubin (haemolysis) or defective conjugation (Gilbert's syndrome).

The first step is to assess whether the elevated bilirubin is predominantly conjugated, in which case it is readily excreted in the urine, or predominantly unconjugated, in which case it is strongly albumin bound and not excreted and the urine will be of normal colour.

▶ **Diagnosing jaundice: questions to ask**

- Is the bilirubin conjugated or unconjugated? (Conjugated if dark urine and high direct serum bilirubin)
- Is there evidence of viral hepatitis? (Markedly raised serum transaminase and positive viral titres)
- Could it be drug- or alcohol-related?
- Could there be a bacterial cause? (e.g. Weil's disease, tuberculosis)
- Could it be an acute presentation of chronic hepatitis? (e.g. autoimmune chronic active or Wilson's disease)
- Could it be due to heart failure? (Check jugular venous pressure)
- Could the hepatic vein be thrombosed? (Consider if ascites is present)
- Could it be due to pregnancy-related liver disease? (Particularly if in the last trimester)
- Are the intrahepatic bile ducts dilated and if so at what level? (Ultrasound followed by cholangiography)

The conjugation of serum bilirubin can be assessed by quantifying bilirubin by the van den Bergh reaction with and without previous alcohol treatment of the sample, the alcohol converting unconjugated (indirect) bilirubin to direct (conjugated) bilirubin.

Gilbert's syndrome

Gilbert's syndrome is an important diagnosis to make since patients with the syndrome become more jaundiced during intercurrent illness or fasting and are frequently misdiagnosed as having hepatitis or gallstones. Liver biopsy, which is normal in Gilbert's syndrome is not necessary as the diagnosis can be confidently made if:

- The excess bilirubin is unconjugated.
- Liver enzyme estimations are normal.
- Haemolysis has been excluded (normal reticulocyte count and plasma haptoglobin).
- There is no hepatosplenomegaly.

Crigler–Najjar syndrome

Crigler–Najjar syndrome is a much rarer and more serious condition in which there is a more marked failure of conjugation. In its milder form (type II) survival into adult life may occur, but bilirubin levels are usually considerably higher than those found in Gilbert's syndrome (where serum bilirubin rarely exceeds 70 μmol/l).

If the hyperbilirubinaemia is conjugated, is it cholestatic or hepatitic?

This is the step where most mistakes occur, usually due to excessive reliance on the inaptly named 'liver function tests'. The serum biochemical profile (i.e. bilirubin, alkaline phosphatase and aspartate transaminase or alanine transaminase) should be used as a screening test for the presence of liver disturbance and at most as a guide to further investigation. Although cholestasis is usually associated with a considerable elevation of serum alkaline phosphatase and hepatitis is usually associated with with a similar elevation of transaminase, there is considerable overlap. Occasionally, biliary obstruction, particularly when caused by gallstones, may be associated with serum aspartate transaminase levels of over 1000 iu/l and hepatitis may be associated with considerable cholestasis and elevation of serum alkaline phosphatase.

A history of itching or the presence of scratch marks is a more reliable feature of cholestasis. Although medical students are almost universally taught that the combination of pale stools and dark urine indicates biliary obstruction, this is a fallacy. Any patient with an elevated serum concentration of conjugated bilirubin will have dark urine and hepatitis, if sufficiently severe, will result in reduced bile secretion and pale faeces.

▶ **Pale stools and dark urine**

- Merely indicate that jaundice has an hepatic cause
- Do not always indicate mechanical bile duct obstruction

If conjugated hyperbilirubinaemia is the only biochemical abnormality, the rare condition **Dubin–Johnson syndrome** should be considered. In this condition the liver biopsy will be deeply pigmented, probably due to excessive melanin in lysosomes and a bromsulphthalein excretion test will show a characteristic second peak with the blood level at 120 minutes greater than the level at 45 minutes. The gallbladder fails to opacify on oral cholecystography and there is an abnormal ration of urine coproporphyrin I to coproporphyrin III (over 4:1 compared to 1:3 normally).

A combination of a careful history, examination and serum biochemical profile will allow most patients to be labelled as 'probably cholestatic' or 'probably hepatitic', but an open mind should be kept until the diagnosis is firmly established.

Probable hepatitic jaundice

Is it due to a drug or toxin?

A careful drug history is extremely important as further exposure to the drug that has initiated hepatitis could be fatal. Many drugs have occasionally been incriminated, but more common causes of hepatitis include methyldopa, anticonvulsants, particularly sodium valproate and phenytoin, isoniazid, rifampicin, co-amoxiclav, flucloxacillin, ketoconasole, oxyphenisatin (a laxative now withdrawn in most countries including the UK) and many of the non-steroidal anti-inflammatory drugs.

A more dramatic picture with a rapid onset of fulminant hepatitis occurs with drug poisoning, and a history should then be taken to exclude exposure to carbon tetrachloride or other organic solvents, wild mushrooms (*Amanita phalloides*) or inadvertent or deliberate paracetamol overdose.

If the patient has recently had a general anaesthetic, **halothane hepatitis** should be considered. This typically, but not always, presents following two or more exposures to halothane, comes on 3–17 days after the anaesthetic and is usually associated with fever and sometimes eosinophilia.

Is it viral hepatitis?

Viruses that may cause hepatitis include the hepatotropic viruses hepatitis A, B, C, D and E. A careful history should be taken enquiring about contact with jaundiced patients, intravenous drug abuse with needle sharing or sexual contact with possible carriers.

Individuals at high risk of acquiring hepatitis B include male homosexuals, intravenous drug abusers, the sexually promiscuous, residents in mental handicap institutions and immigrants from high endemic areas. Similar patients are also at risk of hepatitis C. Recipients of blood products including haemophiliacs, haemodialysis and hypogamma-globinaemic patients are also at risk for hepatitis C, particularly if transfused before the introduction of a reliable serological marker for hepatitis C. Hepatitis D is commoner in patients from the Middle East and Mediterranean countries.

SEROLOGICAL DIAGNOSIS

Diagnosis of viral hepatitis requires some understanding of the serological markers, their time course and limitations.

- For **hepatitis A** the presence of IgM anti-HAV is diagnostic since the test is usually positive from the onset of illness and returns to negative within six months.
- In **hepatitis B**, the surface antigen (HBsAg) is usually present for several weeks after onset of illness. The presence of IgM anti-HBc distinguishes acute hepatitis B from chronic hepatitis. Within a few weeks of the onset of symptoms, HBe antigen usually disappears, signalling virus clearance by the host immune system and anti-HBe appears. Finally, anti-HBs appears, often after several months. In fulminant hepatitis, patients often lose HBsAg and HBeAg positivity as an aggressive host immune system clears the infected hepatocytes and in so doing causes hepatic necrosis, but IgM anti-HBc remains positive.
- Diagnosis of acute **hepatitis C** still partly depends on exclusion of other agents and a history of exposure. This is because antibodies to HCV often do not appear in the serum until after the illness has run its course, which may be 3–6 months after the onset of symptoms. Furthermore the HCV antibody test is not totally specific, some false positive results occurring in other forms of liver disease, particularly those associated with a raised serum globulin. Detection of HCV RNA by the polymerase chain reaction (PCR) is the definitive test for HCV, but is

usually only performed if testing for HCV antibody is positive. The presence of a high titre to the C-100-3 antigen is associated with chronicity. The original C-100-3 'first generation' antibody test is now largely superceded by recombinant immunoblot assay (RIBA) using a range of recombinant HCV antigens.

* **Hepatitis D** infection is diagnosed by a rise in both IgG and IgM anti-HDV. Like HCV infection, this sero-conversion may take several months. Detection of the antigen by western blotting is available in some centres. Hepatitis D (delta agent) infection only occurs in co-existence with hepatitis B.

• **Hepatitis E virus** (HEV) has been detected in stool and serum using PCR, but this is confined to research centres although a serological test has recently become available.

If tests for hepatitis A, B and C are negative further tests should include a monospot or Paul–Bunnell test to exclude infectious mononucleosis and the cytomegalovirus IgM antibody titre. This will still leave occasional patients who have typical viral hepatitis, but no serological markers. It must be remembered though that there is a long list of other viruses that may occasionaly cause significant hepatitis, including varicella, measles, herpes simplex, and coxsackie, and in patients returning from Africa the differential may include Lassa fever, Marburg virus and Ebola virus.

▶ **Serological tests for acute viral hepatitis**

- Hepatitis A IgM antibody
- Hepatitis B surface antigen (sAg)
- Hepatitis B IgM core antibody (may detect sAg-negative fulminant hepatitis B)
- Hepatitis C IgG antibody
- PCR detection of Hepatitis C RNA
- Hepatitis D (delta agent) IgM antibody (only relevant if hepatitis B positive)
- Paul–Bunnell test or monospot
- Cytomegalovirus IgM antibody

Is it non-viral infective hepatitis?

Although non-viral infective causes of hepatitis are relatively uncommon they are important to diagnose and should always be considered if tests for a viral cause prove negative.

Leptospira icterohaemorrhagia infection (Weil's disease), which is usually contracted by contamination of abraided skin by the urine of infected rats, has an initial septicaemic phase, which lasts about one week with rigors, muscular pains and meningism. Jaundice may appear towards the end

of this week and is associated with a polymorphonuclear leucocytosis and thrombocytopenia. The organism is difficult to culture and diagnosis is usually made by finding a rising antibody titre on complement fixation testing.

Other infections that may be associated with a hepatitic illness and for which specific treatment is available include miliary tuberculosis, secondary syphilis and Q fever (*Coxiella burnetti*).

Is it an acute presentation of chronic hepatitis?

It is important to realise that **autoimmune chronic active hepatitis** and **Wilson's disease**, which is histologically similar, may both present as an acute hepatitis that may be fulminant. Liver histology at this stage may be difficult to distinguish from acute viral hepatitis and it is clearly not possible to wait the 3–6 months needed before a repeat biopsy can be interpreted. Diagnosis in this situation usually has to be based on autoantibody status (smooth muscle and antinuclear) and copper status.

In Wilson's disease, the serum concentration of the copper binding protein caeruloplasmin is diminished with a low serum copper as a result and the urine copper and liver copper are increased. Diagnosis of Wilson's disease is more difficult in acute hepatitis since caeruloplasmin behaves as an acute phase reactant so that its serum concentration may rise into the normal range. Morever, copper is released from the liver in hepatic necrosis so that elevated urine copper concentrations may also occur in fulminant hepatitis due to other causes.

The response of urine copper to penicillamine therapy is sometimes useful in determining the diagnosis. An increase of urine copper of more than 500 μg/day after starting on oral penicillamine 10 mg/kg/day is highly suggestive of Wilson's disease. Kayser–Fleischer rings due to copper deposition in the cornea should be sought, but are not reliably present in all patients who present with hepatic rather than neurological features of the disease. Care must be taken to exclude Wilson's disease in any young patient, particularly between 5 and 30 years of age, with biochemical evidence of hepatitis. Neurological disease may present up to 40 years of age.

If viral hepatitis has been excluded and chronic active hepatitis is thought to be a possible diagnosis, a trial of corticosteroid therapy may be the only course with a view to performing liver biopsy as soon as coagulation allows.

ARE THERE CLINICAL SIGNS OF CHRONIC LIVER DISEASE?

Vascular spiders (spider naevi) consist of a central arteriole from which small vessels radiate under the skin resembling the legs of a spider. They are distributed in the drainage region of the superior vena cava, hence are rare below the nipple line. They blanche with pressure over the central arteriole. They may occur in normal subjects, particularly children and in pregnancy although rarely more than a few lesions. They should not be confused with Campbell de Morgan spots, which are red, raised, non-blanching and are age-related. No treatment is usually necessary and they may resolve with improvement of hepatic function. If treatment is required for cosmetic reasons, electrocautery or laser photocoagulation may be helpful.

Palmar erythema is a common non-specific finding in liver disease. The hypothenar and thenar eminences are especially affected with a mottled red discolouration that blanches on pressure. They may be found in normal subjects, pregnancy, rheumatoid arthritis and thyrotoxicosis.

Leuconychia (white nails) is a manifestation of hypo-albuminaemia and is found in many patients with chronic liver disease.

Endocrine changes may be found in patients with cirrhosis particularly when due to alcohol. In the male, it results in feminisation and in the female, it manifests as gonadal atrophy. Hence, the male may experience impotence, sterility and testicular atrophy. There may be gynaecomastia, which may be unilateral or tender. However, gynaecomastia is commonly as a result of spironolactone therapy.

Is it alcoholic liver disease?

Alcoholic liver disease (**Fig. 13.1**) often progresses insiduously and presents late with complications of portal hypertension such as variceal bleeding or ascites. Less commonly a florid alcoholic hepatitis develops. This develops rapidly over a few weeks or months in an alcoholic who has usually been drinking heavily for several years.

The clinician recognises alcoholic hepatitis as a syndrome consisting of jaundice, poor liver function often with portal hypertension and ascites, fever, neutrophil leucocytosis, a hyperdynamic circulation and, commonly, a systolic hepatic

▶ **Typical features of alcoholic hepatitis**

- Jaundice
- Large liver
- Neutrophil leucocytosis
- Macrocytosis (MCV usually over 100)
- Fever (but sepsis needs excluding)
- Hepatic bruit common (but hepatoma needs excluding)
- Serum aspartate transaminase less than 300 iu/l
- 50% three-month mortality

bruit. Approximately 50% of such patients already have cirrhosis. Pathologists often recognise histological evidence of alcoholic hepatitis in much less severe liver disease.

Features that should suggest alcoholic hepatitis as a cause of jaundice apart from a history of excess alcohol therefore include the presence of marked heptomegaly and possibly splenomegaly, spider naevi, a systolic arterial bruit over the liver (although hepatocellular carcinoma will need excluding if present), a persistent neutrophil leucocytosis that is otherwise unexplained and elevation in serum immuno-globulin A, the mechanism of which is unknown. The serum aspartate transaminase is usually only modestly elevated and a level greater than 300 iu/l suggests either an alternative diagnosis or some complicating factor such as paracetamol-induced necrosis in addition.

Is it due to heart failure?

Congestive cardiac failure commonly causes mild to moderate elevation in serum aspartate transaminase and alkaline phosphatase, but occasionally severe jaundice may result, usually with a mixed cholestatic/hepatitic biochemical picture, but without pruritus. Jaundice occurs particularly in patients who have an episode of low cardiac output or 'forward failure' in addition to congestive failure.

Liver function may be severely deranged, but the condition is reversible providing the cardiac status can be improved. Liver biopsy shows intense congestion with centrilobular necrosis, which produces the appearance of 'nutmeg' liver seen at post mortem (**Fig. 13.2**).

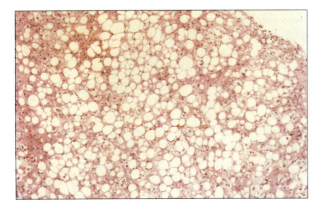

Fig. 13.1 Alcoholic fatty liver showing macrovesicular fat. In the absence of hepatitis or fibrosis this is potentially reversible, but many patients nevertheless slowly progress to cirrhosis.

▶ **Jaundice in heart failure**

- Serum transaminases and alkaline phosphatase modestly elevated
- Usually poor cardiac output ('forward failure') in addition to congestion

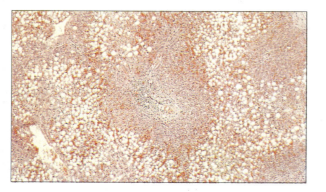

Fig. 13.2 The liver in congestive cardiac failure showing areas of functioning hepatocytes around portal tracts, but extensive necrosis around central veins due to hypoxia. Fatty change, shown here. is often present and gives rise to the resemblance to sliced nutmeg if the liver is sliced into at postmortem examination.

Is the cause hepatic vein thrombosis (Budd–Chiari syndrome)?

Hepatic vein thrombosis causes acute congestion of the liver, resulting in liver failure and ascites, which progress over a period of weeks. Clinical features include marked ascites, which is often resistant to conventional therapy and compensatory hypertrophy of the caudate lobe, which may be felt as an epigastric mass.

Technetium colloid isotope scanning may confirm the preservation of function in the caudate lobe (which results from direct venous drainage from the caudate lobe to the inferior vena cava). Hepatic venography should be performed both to confirm the diagnosis and to exclude a vena cava web as a treatable cause. Liver biopsy, if performed, (poor coagulation often precludes it) shows changes of congestion similar to those found in heart failure.

Is it pregnancy-related liver disease?

Although any form of liver disease, including viral hepatitis, may of course occur in pregnancy, there are three specific pregnancy associated liver problems:

- Acute fatty liver.
- Pre-eclamptic toxaemia.
- Cholestasis of the last trimester.

Fatty liver and pre-eclamptic toxaemia both occur from about 30 weeks onwards and features of the two conditions commonly overlap. Fatty liver classically presents with a rapid onset of jaundice, vomiting and liver failure with markedly deranged coagulation and eventual coma. The liver may be of normal size (whereas most other forms of fulminant failure result in a rapidly shrinking liver) and the serum transaminases are only moderately elevated. It is possible that milder forms of this condition causing vomiting and mild derangement of liver function may occur, but this is unproven.

Some degree of pre-eclampsia often coexists in acute fatty liver of pregnancy, but can in its own right produce liver damage as a consequence of microvascular occlusion. The coagulopathy is then more severe with associated platelet consumption and the liver disease usually milder, but the two conditions may be very difficult to distinguish.

Probable cholestatic jaundice

Is there extrahepatic biliary obstruction?

Some patients present with an almost diagnostic combination of painless jaundice, itching and a palpable gallbladder reflecting low common bile duct obstruction by pancreatic cancer; alternatively, the patient may give a history or rigors and intermittent severe right upper quadrant abdominal pain suggestive of cholangitis due to gallstones.

Experienced clinicians not infrequently disagree about whether a gallbladder is palpable and a history of rigors obtained by one clinician may seem more like a flu-like prodrome of hepatitis to another. Ultrasound and cholangiography (percutaneous or endoscopic) are now widely available and **it is no longer acceptable for any jaundiced patient to undergo laparotomy before the anatomical site of extrahepatic obstruction has been defined.**

Ultrasound scanning has become generally accepted as the best initial test for suspected obstructive jaundice (**Figs 13.3** and **13.4**). It has a reliability of over 90% for detecting dilatation of intrahepatic bile ducts, but is less reliable at defining the site of obstruction.

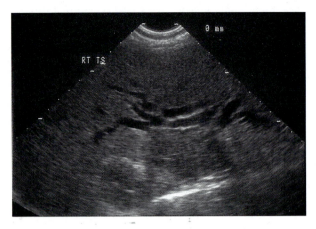

Fig. 13.3 Ultrasound scan showing dilatation of the intrahepatic bile ducts in jaundice due to mechanical bile duct obstruction.

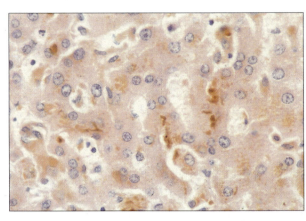

Fig. 13.4 Histological appearances of severe cholestasis with formation of bile plugs. These may be seen in cholestasis of any cause.

Other possible problems with interpretation include the misdiagnosis of portal vein branches as dilated bile ducts and the fact that in some patients with gallstone related cholangitis, the ducts fail to dilate. Despite these reservations ultrasound is non-invasive and should usually be the initial investigation in suspected obstructive jaundice.

▶ **Ultrasound scanning in jaundice**

- Very reliable for detecting mechanical obstruction (indicated by dilatation of intrahepatic bile ducts)
- Less reliable at determining the site of obstruction
- Unreliable for determining the underlying diagnosis

Computerised tomography (CT) scanning has not so far proved superior although modern 'spiral' CT may perform better. If the ultrasound or CT scan confirms dilatation of intrahepatic ducts, a cholangiogram should always be performed to determine the precise level of the obstruction and will usually result in a firm diagnosis. Oral and intravenous contrast agents usually produce inadequate quality cholangiograms and often fail completely in the jaundiced patient.

Percutaneous fine-needle cholangiography is simple in theory and widely available. Care needs to be taken to allow adequate mixing of contrast with bile, either by aspirating bile or by tilting the patient, otherwise a false impression may be gained of a block at the hilum in patients with lower common bile duct obstruction. It also carries an appreciable risk of precipitating cholangitis and for this reason should only be performed after a surgical opinion has been obtained and not late in the day.

▶ **Cholangiography before surgery**

Cholangiography should always be performed before surgery for obstructive jaundice

Endoscopic retrograde cholangiopancreatography (ERCP) is safer, although still carries some risk of precipitating cholangitis, so antibiotic cover should be continued for at least 48 hours afterwards if the bile duct obstruction persists. It usually gives more information than percutaneous cholangiography, particularly if a pancreatogram is obtained and, more importantly, may allow simultaneous endoscopic therapy to relieve the biliary obstruction (**Figs 13.5–13.17**).

Is there intrahepatic biliary obstruction?
Intrahepatic cholestasis is relatively uncommon and, as a result is often not considered until negative ultrasonography or cholangiography has been obtained. As with other causes of obstructive jaundice the liver is likely to be enlarged and itching may be intense.

Commoner causes include drugs, particularly phenothiazines, oestrogens and erythromycin and the cholestatic phase of viral hepatitis, particularly hepatitis A. It may also be the initial presentation of the chronic biliary diseases primary biliary cirrhosis and sclerosing cholangitis. Septicaemia and intravenous feeding may be complicated by jaundice, which is histologically cholestatic although itching is not usually a feature. Intrahepatic cholestasis may occur in the last trimester of pregnancy and there is also a rare congenital disorder of benign recurrent cholestasis.

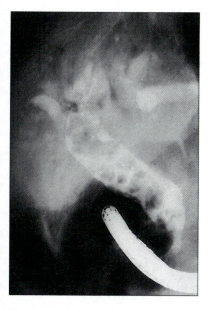

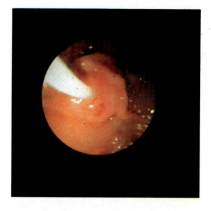

Fig. 13.6 ERCP cannulation of a normal papilla of Vater. The success rate for cannulation should be higher than 90%.

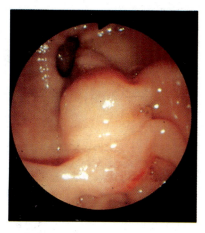

Fig. 13.7 Bulging papilla due to impacted stone. There is also a peri-ampullary diverticulum.

Fig. 13.5 Endoscopic cholangiogram (ERCP) showing the common bile duct containing numerous stones. These were retrieved following endoscopic sphincterotomy.

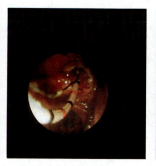

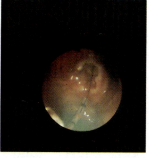

Fig. 13.8 Endoscopic sphincterotomy being performed using a diathermy catheter. There is a 3% risk of significant bleeding, pancreatitis or cholangitis and a mortality of about 0.5%, but this makes it considerably safer than surgical common bile duct exploration, particularly in elderly patients.

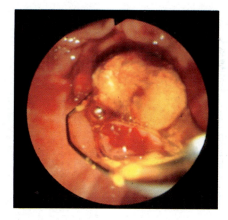

Fig. 13.9 A Dormia basket being used to extract a stone from the common bile duct after endoscopic sphincterotomy. Stones larger than 2cm diameter usually need fragmenting with a lithotripsy basket before removal.

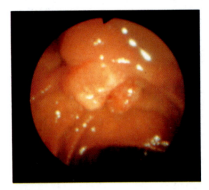

Fig. 13.10 Endoscopic appearance of carcinoma of the papilla. Surgical resection should be considered because this has a much better outlook than pancreatic cancer.

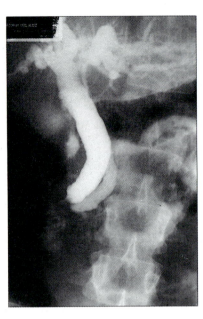

Fig. 13.11 ERCP appearances in ampullary carcinoma with dilatation of both bile and pancreatic ducts.

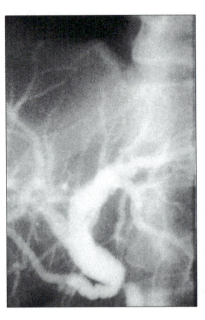

Fig. 13.12 ERCP appearance of post-surgical stricturing of the common bile duct. This can be the result of either inappropriately placed surgical clips or ischaemia following devascularisation. Good long-term results can be achieved by balloon dilatation of the stricture, but surgical revision (usually hepatico-jejunostomy) may be required.

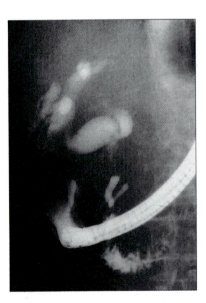

Fig. 13.13 ERCP appearances of carcinoma of the head of pancreas. There is stricturing of both the common bile duct and the pancreatic duct..

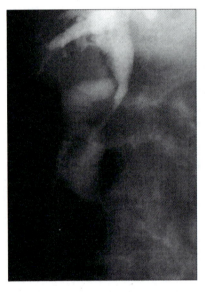

Fig. 13.14 A plastic tube ('stent') has been placed through the bile duct stricture to relieve the jaundice. The jaundice is relieved in about 80% of patients using this technique. The stents remain patent for about six months on average, but there is little if any increase in life expectancy, which remains limited with a median survival of six months, although occasional patients survive up to three years.

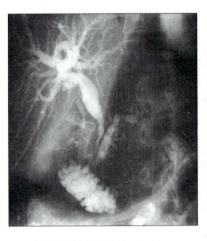

Fig. 13.15 ERCP in alcoholic chronic pancreatitis. The pancreatic duct is dilated and irregular with distended side branches and there is a tapering stricture of the lower common bile duct. Secondary biliary cirrhosis can ensue in this situation if biliary drainage is not improved, usually by surgical hepatico-jejunostomy.

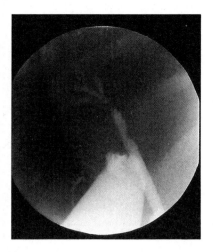

Fig. 13.16 ERCP showing a tight stricture at the bifurcation of the main hepatic ducts due to a cholangiocarcinoma ('Klatskin tumour'). About 10% of such tumours are resectable and they are relatively slow growing: survival up to three years is not uncommon.

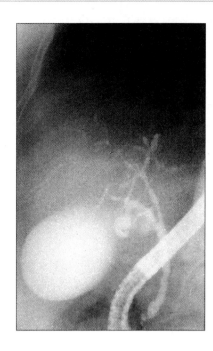

Fig. 13.17 ERCP appearances of sclerosing cholangitis in a patient with ulcerative colitis. There is alternate beading and stricturing of the intrahepatic ducts.

Correct diagnosis depends firstly on awareness that not all patients with painless jaundice and pruritus have obstructed extrahepatic bile ducts.

A careful drug history (including oral contraceptives) is essential. Hepatitis A IgM antibody should be checked and a negative test for antimitochondrial antibody virtually excludes primary biliary cirrhosis.

Liver biopsy should then be performed if coagulation permits and the diagnosis is still uncertain. In severe cholestasis of any cause, bile plugging of canaliculi and extravasation of bile to form bile lakes may occur and is often misconstrued as indicative of large bile duct obstruction. Neutrophil polymorphs in or around bile ducts are, however, suggestive of large duct obstruction and endoscopic cholangiography is then indicated (percutaneous cholangiography has a failure rate of up to 50% if dilated ducts cannot be visualised by ultrasound). Primary biliary cirrhosis is suggested by lymphocytic or granulomatous infiltration of portal tracts with relative paucity of interlobular bile ducts. Proliferation of small bile ductules is non-specific and may occur in cholestasis of any cause. Accumulation of eosinophils in portal tracts possibly associated with focal necrosis or ballooning degeneration of hepatocytes is suggestive of a drug reaction.

ERCP should always be performed when there is any doubt over the diagnosis as there is a considerable overlap between the histological appearances found in cholestatic disorders. Sclerosing cholangitis in particular, cannot be confidently diagnosed or excluded until a cholangiogram has been performed.

CONDITIONS CAUSING JAUNDICE: NATURAL HISTORY AND MANAGEMENT

Gilbert's syndrome

Natural history

Jaundice is mild (bilirubin < 70 μmol/l) and often intermittent, deepening during periods of fasting or intercurrent illness. As a result a mistaken diagnosis of infectious hepatitis is often made. For this reason, it is important to make a firm diagnosis of Gilbert's syndrome and then explain the diagnosis to the patient, preferably writing it down so that the patient can inform other doctors he or she may consult later.

Individuals with the syndrome complain of nausea or right upper quadrant pain more often than controls, but it is not clear whether this may be a consequence of concern about liver disease, for the liver is histologically normal and it is difficult to see why pain should arise.

Pathology

It has been argued that this is not a separate entity, but simply a label applied to the 5% of otherwise healthy people who have a serum bilirubin level above the statistically defined normal range. It does however, have a familial tendency, probably via autosomal dominant inheritance. The excess bilirubin is predominantly unconjugated, and individuals with the syndrome have reduced hepatic levels of the conjugating enzyme UDP glucuronyl transferase. There may also be a clinically unimportant reduction in red blood cell survival, which contributes to the bilirubin load.

Management
Life expectancy is normal and no treatment required.

Crigler–Najjar syndrome
Crigler–Najjar syndrome is a more severe and much rarer form of unconjugated hyperbilirubinaemia. There are two types:

- Type I, in which the conjugating enzyme is absent and death occurs in the first year of life.
- Type II, a milder defect, which behaves like a severe form of Gilbert's syndrome with survival into adult life. Jaundice may be severe, but usually improves if liver enzymes are induced by phenobarbitone therapy.

Dubin–Johnson syndrome
Dubin–Johnson syndrome is a rare congenital jaundice in which the bilirubin is predominantly conjugated, but cannot be normally excreted from the liver as a result of a defect in lysosomal function. Other features of cholestasis such as elevation of serum alkaline phosphatase or itching are absent. Prognosis is excellent and no treatment is required.

Rotor's syndrome
Rotor's syndrome is similar to the Dubin–Johnson syndrome, but not associated with retention of pigment in the liver or a late reflux of bromsulphthalein. Prognosis is excellent and no treatment is required.

Infective hepatitis

Viral hepatitis

NATURAL HISTORY
All the hepatotropic viruses may cause a transient acute hepatitis, but they differ in their risks for fulminant hepatitis or chronic liver disease.

- **Hepatitis A** usually runs a benign course and may be subclinical (**Fig. 13.18**), but may rarely give rise to a fulminant hepatitis. Cholestatic hepatitis is more common in hepatitis A and may persist for up to six months, but it always resolves. Hepatitis A does not give rise to chronic disease.
- **Hepatitis E** infection also gives rise to acute hepatitis and usually runs a benign course except in women in the third trimester of pregnancy when it may cause fulminant hepatitis with high mortality. Hepatitis E does not give rise to chronic disease.
- **Hepatitis B** can cause a typical acute hepatitis, cholestatic hepatitis (rarely), fulminant hepatitis and chronic hepatitis (either chronic persistent or chronic active) (**Fig. 13.19**). Chronicity occurs most frequently in neonates and children and in the immunosuppressed (including patients at risk for multiple viral infections such as drug addicts, the sexually promiscuous and haemophiliacs).
- More than 50% of patients acquiring the **hepatitis C** virus (**Fig. 13.20**) will develop a chronic infection, which is often subclinical.
- **Hepatitis D** infection can occur as a superinfection (in patients already HBsAg positive) or as a co-infection (simultaneous HBV and HDV infection), with the latter being a more severe illness. Hepatitis D superinfection of an HBV-positive individual is associated with a high likelihood of chronic hepatitis.

Acute hepatitis often starts insidiously with nonspecific symptoms of anorexia, malaise, nausea and right upper quadrant pain. Headache and menigism are common in hepatitis A. Arthralgia and urticaria may occur as part of the prodrome of hepatitis B. With the onset of jaundice, nausea and anorexia may become more pronounced, but the flu-like symptoms and general malaise often improve. The length of jaundice varies from a few days to several months. Jaundice

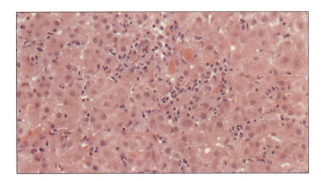

Fig. 13.18 Acute hepatitis A showing focal inflammation and swollen hepatocytes.

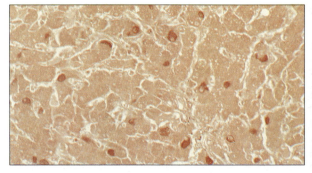

Fig. 13.19 Orcein stain showing hepatitis B-positive cells in acute hepatitis B.

persisting for more than a few weeks is usually due to intrahepatic cholestasis and is likely to be associated with pruritus. Fatigue is often pronounced. Fever is usually low grade or absent. Tender hepatomegaly may be present. Drowsiness is worrying, suggesting impending encephalopathy and a fulminant course. Serum transaminases are usually markedly raised, often 10–50-fold and serum alkaline phosphatase and gammaglutamyltransferase are mildly raised (more so if cholestasis has developed) (**Figs 13.21–13.23**).

Prothrombin time may be prolonged and is a useful indicator of severity.

Acute fulminant hepatitis is arbitrarily defined as the onset of encephalopathy in patients with acute hepatitis within eight weeks of onset of illness. Onset of encephalopathy beyond eight weeks is termed **subacute fulminant**. It carries a grave prognosis and is an indication for immediate transfer to a liver transplant centre. Serological markers for viral hepatitis are often negative in this group.

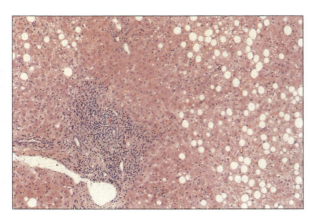

Fig. 13.20 Acute hepatitis C showing patchy inflammation and the typical patchy steatosis.

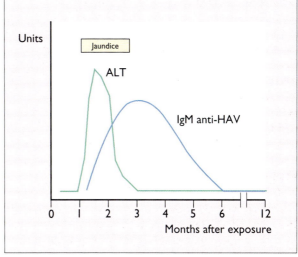

Fig. 13.21 Typical course of hepatitis A with development of transient IgM antibody.

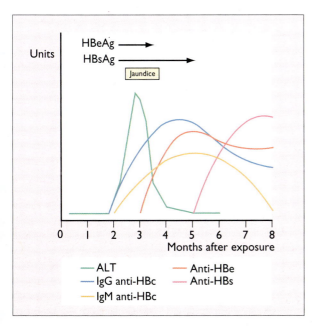

Fig. 13.22 Typical course of hepatitis B in a patient who has acute hepatitis and becomes immune (the commonest consequence of hepatitis B infection).

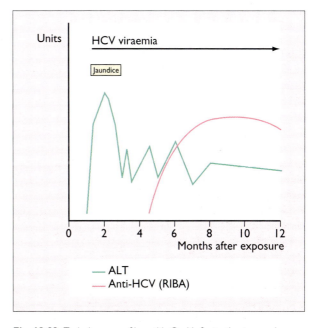

Fig. 13.23 Typical course of hepatitis C with fluctuating transaminase and development of chronic hepatitis.

AETIOLOGY AND PATHOGENESIS

The hepatotropic viruses are by far the commonest and most important cause of viral hepatitis. To date five viruses have been identified and well characterised – hepatitis A, B, C, D and E. Hepatitis F has been postulated for a non-A, non-B, non-C sporadic hepatitis that leads to fulminant hepatic failure and hepatitis G is the putative cause for giant cell hepatitis, but they have not been conclusively identified.

Hepatitis A virus

Hepatitis A (HAV) is a 27 nm picornavirus with a single-stranded RNA genome of 7500 nucleotides. It is transmitted by the orofaecal route with an incubation time of about 28 days. Infection is often subclinical in infants and young children. In developing countries, subclinical childhood infection is the norm, but in most developed countries where many adults have not encountered the virus, at least 65% develop jaundice when they acquire the infection.

Hepatitis B virus

Hepatitis B (HBV) is a more complex virus. The complete virion (Dane particle) is a 40 nm incompletely double-stranded DNA virus. Proteins encoded by the DNA genome include a reverse transcriptase, core and envelope proteins and a regulatory X protein. The genome is enveloped by the core antigen (HBcAg) and the complete virus has a lipoprotein envelope referred to as the surface antigen (HBsAg). It is this surface antigen that was discovered by Blumberg and colleagues in 1965 in serum from an Australian Aborigine, hence its early name of Australia antigen. A subunit of the core antigen is secreted into serum (HBeAg) and is a useful serological marker of infectivity. Viral DNA may be found incorporated into chromosomal DNA of hepatocytes.

Hepatitis C virus

It has long been recognised that a parenterally acquired hepatitis exists, which is seronegative for hepatitis A or B, previously termed non-A, non-B hepatitis (NANB) and responsible particularly for post-transfusional hepatitis. In 1989, Choo and co-workers cloned an RNA virus from an infected chimpanzee and expressed it in *Escherichia coli*. The expressed antigen cross-reacted with serum of patients with NANB hepatitis. Since then the entire genome of this hepatitis C virus (HCV), has been cloned. It is a single-stranded RNA virus with an approximately 10,000 nucleotide genome. It has a lipid nucleocapsid and it shares sequence homology with flaviviruses and pestiviruses.

Hepatitis D virus

Originally designated the 'delta particle', hepatitis D is a defective RNA virus, which requires the presence of HBV to perform a helper function. Its circular single-stranded genome codes for the hepatitis D antigen and the virus is encapsulated with the HBV surface antigen (HBsAg). Like hepatitis B, it is usually acquired parenterally by a hepatitis B-positive individual, but co-infection also occurs. It is rare in Britain except in drug abusers and haemophiliacs, but more prevalent in Brazil, Equatorial Africa the Middle East and the Mediterranean. Co-infection with hepatitis B and D is more likely to lead to either chronic liver disease or fulminant hepatitis than infection with hepatitis B alone.

Hepatitis E virus

An enterically transmitted form of non-A, non-B hepatitis has been recognised for some time and this RNA virus has been cloned. It has been responsible for several epidemics in India, South East and Central Asia. Sporadic cases have been encountered in Britain among travellers returning from affected areas.

MANAGEMENT

Acute hepatitis

Rest, preferably in bed, is the traditional mainstay of treatment and the value of this is reinforced by anecdotal reports of fulminant hepatitis developing in people who have played strenuous sports while in the prodromal illness. The importance of diet has probably been overemphasised, but the diet should be fairly high in protein, providing there is no evidence of encephalopathy, and high in carbohydrate. Fat will not be absorbed well and in any case most patients find fatty foods unappealing when they are ill with hepatitis.

There is no specific effective drug therapy, although corticosteroids are occasionally used to hasten the resolution of cholestasis in hepatitis A. Corticosteroids should be avoided in hepatitis B or C. Alcohol should be avoided as long as the serum transaminases are elevated and abstinence for six months is usually recommended.

The serology of all close contacts of patients with hepatitis B or C, particularly sexual partners, should be checked. Hepatitis B vaccine should be given to seronegative contacts. Hepatitis A vaccine should be given to contacts of patients with hepatitis A. There is as yet no vaccine available for hepatitis C.

Fulminant hepatitis

Patients with fulminant hepatitis should be managed supportively with close monitoring of conscious level, coagulation and blood glucose, and screening for infection, preferably in units where there is availability of hepatic transplant facilities. Prognosis is bad with a mortality rate of more than 70% for patients in hepatic coma. The most important aspects to management are the avoidance of hypoglycaemia or fluid overload. Cerebral oedema is the commonest cause of death. It may respond to intravenous mannitol, but usually does not respond to dexamethasone.

Transplantation offers the best hope in Grade 4 coma due to viral hepatitis, but graft infection with hepatitis B is common despite infusion of hyperimmune globulin during the operation. Other forms of acute liver support such as charcoal haemoperfusion have not been shown to improve survival. (See chapter 15.)

Other forms of viral hepatitis

CYTOMEGALOVIRUS, EPSTEIN–BARR VIRUS (INFECTIOUS MONONUCLEOSIS) AND HERPES SIMPLEX

Cytomegalovirus, Epstein–Barr virus (infectious mononucleosis) and herpes simplex are all herpes type DNA viruses and cause a similar hepatitis. Centrizonal necrosis is absent, but there is patchy focal necrosis. Atypical lymphocytosis in the peripheral blood is common. All three viruses occasionally cause fatal hepatitis, but the hepatitis is usually mild and often subclinical. Diagnosis can be confirmed by serological testing for IgM antibodies to the causative agent (and/or monospot test for infectious mononucleosis).

YELLOW FEVER, MARBURG, LASSA AND EBOLA VIRUSES

Yellow fever is caused by an RNA virus transmitted by mosquitoes. It has an incubation period of 3–6 days with an abrupt onset of flu-like symptoms followed by jaundice. If severe, there may be renal failure, intestinal haemorrhage and encephalitis.

Marburg, Lassa and Ebola viruses are all RNA viruses, which cause similar very severe illnesses. The reservoir for Lassa fever infection is a wild rat, while Marburg and probably Ebola virus, are transmitted by monkeys. The incubation period for Lassa fever ranges from 6–20 days while those for Marburg and Ebola virus are shorter (4–7 days).

Lassa fever causes a severe flu-like illness, which if severe is associated with profound hypotension. Hepatitic involvement is a relatively minor feature of all three diseases, although transaminases may be high. Mortality approaches 50% with all three diseases and is usually due to cardiovascular collapse.

BACTERIAL AND PARASITIC INFECTIONS

Weil's disease (leptospirosis)

Weil's disease was first described in 1886 by Adolph Weil, Professor of Medicine in Heidelberg. The causative organism *Leptospira icterohaemorrhagia* is a spirochaete transmitted by rodents. The main route of entry is thought to be via skin abrasions contaminated by rat urine, although it can probably also be transmitted by ingestion. Sewage workers, farmers and coalminers are amongst those most at risk.

Course

The incubation period lasts 6–15 days. It is followed by abrupt onset of septicaemia with rigors, meningism, conjunctivitis, cough and a haemorrhagic tendency. Jaundice appears towards the end of the first week and is accompanied by neutrophil leucocytosis, which may be a clue to the diagnosis. Renal failure may develop in the second week of the illness and exacerbates the hyperbilirubinaemia. An acute myocarditis may also occur at this stage.

Management and prognosis

Benzylpenicillin therapy may be of help if started very early in the cause of the illness, but after the first week, treatment is supportive. Mortality is about 15% but the disease is usually self-limiting and chronic disease does not result.

Toxoplasmosis

Toxoplasma gondii is a 5 mm long crescent-shaped protozoan, transmitted particularly by cats. In adults it usually causes a mild illness that mimicks infectious mononucleosis with lymphadenopathy, hepatomegaly and sore throat. Congenital toxoplasmosis can be a very severe illness with jaundice developing within a few hours of birth and severe cerebral damage.

Syphilis

Secondary syphilis is one of the many causes of a granulomatous hepatitis and should be excluded when otherwise unexplained hepatic granulomas are found on liver biopsy. The serum alkaline phosphatase is elevated, but jaundice is unusual. Congenital syphilis is nowadays a very rare cause of neonatal jaundice. It usually progresses to cirrhosis.

Tuberculosis

Miliary tuberculosis may occasionally present with jaundice or even hepatic failure, sometimes without the characteristic miliary shadowing on chest radiography. When liver biopsy is performed as part of the investigation of pyrexia of unknown origin an unfixed sample should always be sent for mycobacterial culture.

Brucellosis

Brucellosis occurs worldwide and is caused by a small Gram-negative coccobacillus. Sheep, goats and cattle are the main reservoirs of infection and transmission is via contaminated milk or by direct contact with the products of infectious abortions. The illness is very variable with an incubation period of 1 week to several months. Clinical features include a remittent fever, night sweats, arthralgia and arthritis of large joints, severe depression and hepatosplenomegaly. Jaundice is unusual, but there is granulomatous infiltration of the liver with elevation of serum alkaline phosphatase.

Alpha-1 antitrypsin deficiency

Natural history
The liver disease may present:

- As neonatal hepatitis with jaundice occurring in the first four months of life.
- In adult life with cirrhosis and portal hypertension.
- As an incidental finding at post mortem.

Many patients with alpha-1 antitrypsin deficiency remain well throughout a normal life span. On liver biopsy, the hepatocytes are found to contain globules of trapped alpha-1 antitrypsin, which may be stained with peroxidase labelled specific antibody or by periodic acid–Schiff (diastase-resistant) (**Fig. 13.24**).

Alpha-1 antitrypsin accounts for over 90% of the alpha-1 globulin seen on electrophoresis of serum and inhibits a range of proteolytic enzymes including neutrophil elastase. Homozygotes for alpha-1 antitrypsin deficiency and arguably heterozygotes also are prone to develop liver disease although the most important consequence of the disease is usually emphysema.

Management
Alcohol and cigarette smoking should be avoided, but management is otherwise supportive. Liver transplantation occasionally needs to be considered.

Chronic hepatitis
Chronic hepatitis has been strictly defined as hepatitis lasting longer than six months, but must also be included in the differential diagnosis of patients with much shorter histories since prompt treatment is essential in autoimmune hepatitis and Wilson's disease. Three types are definable histologically:

- Chronic active hepatitis.
- Chronic lobular hepatitis.
- Chronic persistent hepatitis.

CHRONIC ACTIVE HEPATITIS
This is the most severe form of chronic hepatitis and the only form that commonly progresses to cirrhosis. The portal tracts are expanded by an infiltrate of lymphocytes and plasma cells, which spill out into the surrounding hepatocytes causing piecemeal necrosis. Fibrous septa then spread out from the portal tracts to surround groups (rosettes) of liver cells (**Fig. 13.25**). The commonest causes are hepatitis B and C virus infection and autoimmune chronic active (lupoid) hepatitis. Other causes include Wilson's disease, drugs such as isoniazid and methyldopa and alcohol.

CHRONIC LOBULAR HEPATITIS
This resembles acute hepatitis histologically and in some cases may be a sequel of infection with hepatitis C. There is patchy 'spotty' intra lobular inflammation and necrosis, but the necrosis does not extend to 'bridge' between portal tracts and central veins nor is there piecemeal necrosis. The patient has mild symptoms and a fluctuating serum transaminase.

CHRONIC PERSISTENT HEPATITIS
This is simply an increase in lymphocytes and plasma cells within the portal tracts (**Fig. 13.26**). It is a nonspecific finding, but is quite commonly associated with persistent hepatitis B infection. Jaundice is usually absent or very mild and the transaminase only modestly elevated.

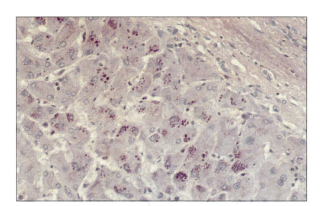

Fig. 13.24 Periodic acid–Schiff stain in alpha-1-antitrypsin deficiency showing the pink stained alpha-1-antitrypsin trapped within hepatocytes.

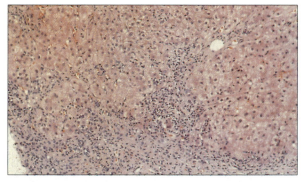

Fig. 13.25 Autoimmune chronic active hepatitis showing inflammatory cells, predominantly lymphocytes, extending beyond the limiting plates of the portal tracts with resulting piecemeal necrosis.

Chronic viral hepatitis

NATURAL HISTORY

Hepatitis B, C and D (but never A) are important causes worldwide, although chronic D infection is rare in Britain. The natural history is towards eventual cirrhosis in a majority of patients and hepatocellular carcinoma is a common late complication, particularly in patients with Hepatitis B.

Patients with chronic hepatitis may be completely asymptomatic and picked up on routine screening with elevated transaminases. Some may give a history of an acute hepatitis with jaundice. Others present with nonspecific symptoms of malaise or fatigue. Older patients may present with late sequelae of cirrhosis or hepatocellular carcinoma.

Physical findings are usually absent except in advanced disease where there may be hepatomegaly, spider naevi, ascites, easy bruising and leuconychia when cirrhosis has developed. Serum transaminase is typically elevated and may fluctuate considerably especially in hepatitis C where patients may experience periodic exacerbations of the disease. Diagnosis is made serologically. In chronic hepatitis B tests for HBeAg and HBV DNA are commonly positive. It is important to follow these markers serially for at least six months after the onset of illness to see if the patient is likely to clear the virus (as evidenced by disappearance of HBV DNA followed by HBeAg). In some patients (particularly from Italy or Greece) HBeAg becomes undetectable, but HBV DNA (and thus viral replication) persists. Disappearance of these markers is accompanied by an exacerbation of the illness followed by complete resolution and no need for further treatment.

MANAGEMENT

Management must include patient education and protection of close contacts. This may be achieved by immunisation against hepatitis B and the practice of 'safe sex' for sexually active individuals. Patients should avoid excess alcohol as there is good evidence that patients with chronic hepatitis and alcohol abuse do badly. Patients should be periodically monitored by serum transaminase and viral markers.

Specific therapy for chronic hepatitis B, C and D in the form of α-interferon is available, but it is expensive and only achieves viral clearance in about 35% of patients (**Fig. 13.27**). Before giving interferon the diagnosis should be confirmed by the presence of HBeAg and HBV DNA (or HCV antibody or HDV antibody positivity for Hepatitis C and D respectively), an elevated serum transaminase and a liver biopsy showing histological evidence of active hepatitis. The main aims of interferon therapy are to prevent cirrhosis and to reduce infectivity.

Treatment with α-interferon may need to be continued for 6–12 months. Monitoring of serum transaminase is performed and patients that respond will have a rise in transaminase followed by clearance of markers of viral replication. α-interferon treatment should be avoided in patients with established cirrhosis, acquired immune deficiency disease (AIDS), thyroid disease and severe neutropenia. Patients with vertically transmitted disease (commonly from the Middle or Far East) are unlikely to respond to α-interferon treatment.

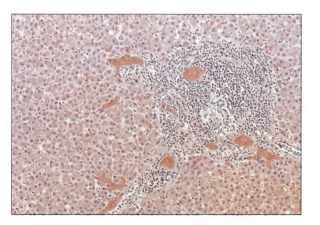

Fig. 13.26 Chronic persistent hepatitis with inflammation confined to the portal tracts.

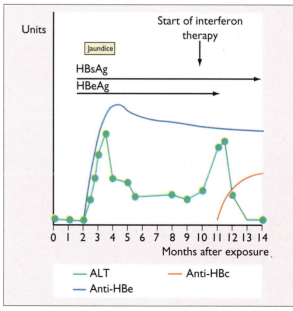

Fig. 13.27 Successful response to interferon therapy for chronic hepatitis B antigenaemia. Note the rise in transaminase following therapy. This may result in fatal hepatic failure if the patient is already cirrhotic.

Autoimmune chronic active hepatitis

Autoimmune chronic active (lupoid) hepatitis has a female:male preponderance of 8:1 and is associated with HLA DR3. Antinuclear and anti-smooth muscle antibodies are commonly found in the serum. Other autoimmune diseases may be associated including thyroiditis, Coombs'-positive haemolytic anaemia, non-erosive migratory polyarthritis and rarely fibrosing alveolitis. LE cells are found in the blood in 15% of patients, but the condition is distinguished from systemic lupus erythematosus by the lack of neurological, cardiac or significant renal involvement.

Diagnosis of autoimmune hepatitis requires the absence of serological markers for viral hepatitis and a careful drug history since serum autoantibody tests are not totally specific.

MANAGEMENT

Corticosteroids have transformed the prognosis of auto-immune chronic active hepatitis from an average life expectancy of only about 3–4 years to well over 10 years. Fairly high doses are needed, usually starting with prednisolone, 30 mg daily. Some patients can come off steroid therapy after a year or so, but at least half will relapse again, sometimes with serious consequences, so many hepatologists feel it is better to continue low-dose maintenance therapy indefinitely. The steroid dosage can be titrated against the serum transaminase, but a repeat liver biopsy should be performed after six months therapy as there is often a discrepancy between the biochemical and histological response. Azathioprine, 1–2 mg/kg, may be added in as a 'steroid-sparing' drug, but is not effective as sole therapy.

If unrelated to hepatitis C, **chronic lobular hepatitis** usually responds promptly to oral corticosteroid therapy, which can usually be discontinued after a few months. **Chronic persistent hepatitis** requires no specific therapy.

Wilson's disease (hepatolenticular degeneration)

NATURAL HISTORY

About 50% of patients present with liver disease and the other half with neurological disorders, which include tremor, dysarthria, psychiatric disturbance and athetosis. A Kayser–Fleischer ring, a brown ring at the periphery of the cornea, is present in most, but not all patients. Presentation is commonly in adolescence, but may be anytime from 5–40 years of age. Associated problems include renal tubular acidosis, premature osteoarthritis and haemolysis.

The liver disease may present either as chronic hepatitis, closely mimicking autoimmune chronic active hepatitis from which it must always be distinguished, or as an acute hepatitis which may be fulminant.

Liver histology shows the usual features of chronic active hepatitis with or without established cirrhosis, but in addition there is usually microvesicular fat and vacuolation of nuclei (**Fig. 13.28**). Histochemical stains for copper (e.g. rubeanic acid) or copper-associated protein (e.g. orcein, **Fig. 13.29**) usually show periportal copper accumulation, but are not sufficiently reliable for diagnosis, which necessitates chemical quantification of liver copper.

PATHOGENESIS

Wilson's disease is inherited as an autosomal recessive disorder and has a prevalence of 1 in 30,000. Copper is deposited in tissues resulting in degeneration of the basal ganglia and cirrhosis. The underlying defect is poorly understood, but serum concentration of the alpha-2-globulin caeruloplasmin, a copper-binding protein, is low and the serum copper is low as a consequence. Liver and urine copper concentrations are high.

MANAGEMENT

The chelating agent penicillamine is highly effective. Treatment is started with 300 mg four times daily and monitored by annual liver copper estimation.

The prognosis is usually good if the disease is recognised early, but poor in fulminant hepatitis or if there is dystonia. Close relatives need screening by serum caeruloplasmin and urine copper, and asymptomatic patients with proven disease should be treated.

Haemochromatosis

Natural history

The excessive iron deposition in tissues results in cirrhosis, diabetes, hypopituitarism, cardiomyopathy and pseudogout. These manifest as signs of chronic liver disease, loss of secondary sexual hair and loss of libido, congestive heart failure and arthritis affecting particularly the metacarpophalangeal joints and knees. Chondrocalcinosis affecting the menisci may be visible on an X-ray of the knee. Increased

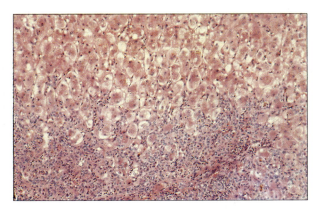

Fig. 13.28 Wilson's disease (haematoxylin and eosin stain) showing the typical microvesicular fat accumulation and features of chronic active hepatitis with lymphocytes infiltrating beyond the portal tracts and accompanying piecemeal necrosis. Courtesy of Dr S Hubscher.

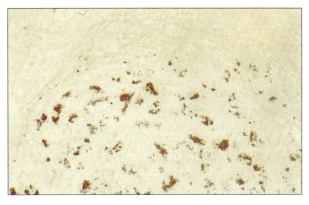

Fig. 13.29 Wilson's disease (Orcein stain) showing accumulation of copper. Courtesy of Dr S Hubscher.

skin pigmentation occurs due to a combination of iron and melanin resulting in the description 'bronze diabetes'.

- Serum iron is increased and iron binding capacity is over 90% saturated.
- Serum ferritin is markedly elevated, but is also elevated in acute liver disease due to other causes.
- Liver iron is easily seen histochemically using Perls' stain (**Fig. 13.30**) and this is fairly reliable for diagnosis, although direct quantification of liver iron may sometimes be needed, particularly in alcoholics who often have a moderate increase in liver iron.

If untreated the disease progresses over 12 years and hepatoma is common.

Pathogenesis
Haemochromatosis has an autosomal recessive pattern of inheritance. Its inheritance is strongly linked with HLA status, particularly A3. Expression of the gene is variable and is more likely if the patient has at least a moderately heavy alcohol intake, but may occur in complete teetotallers. The basic defect seems to be disordered regulation of intestinal iron absorption.

Management
Avoidance of alcohol is essential. Venesection of one pint should be carried out weekly until the haemoglobin starts to fall. Up to 100–150 pints of blood may have to be removed to lower tissue iron stores to a normal level. First degree relatives should be screened by HLA typing and by estimation of serum iron and iron binding capacity or serum ferritin. The iron studies should be repeated at two-year intervals in patients at risk and liver iron estimated if the serum studies are abnormal.

Alcoholic liver disease

Natural history
The commonest mode of presentation is in the young heavy drinker who is found to have hepatomegaly and a modestly elevated serum transaminase. The majority of such patients have a fatty liver without cirrhosis and the initial prognosis for the liver is good although the long-term prognosis will depend entirely on successful abstinence. Next common is the patient, often a middle-aged 'social drinker,' who presents with established cirrhosis with complications of portal hypertension or liver failure and often denies an excessive alcohol intake.

Aetiology and pathogenesis
The link between excessive alcohol consumption and liver disease is undisputed, but the mechanism quite unclear. It has proved surprisingly difficult to produce alcoholic cirrhosis experimentally in animals. Postulated mechanisms have included a direct toxic effect of the major metabolite acetaldehyde, malnutrition, depletion of hepatic ATP and

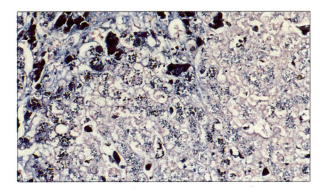

Fig. 13.30 Perls' stain showing massive iron accumulation within hepatocytes and Kuppfer cells in haemochromatosis.

free radical-mediated damage. Free radicals are highly reactive chemical species with an unpaired (and therefore unstable) electron in their outer orbit. They are responsible, among other actions, for rancidification of fats. None of these mechanisms for alcoholic liver damage has been firmly established.

There is a definite correlation between the volume of alcohol consumed and the risk for liver disease and this is reflected by a much higher rate of death due to cirrhosis in countries with a high alcohol consumption. It has however, proved difficult to identify the maximum safe level for any individual. The risk seems greater for women than for men, even after allowing for differences in body weight. This may be due to the reported lower levels of alcohol dehydrogenase in the gastric mucosa of women. Successive publications have gradually lowered the 'safe' level, which currently stands at about 40 g alcohol (two pints of beer or four glasses of wine) daily for men and 20 g daily for women.

It has been suggested that there may be an HLA-linked risk for susceptibility to alcoholic liver disease, but this has been disputed.

Pathology

The main histological features of alcoholic liver disease are fatty infiltration, hepatitis and cirrhosis (**Fig. 13.31**). A characteristic feature is Mallory's hyaline, which is amorphous material seen in the cytoplasm of hepatocytes and staining red with eosin. It is thought to represent degraded cytokeratin and can be shown by electron microsopy to consist of randomly orientated filaments.

Inflammation (hepatitis) is predominantly polymorphonuclear with polymorphs seen around and even within the damaged hepatocytes although a lymphocytic infiltrate with other histological features of chronic active hepatitis may less commonly be seen.

It is intriguing that in severe obesity, particularly if associated with mild diabetes mellitus, the fatty infiltration of the liver may also be associated with Mallory's hyaline,

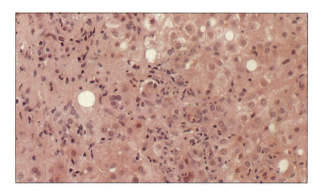

Fig. 13.31 Alcoholic hepatitis showing steatosis and neutrophils infiltrating the hepatic parenchyma and Mallory's hyaline.

neutrophil polymorph infiltration and increased fibrosis. It is quite likely therefore that simple fatty infiltration of the liver is not such a benign condition as previously thought, and recent long-term follow-up studies of patients with alcoholic fatty liver have shown a high incidence of subsequent cirrhosis even when fibrosis and inflammation were absent from earlier biopsies.

Fibrosis is perisinusoidal and initially is predominantly centrizonal rather than periportal. Fibrous strands eventually link up with loss of the normal relationship between central veins and portal tracts, development of regeneration nodules (identifiable by displaced or absent central veins) and establishment of irreversible cirrhosis.

It is likely that most patients insidiously pass from fatty liver via fibrosis to cirrhosis, but in a minority the florid clinical syndrome of acute alcoholic hepatitis develops. This is characterised by jaundice (which is otherwise uncommon in alcoholic liver disease except in the end stage) neutrophil leucocytosis, fever and a hypermetabolic state with a high cardiac output and a hepatic blood flow sufficient to generate a systolic hepatic bruit.

Only approximately 50% of patients with florid alcoholic hepatitis have established cirrhosis, but the mortality is high nevertheless, approximately 50% dying within three months of presentation.

Management

The prognosis for patients with alcoholic liver disease depends almost entirely on their success at abstinence. In one study of patients with established alcoholic liver disease survival at five years was 34% for those who continued to drink and 69% for those who stopped.

Unfortunately hypnosis, group psychotherapy and the acetaldehyde dehydrogenase inhibitor disulfuram (antabuse) have all failed to show consistent efficacy in helping patients to abstain.

The main factors are the patient's ability to recognise the problem and a determination to cope with it. It is important to offer sympathetic follow-up for one approach that is certain to result in failure is a one-minute admonition followed by a prompt discharge from medical supervision. In some centres day attendance facilities have proved very successful and a motivated social support team is essential.

Patients suffering from acute alcoholism should be offered hospital in-patient 'drying-out' providing they show some intentions of abstaining permanently. Alcohol withdrawal commonly results in convulsions and psychosis if not carefully managed and may even result in death from cardiovascular collapse. Withdrawal symptoms should be anticipated and prevented by prophylactic administration of chlormethiazole or chlordiazepoxide given in reducing doses over about five days with adjustment of the dose according to tremor and tachycardia.

Vitamin deficiency states
Another very important aspect of the initial care is the prevention of vitamin deficiency states, particularly thiamine deficiency with its disastrous consequences of **Wernicke's** encephalopathy and **Korsakoff's** psychosis. This is recognised clinically as a combination of:

- Defects of visual gaze (usually lateral, but sometimes vertical).
- Nystagmus.
- Ataxia.
- Confusion.

It requires prompt diagnosis and treatment with thiamine otherwise the damage quickly becomes irreversible.

Deficiency of vitamin C and folate are almost universal and the dietary intake of protein is often minimal. A high protein diet should be encouraged providing there is no evidence for hepatic encephalopathy and multivitamin supplements should be prescribed. The appetite is usually very poor and enteral feeding may be required.

Florid alcoholic hepatitis
In the rarer patients with florid alcoholic hepatitis, attempts have been made to reduce the hypermetabolic state. In experimental animals hepatic oxygen consumption can be reduced by pre-treatment with the antithyroid drug propylthiouracil. This drug has been used in alcoholic liver disease with conflicting results.

One double-blind controlled trial showed no benefit in severe alcoholic hepatitis, but a recent large trial in patients with all forms of alcohol-related liver disease showed a reduced mortality over a two year period. Its cautious use in combination with regular blood count and thyroid function test monitoring may therefore be justified. A simpler alternative, which has also proved effective in controlled trials is to prescribe a one-month course of corticosteroid (prednisolone, 30 mg/day). Drug therapy must not be seen as an alternative to abstinence.

Drugs and jaundice
Some drugs, such as paracetamol, predictably cause liver damage in all patients if taken in sufficient dosage, while many others cause unpredictable (idiosynchratic) reactions in a minority of patients.

Drug-induced acute hepatitis
Abnormalities may range from mild elevation of serum transaminase to fulminant hepatitis. Mechanisms of toxicity vary considerably, but it is thought that one common mechanism is oxidation of the drug by the cytochrome p450 enzyme system resulting in the formation of a reactive metabolite. This metabolite is then electrophilic and liable to form covalent bonds with proteins or nucleic acids and to affect their structure and function as a result. Covalent binding occurs particularly to sulphhydryl (SH) groups so if an alternative source of sulphhydryl groups such as N-acetylcysteine or methionine can be provided, toxicity is greatly reduced. Conversely if the liver content of glutathione (which is SH-rich) becomes depleted, damage is increased.

Damage is usually most marked in centrizonal areas. Drugs that predictably cause an acute hepatitic reaction include paracetamol (acetaminophen) and carbon tetrachloride, but many drugs cause occasional idiosyncratic reactions.

Microvesicular fat deposition
Adults are susceptible to Reye's syndrome, in which there is a rapid accumulation of microvesicular fat within the liver (**Fig. 13.32**) accompanied by elevated serum transaminase and a high risk of acute liver failure.

Reye's syndrome has been well known for some time as a rare cause of liver failure in children in whom it usually follows a viral illness particularly if aspirin has been used. Aspirin has been withdrawn from general use in childhood ailments as a result. Intravenous tetracycline was the first drug shown to cause this condition in adults, but the commonly used antiepileptic sodium valproate may also cause severe liver damage via this mechanism.

Alcohol-mimicking hepatotoxic drugs
Perhexilene and amiodarone both occasionally cause a hepatitis, which closely mirrors alcoholic hepatitis with Mallory's hyaline and a neutrophil polymorph reaction.

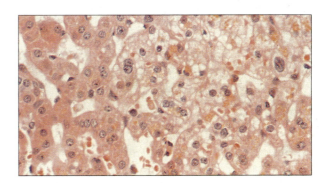

Fig. 13.32 Microvesicular fat in Reye's syndrome.

Immune-mediated damage

Most drug-related acute hepatitis is thought to result from a direct toxic effect of the drug itself or more commonly a reactive metabolite. However, in halothane hepatitis there is good evidence for an immunological component since the patients serum can be shown to contain antibodies directed against halothane altered liver cell membranes.

Chronic hepatitis and fibrosis

Some forms of drug-related hepatitis follow a more indolent chronic course that mimicks autoimmune chronic active hepatitis clinically, histologically and biochemically. As a result, the drug aetiology can easily be overlooked with progression to cirrhosis or liver failure as a result. Drugs that may cause this form of hepatitis include methyldopa, isoniazid and the laxative agent oxyphenisatin.

Sometimes a chronic fibrotic reaction with consequent portal hypertension occurs without significant hepatitis; this is particularly the case with the cytotoxic drugs azathioprine, methotrexate, 6-mercaptopurine and cyclophosphamide.

Cholestasis

In some forms of drug-related hepatitis, there may be marked intrahepatic retention of bile (cholestasis) with little or no inflammation. Oestrogens taken as oral contraceptives may cause a pure cholestasis, which is dose related. The risk for oestrogen cholestasis is familial and susceptible individuals may also develop jaundice in the last trimester of pregnancy. Other drugs that cause cholestasis, usually with a mild hepatitic element include all the phenothiazines, noteably chlorpromazine as well as erythromycin , co-amoxiclav and nitrofurantoin. Chlorpromazine jaundice may be prolonged for six months or more after cessation of therapy, but chronic liver damage is rare.

Management of drug-related jaundice

The first vital step is to be alert to the possibility of drug-related liver damage and to stop any potentially toxic drug immediately. With the exception of acute drug overdose with paracetamol when administration of sulphhydryl donors such as N-acetylcysteine or methionine may be life-saving, there is rarely any specific therapy. In chronic hepatitis due to methyldopa where there is probably an autoimmune component, corticosteroid therapy may be helpful, but the most important aspect of treatment is still cessation of the offending drug.

In patients receiving multiple therapy, it may be impossible to be certain which drug is the culprit. Re-challenge with a small dose of the potentially harmful drug may produce a severe reaction and is probably best avoided. It is safest to find alternative drugs if possible, but if this is impracticable then those essential drugs that have a low rate of reported hepatotoxicity (e.g. digoxin or diuretics) should be reintroduced, one at a time and as a single dose initially.

Pregnancy-associated liver disease

Acute fatty liver

The best-known and most serious hepatic complication of pregnancy is acute fatty liver. It is thought to have an incidence of approximately 1 in 13,000 deliveries, but it is quite likely that milder disease is undiagnosed. It always occurs in late pregnancy, usually after 35 weeks' gestation, but occasionally after 30 weeks.

Clinical features include vomiting and, in more serious illness, jaundice and coma. Abdominal pain may be present. Features of pre-eclampsia such as oedema, hypertension and proteinuria are often, but not invariably present. The degree of coagulation disturbance and coma often seem out of proportion to the relatively modest rise in serum transaminase (rarely more than 500 iu/l).

In established fatty liver of pregnancy with coagulopathy and encephalopathy, mortality is high: at least 33% for the mother and higher for the fetus.

There is microvesicular fat accumulation in the liver similar to Reye's syndrome, but subtle differences in mitochondria have been documented and it seems likely that the two mechanisms are different. Elevation of serum uric acid is usual and may help in the diagnosis.

MANAGEMENT

The most important aspect of treatment is early delivery, which should probably be by Caesarean section. Subsequent pregnancies do not seem to carry a significant risk of recurrence, although there are relatively few reported cases.

Pre-eclampsia

Features of preeclampsia are common in patients with acute fatty liver of pregnancy, but pre-eclampsia itself can cause a separate liver problem. Focal periportal necrosis with fibrin plugging of sinusoids may occur in association with other features of disseminated intravascular coagulation (e.g. microangiopathic haemolytic anaemia with fragmented red cells, thrombocytopenia, prolonged prothombrin time, reduced fibrinogen concentration and increased concentration of fibrin degradation products). Transaminase elevation is usually modest and jaundice is rare, but bleeding problems may be severe due to the coagulopathy and may necessitate early delivery.

Hyperemesis gravidarum

Severe hyperemesis in the first trimester may be associated with jaundice. The mechanism for this is unclear since liver biopsies have generally not been performed. The bilirubin is often predominantly unconjugated and may partly reflect the effects of fasting and 'stress' on hepatic conjugation as in Gilbert's syndrome.

MANAGEMENT
Oral pyridoxal phosphate is sometimes effective if anti-emetic therapy (usually chlorpromazine) fails, but its mechanism of action is unknown.

Cholestasis of pregnancy
Cholestasis of pregnancy is generally a benign condition occurring in the last trimester and presenting as itching, either alone or in combination with jaundice. It is genetic-ally transmitted together with oestrogen cholestasis, probably by autosomal dominant inheritance. There is a slightly increased risk of premature delivery.

Treatment of cholestasis in preganancy includes oral cholestyramine for relief of itching and intramuscular vitamin K to correct prothrombin deficiency.

Miscellaneous causes of intrahepatic cholestasis
Intrahepatic cholestasis is usually due to drugs, oestrogens or previous viral hepatitis, but in the absence of these, a number of less common causes should be considered. These include sepsis, neoplasia, intravenous feeding and benign recurrent cholestasis.

Sepsis due to any organism may occasionally be followed by a period of intrahepatic cholestasis, which may take several weeks to resolve, but has a good prognosis providing the underlying cause for sepsis has resolved. The mechanism is unclear. Neoplasia, particularly lymphoproliferative diseases such as Hodgkin's disease, and occasionally hypernephroma, causes non-metastatic cholestasis. One theory is that the malignant tissue releases oestrogen-like humoral factors, which cause the cholestasis.

▶ **Causes of intrahepatic cholestasis**

- Post-viral (particularly hepatitis A)
- Oral contraceptives (oestrogen)
- Pregnancy
- Drugs (chlorpromazine and many others)
- Malignancy without metastasis (e.g Hodgkin's or hypernephroma)
- Sepsis
- Intravenous feeding
- Chronic liver disease (primary biliary cirrhosis, sclerosing cholangitis)

Jaundice in patients receiving intravenous feeding is often multifactorial and may be due to a combination of drugs, sepsis, heart failure and haemolysis. The feeding solution itself does sometimes seem to contribute to the jaundice. The mechanism is unclear. It may be related to the amino acid or fat emulsion or both. There is some evidence that it may be preventable by prophylactic metronidazole therapy, which is thought to result in reduced production of cholestatic fatty acid metabolites by intestinal bacteria. The prognosis depends on the underlying condition but hepatic dysfunction, apart from hyperbilirubinaemia, is usually mild. Benign recurrent cholestasis is a very rare familial disorder, which usually presents by 10 years of age and requires no specific therapy. The mechanism is unknown.

Primary biliary cirrhosis

Natural history
Primary biliary cirrhosis is an unfortunate label for a condition in which the majority of patients present at a non-cirrhotic stage. The more accurate alternative 'chronic non-suppurative destructive cholangitis' has not gained acceptance for obvious reasons. There are three common forms of presentation:

- The chance finding of elevated serum alkaline phosphatase and/or mitochondrial antibody.
- Itching with or without jaundice.
- End-stage liver disease with features of portal hyper-tension such as ascites or bleeding oesophageal varices.

About 90% of patients are women, a fact that still eludes explanation. Onset of symptoms typically occurs between 30 and 65 years of age and the estimated incidence ranges from 6–15/million/year. Prognosis depends very much on the mode of presentation. In symptomatic patients there is a reported mean survival of 6–11 years, while asymptomatic patients may even have a normal life expectancy.

The hallmark of the disease is the presence in the serum of an antibody against an antigen on the inner membrane of mitochondria. This antibody is detectable in at least 95% of patients and the diagnosis can rarely be made with certainty in its absence. It has recently been shown that the antigen (M2) for this antibody is part of the pyruvate dehydrogenase complex. The same antigen is also present in some bacteria and yeasts.

This leads to the intriguing possibility that it may reflect an immune reaction to the bacteria, which have been reported more frequently to colonise the urinary tract of women with this disease. This might also explain the female preponderance, although there are other possible explan-ations for this including the general tendency for women to be more prone to autoimmune disease as well as possible hormonal factors.

The mitochondrial antibody is unlikely to be directly involved in hepatic damage, which seems to be lymphocyte mediated. Early in the course of the disease there is an increase of lymphocytes in the portal tracts and non-caseating granulomas form by coalescence of macrophages in the portal tracts (**Fig. 13.33**). As the disease progresses interlobular bile ducts become damaged and finally disappear resulting in intense cholestasis with proliferation of the small ductules. Fibrosis develops and extends to bridge between portal tracts with the eventual development of cirrhosis. Progression is patchy, however, so histological staging based on a needle biopsy usually gives a less reliable guide to the prognosis than the serum bilirubin concentration.

As a consequence of the cholestasis, the serum cholesterol is markedly elevated and xanthelasmata are often prominent. Palmar xanthomas may occur and are sometimes associated with a debilitating painful peripheral neuropathy.

Fat malabsorption is severe in advanced disease and deficiency of the fat-soluble vitamins A, D, K and E becomes clinically important.

- Vitamin A deficiency leads to night blindness, vitamin D deficiency to osteomalacia, and vitamin K deficiency to prothrombin deficiency, all of which occur commonly in advanced primary biliary cirrhosis.
- Vitamin E used to be thought of as an unimportant curiosity that improved the virility of rats, but was of no importance in man. It is now known to be essential for the development of the nervous system and its deficiency in the neonatal period and in early childhood results in severe spinocerebellar degeneration. Although this

problem mainly affects children with malabsorptive conditions such as cystic fibrosis and abetalipoproteinaemia, milder versions have been reported in primary biliary cirrhosis.

The chronic cholestasis also results in skin pigmentation (due mainly to increased melanin). Itching may be debilitating. It is presumably related to bile acid accumulation because it is improved by cholestyramine, but there is no good correlation with serum or tissue concentrations of bile acid. Osteoporosis may be very severe and is not fully understood, although vitamin D and calcium deficiency may be contributory factors.

Biochemical features of cholestasis are universal and include elevation of serum alkaline phosphatase, variable elevation of bilirubin concentration and modest elevation of serum transaminase. Sometimes, however, there may be overlap with chronic active hepatitis with piecemeal necrosis extending into the parenchyma from the portal tracts and an accompanying greater elevation in serum transaminase.

Serum Ig M concentration is usually elevated, but this seems to be a nonspecific feature of most chronic cholestatic disorders. One or more of the other autoimmune diseases commonly coexist including the sicca syndrome, thyroid disease, sclerodactyly, fibrosing alveolitis and renal tubular acidosis.

Management

In primary biliary cirrhosis, as in other chronic progressive illnesses, the patient needs careful and sympathetic handling. If cirrhosis is not yet established the patient should be made aware of this and the misleading nature of the name of the disease explained.

Many different approaches to therapy have been tried, but so far, none of them has been reproducibly shown to affect the prognosis. It seems unlikely that any drug will significantly effect the outcome once the majority of the interlobular bile ducts have disappeared.

Most of the trials of therapy have included patients with advanced disease, which may have obscured a favourable response in patients with earlier disease. Corticosteroid therapy was felt to be contraindicated after it was shown to accelerate osteoporosis in patients with advanced disease, however reports of beneficial effects suggest a need for further evaluation in patients with early disease.

Because of the immunological and histological similarities between primary biliary cirrhosis and the graft versus host disease seen in liver transplant recipients cyclosporin has been tried, but without convincing benefit. Pencillamine was tried extensively, partly because of its immunosuppressive effects and partly because primary biliary cirrhosis, like all cholestatic liver diseases, is associated with accumulation of copper in the liver. The copper may be potentially harmful

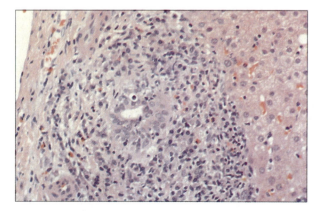

Fig. 13.33 Primary biliary cirrhosis showing a bile duct surrounded by an early granulomatous reaction with inflammatory cells invading the wall of the duct. Eventually the duct is likely to be destroyed completely leaving only hyperplastic ductules visible within the portal tract.

(see Wilson's disease) and can be removed by chelation with penicillamine. After initial promising results it now looks as though this form of treatment does not improve the prognosis. More recently, promising results have been obtained with oral colchicine, a drug that inhibits collagen synthesis. Further studies are needed to evaluate this.

The most promising medical therapy at present is **ursodeoxycholic acid**, 250 mg three times daily, which seems to improve all forms of chronic cholestasis.

Regular supplements of fat-soluble vitamins should be given to all jaundiced patients (i.e. 100,000 iu of vitamin A, 100,000 iu of vitamin D and 10 mg of vitamin K every four weeks by intramuscular injection).

If steatorrhoea is present, a low fat intake should be advised and additional calcium supplements prescribed.

Itching usually responds initially to cholestyramine (up to 12 g/day), but 'breakthrough' often occurs. One of the relatively non-sedating antihistamines, such as terfenadine, may then be tried, but relief is often only partial.

Many patients with primary biliary cirrhosis eventually develop deteriorating liver function with resulting lethargy, altered sleep pattern and encephalopathy, often compounded by intense itching. This state may persist for many months, until an intercurrent event such as variceal haemorrhage or septicaemia precipitates terminal liver failure.

Liver transplantation is now offering a realistic chance of restoring normal, or near normal, health for these patients, many of whom are mothers with young families.

Liver transplantation

Primary biliary cirrhosis is the commonest benign disease indication for transplantation.

The risk of the operation itself depends very much on the condition of the patient at the time of surgery. Severely abnormal coagulation combined with portal hypertension and adhesions from previous abdominal surgery can result in a very difficult operation with massive transfusion requirements and a considerable mortality, while in the relatively 'fit' patient, the operation can be reasonably straightforward.

After the immediate operative period, the main problems are rejection, renal failure and sepsis, but these have diminished considerably since the introduction of cycloporin A and improved management of the immunosuppression.

Careful patient selection is crucial. Most centres try to select adults with a life expectancy of under one year and a poor quality of life, but these are both difficult points to judge. Primary biliary cirrhosis is relatively easy in that there is a fairly good inverse correlation between serum bilirubin and prognosis. A serum bilirubin greater than 100 μmol/l that continues to rise on follow-up in conjunction with lethargy, is a reliable indication of a poor prognosis without transplantation. Sclerosing cholangitis is another relatively common indication for transplantation.

Children with primary biliary atresia also make good candidates since they have a universally hopeless prognosis without transplantation and have a postoperative survival of up to 95% following transplantation. Storage diseases and other inherited metabolic diseases such as alpha-1 antitrypsin deficiency are also successfully treated by transplantation.

Transplantation for carcinoma

Transplantation for carcinoma is a difficult area. Metastatic carcinoma is definitely not appropriate for transplantation, but patients with primary liver cancers, either hepatocellular or cholangiocarcinoma, occasionally do well following transplantation. Many centres now feel that the recurrence rate after transplantation for cholangiocarcinoma (approximately 80%) is too high to make the procedure worthwhile. Results for hepatocellular carcinoma are generally slightly better and the prognosis in that condition is so bleak without transplantation (median survival under three months), that the small proportion of excellent results make it worthwhile in selected patients, particularly those with fibrolamellar tumours, providing a careful search before transplantation has failed to show evidence of metastatic spread.

Transplantation for alcoholic liver disease

Transplantation for alcoholic liver disease is increasing. It used to be avoided on the grounds that the alcoholism itself has a poor prognosis and compliance with chemotherapy and follow-up are likely to be poor. There is probably also at least a subconscious feeling that resources are limited and that self-inflicted disease should have a low priority. It is now widely felt that transplantation is reasonable in a small group of patients under 60 years of age who have abstained from alcohol for at least six months, but are debilitated by end-stage liver disease. Long-term prognosis in these patients seems to be at least as good as for transplant performed for other indications.

▶ **Consequences of chronic cholestasis**

- Itching
- Pigmentation
- Malabsorption of fat-soluble vitamins, leading to:
  Osteomalacia (D)
  Coagulopathy (K)
  Night blindness (A)
  Spinocerebellar degeneration (rare in adults) (E)
- Hypercholesterolaemia
- Xanthomatosis
- Increased serum immunoglobulin M

Transplantation for acute liver failure

Acute liver failure is another major indication for transplantation. Here patient selection is particularly difficult. Many patients make a complete recovery from fulminant hepatic failure and predicting the patients who will not recover is very difficult.

One group that can be identified with some certainty are those with subacute hepatic necrosis in whom an acute hepatitis, often non-A, non-B and non-C, has progressed over eight weeks or more, to liver failure and encephalopathy. Mortality in such patients is over 80% and good results are now being reported for transplantation. (See Chapter 15.)

Overall results

Overall results have been steadily improving and transplantation is now an established form of therapy. Approximately 80% of transplant patients survive the first year. Problems (**Fig. 13.34**) tend to become less frequent after the first post-transplant year and the outlook is then good, although immunosuppression needs to be continued indefinitely. Results in children are even better.

All aspects of transplantation, the pre-transplant assessment, the operation and the follow-up are extremely stressful for the patients and their relatives. Care should be taken not to mention the subject of transplantation unless preliminary enquiries with the appropriate transplant centre suggest that the patient would probably be accepted.

Sclerosing cholangitis

Natural history

In primary sclerosing cholangitis there is a slight male preponderance and the majority of patients present between 25 and 45 years of age. As with primary biliary cirrhosis, presentation may vary from asymptomatic elevation of serum alkaline phosphatase to cholestatic jaundice and symptoms of portal hypertension.

Liver histology typically reveals a paucity of interlobular bile ducts associated with periductal fibrosis and portal inflammation (**Fig. 13.35**). It is, however, usually difficult to make a definite diagnosis from the liver histology alone. Autoimmune chronic active hepatitis may also be associated with ulcerative colitis and in some patients the two conditions overlap.

Pericholangitis (infiltration by polymorphonuclear leucocytes in and around bile ducts) is not a specific finding and is a common abnormality in inflammatory bowel disease where it usually has a completely benign prognosis.

Diagnosis of sclerosing cholangitis is usually based on the typical radiological appearances of beading and stricturing of extrahepatic and/or intrahepatic bile ducts.

The prognosis is extremely variable and depends on the mode of presentation. In a jaundiced patient the mean survival is about five years, but asymptomatic patients may continue untroubled for many years.

AETIOLOGY AND PATHOGENESIS

Primary sclerosing cholangitis is a chronic progressive condition in which there is inflammation, fibrosis and irregular stricturing of bile ducts both within the liver and in the extrahepatic biliary system.

There is a striking association with ulcerative colitis, which is present in approximately 70% of patients. The ulcerative colitis is often mild and colectomy seems to have no effect on the course of the biliary disease.

Other conditions rarely associated with sclerosing cholangitis include fibrosing conditions such as Riedel's thyroiditis and retroperitoneal fibrosis.

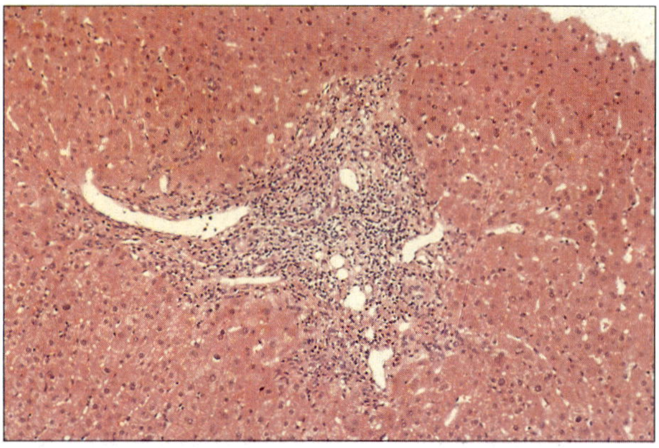

Fig. 13.34 Transplant rejection. Features very similar to those in primary biliary cirrhosis are seen, with destruction of the main bile duct within the portal tract and ductular hyperplasia. In rejection, most of the immunological attack is directed against bile ducts and blood vessels rather than against the hepatocytes themselves.

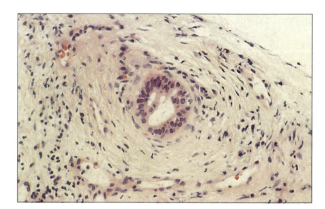

Fig. 13.35 Primary sclerosing cholangitis. A bile duct is seen being infiltrated by inflammatory cells and surrounded by a typical whorl of fibrosis.

There is a statistical link with HLA DR3, an HLA type that is also linked with autoimmune diseases. Over 70% of patients with colitis-associated disease have anti-neutrophil antibody (pANCA) detectable in the serum.

Similar radiological appearances of alternating beading and stricturing are seen:

- Following severe cholangitis in association with gallstones (secondary sclerosing cholangitis).
- In patients with human immunodeficiency virus-I (HIV-I) disease. (See Chapter 17.)
- Following infusion of cytotoxic agents via the hepatic artery.

Management

Many forms of treatment have been tried without convincing benefit including corticosteroids, azathioprine, penicillamine and broad-spectrum antibiotics. Promising results are being obtained with ursodeoxycholic acid, 250 mg three times a day.

The most impressive results have come from surgical or endoscopic dilatatation and stenting of large duct strictures. The cholangiograms should be reviewed carefully and stenting considered particularly if there are tight extrahepatic bile duct strictures in association with relatively mild abnormalities of the intrahepatic bile ducts.

In end-stage liver disease the clinical consequences and management are similar to primary biliary cirrhosis with symptomatic treatment of pruritus, replacement of fat-soluble vitamins and ultimately liver transplantation in selected patients.

Bile duct carcinoma

Natural history

Adenocarcinoma may develop at any point in the intra-hepatic or extrahepatic bile ducts, but the most common site is at the junction of the main right and left hepatic ducts. Presentation is almost always with obstructive jaundice. Histology usually shows a mucin-secreting adenocarcinoma with a dense fibrous stroma. Differentiation from carcinoma of the pancreas cannot usually be made on histological grounds alone and is made on the basis of the site as determined by radiology or surgery. There are a number of interesting disease associations including:

- Ulcerative colitis for which there is a 25-fold increase in relative risk for bile duct carcinoma.
- Infestation by the liver fluke *Clonorchis sinensis*, which occurs typically in areas of the Far East where raw fish are commonly eaten.
- The congenital anomaly, choledochal cyst.

Management

This condition emphasises the importance of pre-operative diagnosis in obstructive jaundice. Too often patients have undergone laparotomy, often by a relatively inexperienced surgeon who finds a collapsed gallbladder and extrahepatic bile duct and either misses the diagnosis or is confronted by a hilar tumour with inadequate information to determine resectability.

Surgery offers the only chance of cure, but should be preceded by a thorough assessment, which should include a good demonstration of the intrahepatic bile ducts via percutaneous or endoscopic cholangiography, CT scanning to assess tumour extent and angiography to assess the anatomy of the hepatic circulation (which varies considerably) and to exclude invasion of the main hepatic or portal veins. Approximately 10–20% of tumours are resectable.

The tumour metastasises late and even without resection the prognosis is relatively good with a median survival over one year and some patients surviving up to five years. Palliation can now often be achieved by endoscopic or percutaneous stenting without the need for surgery.

Chemotherapy has not so far proved of value, but radiotherapy by temporary insertion of [192]Iridium wire has produced promising results.

Transplantation is not usually indicated because of a very high rate of tumour recurrence, but occasional patients have survived more than five years after transplant.

Carcinoma of the gallbladder

Natural history

Presentation is usually either with advanced intra-abdominal tumour or as obstructive jaundice and successful resection is achieved in under 25%. There is only a 5% five-year survival.

AETIOLOGY AND PATHOGENESIS

Most carcinomas of the gallbladder are papillary adenocarcinomas, but squamous carcinomas are occasionally found. At least 75% occur in association with gallstones and there is a female to male ratio of 4:1 similar to gallstones. This has been used as an argument to support cholecystectomy for patients with asymptomatic gallstones, but the tumour is fortunately rare and even the low risks of elective cholecystectomy are usually thought to outweigh any benefit from a reduced risk for gallbladder carcinoma.

The uncommonly seen calcified gallbladder visible on a plain abdominal radiograph does however have a high risk for carcinoma and is an indication for prophylactic cholecystectomy. In some fortunate patients a gallbladder containing early foci of carcinoma is resected at routine cholecystectomy in which case the chances of a cure are good.

Benign stricturing of bile ducts

The commonest cause of benign stricturing of the extra-hepatic bile ducts is iatrogenic and is due either to mistaken identification of the common bile duct as the cystic duct or the placement of surgical clips or sutures too close to the origin of the cystic duct. Some other causes have already been discussed (see sclerosing cholangitis) and include *Clonorchis sinensis* infestation and infusion of cytotoxic agents such as 5-fluorouracil via the hepatic artery. Cholangitis due to stones in the common bile duct may also result in stricturing. Chronic pancreatitis may cause a characteristic tapering 'rat tail' stricture of the lower common bile duct.

Management

Relief of the biliary obstruction is important, not only to relieve jaundice, but also to prevent secondary biliary cirrhosis, which may develop insidiously, sometimes even without obvious jaundice. Even if secondary biliary cirrhosis has already developed, the obstruction should be relieved as there is often a striking improvement in liver histology, even in advanced disease.

Complete obstruction or stricturing due to extensive compression by chronic pancreatitis will require formal surgical treatment usually by construction of a choledocho-jejunostomy. High stricturing of the common hepatic duct may require anastomosis of a Roux loop to a dilated peripheral duct in the left or more rarely the right lobe of the liver. Restenosis at the anastomosis may be a problem after a few years, but can sometimes be successfully treated by percutaneous balloon dilatation.

Partial obstruction can sometimes be treated successfully by endoscopic or percutaneous dilatation with a balloon catheter, sometimes coupled with stenting, but the patient needs careful follow-up to exclude restenosis.

Congenital abnormalities of the biliary tree

Extrahepatic biliary atresia

This is a congenital condition affecting 1/10,000 live births, but is not familial. The severity of the defect varies considerably ranging from involvement of the cystic duct alone (which has an excellent prognosis) through to hypoplasia of the extrahepatic ducts (which usually has a good prognosis) and absence of the extrahepatic ducts (complete atresia). (See also chapter 18.) In complete atresia, jaundice occurs by the end of the first week of life and progresses relent-lessly. Xanthomatous deposits in the skin and all the other consequences of biliary stasis, including pruritus result. If untreated death usually results before three years of age. (See also Chapter 18.)

MANAGEMENT
In complete atresia there are two main options, both surgical. The Kasai operation in which the portal region of the liver is laid bare and anastomosed to jejunum produces remarkably good results in about 50% patients with 33% surviving to five years with a normal serum bilirubin. Transplantation also produces relatively good results, but is made more difficult by a previous failed Kasai procedure.

Intrahepatic biliary atresia

Intrahepatic biliary atresia is usually thought to result from viral infection either in the neonatal period or *in utero*. Presentation is variable with jaundice occurring at any time between three days and six years and followed by inexorable progression to biliary cirrhosis. (See also Chapter 18.)

Arteriohepatic dysplasia (Watson–Alagille syndrome)

Arteriohepatic dysplasia is a rare autosomal dominant inherited condition in which there is a combination of pulmonary stenosis and paucity of intrahepatic bile ducts. Cholestasis may be severe, but patients survive into adult life.

Choledochal cyst

Polycystic liver disease, congenital hepatic fibrosis, Caroli syndrome and choledochal cyst are conditions that some-times coexist (particularly polycystic disease and hepatic fibrosis) and probably all represent different expressions of a similar developmental anomaly.

Cystic dilatation of the common bile duct or choledochal cyst, may occur either as dilatation of the entire common bile duct or as a cyst coming off the side of the duct. Presentation can be extremely variable. It may present in the infant with a combination of obstructive jaundice and abdominal mass, but may be asymptomatic. There is a high risk of complication by adenocarcinoma, which may be the mode of presentation in the adult. (See also Chapter 18.)

MANAGEMENT
Treatment should always be by complete excision of the cyst and biliary reconstruction because of the high risk of adenocarcinoma if a remnant is left.

Caroli syndrome

Caroli syndrome is a very rare congenital abnormality of the intrahepatic bile ducts, which are cystically dilated. Congenital hepatic fibrosis coexists in about 35% of patients. In the absence of hepatic fibrosis, the main consequence is episodic cholangitis associated with mild jaundice and painful hepatomegaly. Most patients live into adult life, but the prognosis is not very good because of recurrent septicemia. (See also Chapter 18.)

Cholangitis

Natural history

Cholangitis is a clinical syndrome consisting of septicemia in association with biliary obstruction. A high fever and rigors are typical. Biliary obstruction is often only partial and jaundice may be absent. Any lesion that causes biliary obstruction may be complicated by cholangitis, but it is particularly common in association with common bile duct stones and uncommon in malignant biliary obstruction unless instrumentation of the bile ducts (e.g. at cholangiography) has introduced infection.

In its more severe form, 'suppurative' cholangitis, profound endotoxaemia occurs with resultant hypotension, disseminated intravascular coagulation and acute tubular necrosis leading to renal failure.

In the absence of jaundice the diagnosis is often missed. Bacteruria is common and may be misinterpreted as indicating a primary urinary infection as the cause of fever. Common organisms include coliforms and other faecal bacteria.

Management

In all but its mildest forms, cholangitis constitutes a surgical emergency. Broad-spectrum antibiotics, such as a cephalosporin or ciprofloxacin should be started as soon as blood culture samples have been taken, but often have little effect unless the biliary obstruction is relieved. This is probably because much of the damage results from endotoxaemia.

If the patient has a high fever (higher than 38.5°C), hypotension or renal failure, biliary drainage needs to be established within hours. Failure to achieve this results in a high mortality. Adequate biliary drainage may be established endoscopically, percutaneously or surgically depending on the aetiology. If common bile duct gallstones are present endoscopic sphincterotomy is the safest approach. It should be possible to remove the stones from the common bile duct in at least 95% of patients and the risk of the procedure itself is low (mortality approximately 0.5% in averagely fit patients, but will, of course, be higher if endotoxaemic shock has already resulted). Even if the stones cannot be removed establishment of drainage by placement of a biliary stent or nasobiliary tube may be life-saving.

Malignant strictures may be stented either endoscopically or percutaneously with approximately 90% sucess and, if this fails, temporary relief of biliary pressure by percutaneous biliary drainage may improve the cholangitis, but should only be considered as a short-term measure.

Supportive management includes the use of intravenous plasma or plasma expanders and dopamine infusion to maintain renal profusion, monitoring of blood gases and oxygen therapy and correction of coagulation defects. Intravenous mannitol (e.g. 200 ml 10% mannitol over four hours) may help to prevent acute renal failure. The importance of establishing prompt relief of biliary obstruction however cannot be overemphasised as the prognosis depends largely on the speed with which this is achieved.

▶ **Treatment of cholangitis**

- Rapid establishment of biliary drainage is crucial
- Antibiotics should be given, but will have little effect without established biliary drainage

Carcinoma of the pancreas

Natural history

About 60% of tumours arise in the head of the pancreas, which results in jaundice in over 80% of patients, whereas tumours of the body or tail cause jaundice in less than 10% of patients. Weight loss is almost universal and over 80% of patients have severe pain. It is typically a relentless epigastric pain with radiation to the back, worse on lying down and eased by sitting up.

The prognosis is poor. Even with an aggressive surgical approach, the five-year survival is only 3% overall. Median survival is about three months and the one-year survival is 8%. This is reflected by the fact that 90% of patients have detectable lymph mode metastases at presentation and 80% have detectable liver metastases. This implies either that the tumour is particularly prone to invade and metastasise early or that symptoms do not develop until disease is advanced.

Aetiology and pathogenesis

Pancreatic cancer is becoming more common. It is the fourth commonest cause of death from cancer (after lung, colorectal and breast). Age-adjusted mortality rates in the USA have risen from 3/100,000 in 1920 to 9/100,000 in 1970. The explanation for this increase is unclear, but there is some evidence that tobacco smoking and a high dietary intake of polyunsaturated fatty acids are risk factors. Reported associations with heavy consumption of coffee are unconvincing, but animal studies suggest that soy products, particularly if taken in infancy, may act as promoters by inhibiting intraluminal trypsin and inducing pancreatic hyperplasia. There is also association with the rare condition of hereditary pancreatitis, but curiously little, if any, link with alcoholism.

- The tumour is thought to arise from ductal tissue in at least 75% of patients, but this is often difficult to determine with certainty and some workers have suggested that carcinogens may stimulate acinar cells to dedifferentiate to ductal type cells (**Fig. 13.36**).
- Most of the remainder are giant cell or adenosquamous carcinomas whose cell of origin is uncertain.
- Acinar cell carcinomas are thought to account for only 1% of the cancers.
- The relatively slow-growing cystadenocarcinomas are even rarer.
- Malignant tumours of peptide-secreting cells are discussed elsewhere, but include insulinoma, gastrinoma, glucagonoma and vipoma.

Management

Chemotherapy and radiotherapy have so far not been proven to have any convincing beneficial effect. Surgery offers the only hope, but the chance of achieving cure is statistically so low that patients should be selected very carefully to avoid unnecessary laparotomies in the presence of obvious metastases.

Assessment should include ultrasound and CT scanning of the liver and pancreas and if this shows no evidence of metastasis angiography should be performed to exclude invasion of the superior mesenteric artery or the portal vein. If possible a histological or cytological diagnosis should be made by fine needle ultrasound-guided aspiration biopsy. Even with an enthusiastic approach, only about 35% of tumours prove resectable and of these only 35% are macroscopically non-invasive.

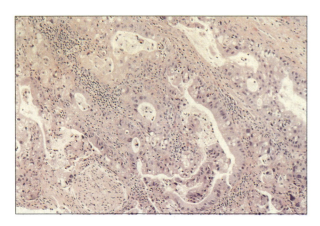

Fig. 13.36 Pancreatic carcinoma showing malignant glandular structures with dark-staining irregularly-shaped nuclei.

The commonest operation for resection is Whipple's pancreaticoduodenectomy in which the head and neck of the pancreas are removed along with the duodenum, the lower common bile duct, gallbladder and a variable portion of distal stomach. The remaining pancreas is anastamosed to jejunum, but because of leakage at this anastamosis, some surgeons advocate total pancreatectomy despite the inevitable complication of insulin-dependent diabetes. Operative mortality for Whipple's procedure for pancreatic cancer is approximately 20%, but the expected survival following successful resection is improved to 16 months.

If the tumour proves non-resectable at laparotomy, a double bypass (i.e. cholecyst-jejunostomy and gastrojejunostomy) is performed. Duodenal obstruction develops subsequently in about 35% of patients if only a biliary bypass is performed.

Because of the high mortality and morbidity and low cure rate of surgery, there has been a general move towards nonoperative palliation in all except the carefully selected few who have a reasonable chance of resection.

Endoscopic stenting for the relief of obstructive jaundice is rapidly becoming more available with success rates of over 90% commonly achieved. The procedure requires an endoscopic cholangiogram (ERCP). A fine guide wire is then placed via the endoscope through the stricture under radiological control. A 10 or 12 French stent tube made from a synthetic polymer is then placed across the stricture (size in French is the circumference in mm). The stents sometimes block after about six months, but can be relatively easily replaced. Stenting has little effect on the survival, but at least ensures that the patient's final months are free from the discomfort of either pruritus or a non-curative laparotomy.

Pain can be very difficult to manage. A coeliac ganglion block is usually worth trying, either at surgery if the patient is undergoing a palliative operation or by injection of alcohol or phenol under radiological control. Indomethacin may be effective, but regular opiates are often required. Sympathetic nursing of the patient in cheerful surroundings, preferably at home, is probably the most important aspect of the terminal care.

Carcinoma of the ampulla of Vater

Natural history

Tumours of the ampullary mucosa present early because of their site and have a very much better prognosis than pancreatic cancer. Jaundice is the commonest presentation, but blood loss due to superficial ulceration is also common and a combination of fatty stools due to biliary obstruction and altered blood may result in the classic 'silver' stool. Occasionally the patient may present with iron-deficiency anaemia without jaundice. Benign adenomas of the ampulla occur occasionally and may become polypoid. Both benign and malignant tumours (**Fig. 13.37**) of the ampulla may be associated with polyposis syndromes.

Management

The results of surgical resection are much better than for pancreatic cancer with an operative mortality of 2.5% and a 35% five-year survival. Metastasis occurs late.

Patients are often elderly and, if considered too frail for surgery, may be palliated by endoscopic sphincterotomy or endoscopic stenting. The tumour is usually slow growing and sphincterotomy will often produce relief of jaundice for up to one year, even without stenting. Duodenal obstruction may eventually necessitate surgery, however, and in view of the reasonable chance of cure, all except the most frail of patients should be treated surgically. A Whipple's procedure is usually necessary to ensure complete excision of tumour.

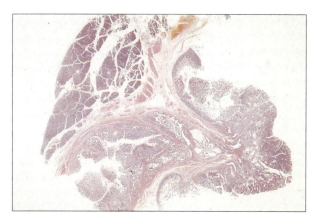

Fig. 13.37 Carcinoma of the ampulla. The histological appearances and behaviour of these tumours are similar to those of malignant change occurring in a colonic adenoma, and carcinoma of the ampulla is common in patients with familial adenomatous polyposis of the colon.

FURTHER READING

Gilbert's syndrome

Watson KJ, Gollan JL. Gilbert's syndrome. *Baillières Clin Gastroenterol* 1989r; **3**(2): 337–55.

Hepatitis (viral)

Brown JL, Carman WF, Thomas HC. The hepatitis B virus. *Baillières Clin Gastroenterol* 1990; 4(3): 721–47

Brown JL, Carman WF, Thomas HC. The clinical significance of molecular variation within the hepatitis B virus genome. *Hepatology* 1992; **15**(1): 144–8.

Carman WF, Thomas HC. Hepatitis viruses. *Baillières Clin Gastroenterol* 1990; **4**(1): 201–32.

Flehming B. Hepatitis A. *Baillières Clin Gastroenterol* 1990 ; **4**(3): 707–20.

Gerin JL. Antiviral agents for hepatitis B. *Hepatology* 1991; **14**: 198–9.

Hoofnagle JH. Alpha-interferon therapy of chronic hepatitis B. Current status and recommendations. *J Hepatol* 1990; **11** Suppl. I: S100–7.

Jacyna MR, Thomas HC. Antiviral therapy: hepatitis B. *Br Med Bull* 1990; **46**(2): 368–82.

Krawczynski K. Hepatitis E *Hepatology* 1993; **17**: 932–939.

Lemon SM. Inactivated hepatitis A virus vaccines. *Hepatology* 1992; **15**: 1194–1197.

Lenzi M Autoimmune hepatitis and hepatitis C. *FEMS Microbiol Rev* 1994; **14**: 247–52.

Mishra L, Seeff LB. Viral hepatitis, A though E, complicating pregnancy. *Gastroenterol Clin North Am* 1992; **21**(4): 873–87.

Sheron N, Alexander GJ. Hepatitis C, D and E virus infection. *Baillières Clin Gastroenterol* 1990; **4**(3): 749–74.

Rizzetto M. Hepatitis delta: the virus and the disease. *J Hepatol* 1990; **11** Suppl. I: S145–8.

Tine F, Liberati A, Craxi A, Almasio P, Pagliaro L. Interferon treatment in patients with chronic hepatitis B: meta-analysis of the published data. *J Hepatol* 1993; **18**: 154–163.

Zuckerman AJ. Vaccines against hepatitis A and B. *Baillières Clin Gastroenterol* 1990; **4**(3): 775–88.

Congenital biliary disorders

Desmet VL. Congenital diseases of intrahepatic bile ducts: variation on the theme 'Duct Plate Malformation.' *Hepatology* 1992; **16**: 1069–84.

α1-antitrypsin deficiency

Perlmutter DH. The cellular basis for liver injury in alpha 1-antitrypsin deficiency. *Hepatology* 1991; **13**(1): 172–85.

Chronic active hepatitis

Desmet VJ, Ferber M, Hoofnagle JH, et al. Classification of chronic hepatitis:diagnosis, grading and staging. Hepatology 1994; **19**:1513–20.

Donaldson P, Doherty D, Underhill J, Williams R The molecular genetics of autoimmune liver disease. Hepatology 1994; 20: 225–39.

Mitchison HC, Bassendine MF. Rolling review: autoimmune liver disease. *Aliment Pharmacol Ther* 1993; **7**(1): 93–109.

Vierling JM. Immune disorders of the liver and bile duct. *Gastroenterol Clin North* Am 1992; **21**(2): 427–49.

Wilson's disease

Sternlieb I. Perspectives on Wilson's disease. *Hepatology* 1990 Nov; **12**(5): 1234–9.

Sternlieb I. The outlook for the diagnosis of Wilson's disease. *J Hepatol* 1993; **17**: 263–4.

Haemochromatosis

Brind AM, Bassendine MF. Molecular genetics of chronic liver diseases. *Baillières Clin Gastroenterol* 1990; **4**(1): 233–53.

Edwards CQ, Kushner JP. Screening for hemochromatosis. *N Engl J Med* 1993; **328**(22): 1616–20.

Powell LW. Does transplantation of the liver cure genetic hemochromatosis? *J Hepatol* 1992; **16**: 259–261.

Alcoholic liver disease

Blendis LM. Review article: the treatment of alcoholic liver disease. *Aliment Pharmacol Ther* 1992; **6**(5): 541–8.

Derr RF, Porta EA, Larkin EC, Rao GA. Is ethanol *per se* hepatotoxic? *J Hepatol* 1990; **10**(3): 381–6.

Lieber CS Alcohol and the liver:1994 update. Gastroenterology 1994:106:1085–1105.

Lumeng L, Crabb DW Genetic aspects amd risk factors in alcoholism and alcoholic liver disease. Gastroenterology 1994; 107: 572–8.

Tsukamoto H, Gaal K; French SW. Insights into the pathogenesis of alcoholic liver necrosis and fibrosis: status report. *Hepatology* 1990; **12**(3 Pt 1): 599–608.

Liver problems in pregnancy

Abell TL, Riely CA. Hyperemesis gravidarum. *Gastroenterol Clin North* Am 1992; **21**(4): 835–49.

Barron WM. The syndrome of preeclampsia. *Gastroenterol Clin North* Am 1992; **21**(4): 851–72.

Barton JR, Sibai BM. Care of the pregnancy complicated by HELLP syndrome. *Gastroenterol Clin North* Am 1992; **21**(4): 937–50.

Lee WM. Pregnancy in patients with chronic liver disease. *Gastroenterol Clin North* Am 1992; **21**(4): 889–903.

Mabie WC. Acute fatty liver of pregnancy. *Gastroenterol Clin North* Am 1992; **21**(4): 951–60.

Mabie WC. Obstetric management of gastroenterologic complications of pregnancy. *Gastroenterol Clin North* Am 1992; **21**(4): 923–35.

Reyes H. The spectrum of liver and gastrointestinal disease seen in cholestasis of pregnancy. *Gastroenterol Clin North* Am 1992; **21**(4): 905–21.

Primary biliary cirrhosis

Bassendine MF, Yeaman SJ. Serological markers of primary biliary cirrhosis: Diagnosis, prognosis and subsets. *Hepatology* 1992; **15**: 545–548.

Berg PA, Klein R. Antimitochondrial antibodies in primary biliary cirrhosis. A clue to its etiopathogenesis? *J Hepatol* 1992; **15**: 6–9.

Beukers R, Schalm SW. Immunosuppressive therapy for primary biliary cirrhosis. *J Hepatol* 1992; **14**(1): 1–6.

Christensen E. Prognostication in primary biliary cirrhosis: relevance to the individual patient. Hepatology 1989 Jul; **10**(1): 111–3.

Luketic VA, Sanyal AJ The current status of ursodeoxycholate in the treatment of chronic cholestatic liver disease. *Gastroenterologist* 1994; **2**: 74–9.

Vierling JM. Immune disorders of the liver and bile duct. *Gastroenterol Clin North* Am 1992; **21**(2): 427–49.

Warnes TW. Colchicine in primary biliary cirrhosis. *Aliment Pharmacol Ther* 1991; **5**(4): 321–9.

Drug-induced liver disease

Lee WM. Review article: drug induced hepatotoxicity. *Aliment Pharmcol Ther* 1993; **7**: 477–485.

Neuberger J. Drug-induced jaundice. Baillières Clin Gastroenterol 1989; **3**(2): 447–66.

Primary sclerosing cholangitis

Chapman RW. Aetiology and natural history of primary sclerosing cholangitis—a decade of progress? *Gut* 1991; **32**(12): 1433–5.

Sherlock S. Pathogenesis of sclerosing cholangitis: the role of nonimmune factors. *Semin Liver Dis* 1991; **11**(1): 5–10.

Vierling JM. Immune disorders of the liver and bile duct. *Gastroenterol Clin North* Am 1992; **21**(2): 427–49.

Pancreatic and bile duct cancer

Adam A, Benjamin IS. The staging of cholangiocarcinoma. *Clin Radiol* 1992; **46**(5): 299–303.

Arbuck SG. Chemotherapy for pancreatic cancer. *Baillières Clin Gastroenterol* 1990; **4**(4): 953–68.

Brambs HJ, Claussen CD. Pancreatic and ampullary carcinoma. Ultrasound, computed tomography, magnetic resonance imaging and angiography. *Endoscopy* 1993; **25**(1): 58–68.

acyna MR, Summerfield JA. Endoscopic management of biliary tract obstruction in the 1990s. *J Hepatol* 1992; **14**: 127–132.

Niederau C, Grendell JH. Diagnosis of pancreatic carcinoma. Imaging techniques and tumor markers. Pancreas 1992; **7**(1): 66–86.

Rhodes JM, Ching CK. Serum tests in the diagnosis of pancreatic cancer. *Baillières Clin Gastroenterol* 1990; **4**(4).

Rosen CB, Nagorney DM. Cholangiocarcinoma complicating primary sclerosing cholangitis. *Semin Liver Dis* 1991; **11**(1): 26–30.

Warshaw AL, Fernandez del Castillo C. Pancreatic carcinoma. *N Engl J Med* 1992; **326**(7): 455–65.

Yeo CJ, Pitt HA, Cameron JL. Cholangiocarcinoma. *Surg Clin North Am* 1990; **70**(6): 1429–47.

Stain SC, Baer HU, Dennison AR, Blumgart LH. Current management of hilar cholangiocarcinoma. *Surg Gynecol Obstet* 1992; **175**(6): 579–88.

Liver transplantation

Advances in liver transplantation. *Gastroenterol Clin North Am* 1993; **22**(2): 213–473.

Benhamon JP Indications for liver transplantation in primary biliary cirrhosis. Hepatology 1994; 20: 115–135.

Lautz HU, Pichlmayr R. Special aspects of timing of liver transplantation in patients with liver cirrhosis. *Baillières Clin Gastroenterol* 1989; **3**(4): 743–56.

Samuel D, Bismuth H. Liver transplantation for hepatitis B. *Gastroenterol Clin North Am* 1993; **22**(2): 271–83.

Wiesner RH, Porayko MK, Dickson ER, Gores GJ, LaRusso NF, Hay JE, Wahlstrom HE, Krom RAF. Selection and timing of liver transplantation in primary biliary cirrhosis and primary sclerosing cholangitis. *Hepatology* 1992: **16**: 1290–9.

Wright TL. Liver transplantation for chronic hepatitis C viral infection. *Gastroenterol Clin North* Am 1993; **22**(2): 231–42.

Miscellaneous

Harinasuta T, Pungpak S, Keystone JS. Trematode infections. Opisthorchiasis, clonorchiasis, fascioliasis, and paragonimiasis. (Review.) *Infect Dis Clin North Am* 1993; **7**(3): 699–716.

14
ABDOMINAL MASSES AND SWELLING

REACHING A DIAGNOSIS

Generalised swelling: 'fat, fluid, flatus, faeces or fetus'

Is it gas, liquid or solid?

Percussion should readily distinguish gas (tympanic) from liquid or solid (dull), but many patients with ascites also have increased intestinal gas ('le vent avant la pluie'), so it is important to check for ascites in any patient with abdominal distension.

This is best done by checking for shifting dullness, which depends on the presence of gas in loops of intestine that float to the top. The lateral border of the area of resonance is carefully defined, a finger kept on this point, and the patient turned onto his/her side away from the examiner and the lateral border of resonance redefined.

This is a much more reliable test than searching for a fluid thrill, which requires a third hand and often produces a false-positive response in the obese patient. It is usually necessary to have at least 2 litres of fluid before ascites can be confidently demonstrated.

Is it ascites or an ovarian cyst?

Complete absence of central resonance (with the patient supine) suggests that the swelling is more likely to be due to a large ovarian cyst or other tumour.

Transmission of aortic pulsations also suggests that distension is due to an ovarian cyst rather than ascites.

If there is ascites, what is its cause?

Clues to the cause of ascites are often present. Stigmata of chronic liver disease may include palmar erythema, spider naevi, leuconychia and signs of feminisation in the male.

Examination of the ascitic fluid is also very helpful. Ascitic protein content differentiates transudates from exudates. It is better to be guided by the ratio of ascitic fluid protein to serum protein rather than the absolute concentration. Ascitic fluid protein concentration that is higher than 60% of serum concentration suggests exudate.

▶ **Causes of ascites**

Transudate

- Cirrhosis
- Hypoproteinaemia (e.g. nephrotic sydrome)

Exudate

- Heart failure (may also be transudate)
- Budd–Chiari syndrome (may also be transudate)
- Infection
- Malignancy
- Systemic lupus erythematosus
- Chronic pancreatitis (high amylase content)

- Ascites due to cirrhosis should be a transudate unless complicated by infection, tumour or hepatic vein occlusion.
- Congestive cardiac failure may result in either a transudate or exudate and needs excluding in any patient with ascites.

Constrictive pericarditis may also cause substantial ascites and can be particularly difficult to diagnose since the heart shadow may be normal on routine chest radiography. It should be suspected in the presence of a particularly high jugular venous pulse (JVP) when the patient is upright. An echocardiogram is usually diagnostic.

Tuberculous ascites: The abdominal distension is usually not marked and has a doughy feel. The fluid is high in protein content. Yield from ascitic culture is relatively low and takes several weeks. If the diagnosis is considered likely laparoscopy, which allows direct visualisation of peritoneal nodules and peritoneal biopsy, gives the best chance of rapid diagnosis.

Malignancy: Ascitic cytology should be performed to exclude malignancy. The yield is greater if a large volume of fluid is centrifuged before examination.

Pancreatic ascites is a rare complication of chronic pancreatitis. There is usually a history of abdominal pain and a very high amylase content (several thousand iu/ml) can be demonstrated in the ascitic fluid. Treatment is usually by prolonged intravenous feeding, but may require partial pancreatic resection if the fistulous communication between the pancreatic duct and abdominal cavity persists.

Chylous ascites (milky due to the presence of lymph) is easy to recognise with naked eye inspection. It usually implies obstruction of the thoracic duct by malignant disease, either carcinoma or lymphoma, but may occasionally result from trauma or tuberculosis.

Systemic lupus erythematosus is a rare cause of high protein ascites. As with most other forms of high protein ascites, glucose content will be low, and diagnosis depends on the demonstration of a high titre of antinuclear antibody in the blood.

What does auscultation reveal?

Omitting auscultation of the abdomen is a common error. It can often yield diagnostic information.

IS THERE A TUMOUR BRUIT?

Auscultation should always be performed over any mass. The presence of a systolic bruit is highly suggestive of a tumour circulation. A hepatic bruit suggests hepatocellular carcinoma. It may more rarely indicate the presence of a benign haemangioma and is also common inpatients with alcoholic hepatitis.

A bruit may be a useful sign even in the absence of a mass. About 60% of patients with carcinoma of the body of the pancreas have a bruit due to encasement of the superior mesenteric or splenic arteries.

IS THERE A VENOUS HUM?

In a patient with ascites the presence of a venous hum between the umbilicus and xiphisternum is a valuable physical sign. It is due to retrograde flow from the portal vein, through the umbilical vein into collaterals. It indicates not only that there is portal hypertension, but that the portal vein is patent.

Is there intestinal obstruction?

Intestinal obstruction usually presents with a history of abdominal pain and vomiting and in such a patient the presence of high-pitched, tinkling bowel sounds in a distended abdomen is diagnostic.

Radiology will then be required to determine the site of the obstruction. Plain abdominal radiography will usually determine whether this is in the colon or small intestine. If the probable site is colonic a barium enema examination should then be performed. If small bowel obstruction is suspected supine and erect plain films should first be obtained. Distension of both small and large intestine with gas-filled rectum suggests ileus whereas distension of small intestine without colonic distension suggests small bowel obstruction. If there is doubt, a barium enema should be performed. If barium can be refluxed through the ileocaecal valve it may be possible to outline a distal ileal obstruction.

If there remains a strong suspicion of small bowel obstruction, particularly if the patient has Crohn's disease or has had recent abdominal surgery, a **small bowel barium enema** should be peformed. A nasoduodenal tube is passed under radiological control. The stomach and duodenum are aspirated and up to 200 ml of dilute barium are instilled through the tube directly into the distal duodenum. Water-soluble contrast is generally ineffective in this situation. It becomes diluted by the small bowel contents and also increases fluid and electrolyte losses as a consequence of its hyperosmolarity. It is now generally accepted that previous worries that barium would become inspissated proximal to a lesion and convert a partial obstruction into a complete obstruction are unfounded.

Is there gastric outlet obstruction?

A succussion splash should be sought providing that the patient has fasted for four hours. It suggests gastric outlet obstruction. Very occasionally, visible peristalsis may occur. If a splash is present then nasogastric aspiration should be performed before further investigation by endoscopy or barium meal examination. Endoscopy in gastric outlet obstruction without previous aspiration is at best unpleasant and unrewarding, but also carries a high risk of aspiration.

Is there portal hypertension?

The presence of dilated periumbilical veins (caput medusae) with the venous flow away from the umbilicus is a sign (usually late) of portal hypertension. Vena cava obstruction also results in dilated veins, but in this situation flow of blood in the lower abdominal wall veins is upwards whereas in portal hypertension the flow is in the normal direction (i.e. downwards in the lower abdomen and upwards in the upper abdomen).

▶ **Causes of hepatic bruit**

- Hepatocellular carcinoma
- Haemangioma
- Alcoholic hepatitis

▶ **Gastric outlet obstruction**

Nasogastric aspiration should be performed before endoscopy or barium meal

Is there faecal loading?

Faecal loading may present as generalised abdominal swelling, often more prominent in the flanks. In untreated Hirschsprung's disease and acquired megacolon, this may be quite dramatic. A plain abdominal film is helpful to confirm faecal loading in the proximal colon.

Hepatomegaly

It is important to start palpation in the right iliac fossa to avoid missing a very large liver. It is also important to start palpation lateral to the rectus abdominis muscle as it may be mistaken for the liver. Other features that characterise the liver edge are movement with respiration, inability to get above the mass and dullness to percussion. A liver edge may be palpable in the absence of hepatomegaly if the diaphragm is displaced inferiorly by emphysema or fluid. Percussion is then very helpful to assess liver size.

A Riedel's lobe may be mistaken for an enlarged liver. It is commoner in women and is an anatomical variant of the right lobe extending down the right hypochondrium and occasionally into the iliac fossa.

Having felt an enlarged liver, the examiner should decide if it is smooth or nodular by feeling the liver surface and not merely its lower edge. Any parenchymal liver disease may present as a smooth hepatic enlargement. This includes:

- Chronic liver diseases such as primary biliary cirrhosis and chronic active hepatitis.
- Haematological disorders.
- Cirrhosis from any cause.

Hepatic enlargement from chronic conditions is usually non-tender. A tender smooth enlarged liver suggests acute stretching of the Glisson's capsule and may occur in acute hepatitis, right heart failure, liver abscess and Budd–Chiari syndrome (hepatic vein thrombosis).

In acute **Budd–Chiari syndrome**, the pain may be considerable. In post-acute or chronic Budd–Chiari syndrome, an enlarged caudate lobe is felt anteriorly. This is because the venous outflow of the caudate lobe is direct into the vena cava and not via the hepatic veins.

Is the hepatomegaly due to a metabolic disorder?

Metabolic causes of hepatomegaly may need consideration.

- A common cause of a very enlarged liver is **alcoholic liver disease** where there is fatty change.
- Poorly controlled **diabetes** may also result in massive hepatomegaly, particularly in children. The hepatomegaly then is usually due chiefly to accumulation of glycogen rather than fat.
- Glycogen storage diseases and mucopolysaccharidoses are also associated with hepatomegaly

Is there a hepatic cyst?

Simple hepatic cysts are usually small, impalpable and asymptomatic, but may occasionally be large and palpable (**Fig. 14.1**). Hydatid cysts present as asymptomatic hepatomegaly and should be suspected in patients who come from sheep farming areas. Ultrasound scanning usually shows typical daughter cysts around the rim of the cyst and calcification is usually present. Plain abdominal radiography may also show the calcification, but scanning will usually be required to exclude a calcified tumour (**Figs 14.2 and 14.3**). Serology (hydatid complement fixation test) is usually positive unless the cyst is longstanding and has become inactive.

▶ **Benign causes of hepatomegaly**

- Fatty infiltration (alcohol, diabetes, obesity)
- Glycogen (diabetes, glycogen storage disease)
- Congestion (heart failure, constrictive pericarditis)
- Granulomatous disease (sarcoid, tuberculosis)
- Other storage disorders (Gaucher's disease, mucopolysaccharidoses)
- Extramedullary haemopoiesis (myelofibrosis)
- Amyloidosis
- Cysts (polycystic disease, hydatid cyst)
- Abscess

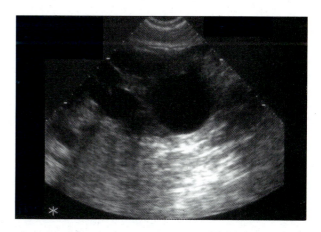

Fig. 14.1 Ultrasound scan of a large 'simple' hepatic cyst.

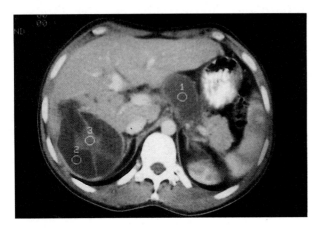

Fig. 14.2 CT scan showing hydatid cysts affecting the liver and pancreas. Typical 'daughter' cysts can be seen.

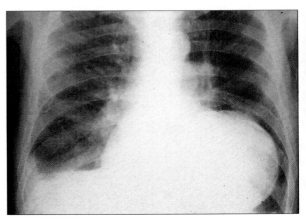

Fig. 14.3 Chest radiograph showing a large hydatid cyst. Courtesy of Dr R Evans.

Is there an hepatic abscess?

The combination of pyrexia, hepatomegaly and an elevated right diaphragm suggests hepatic abscess. Abscesses caused by pyogenic organisms are accompanied by systemic signs of weight loss, malaise, fever and right upper quadrant pain. Abdominal ultrasound may be diagnostic, but CT is probably more sensitive, particularly for lesions close to the diaphragm.

Amoebic abscess should be considered if the patient has been to the tropics. Amoebic serological testing is positive in about 95% and stool should be examined for pathogenic amoebae although these are often not found. Aspiration of the abscess will reveal thick brown 'anchovy-sauce' pus, but should be avoided if possible because of the risk of introducing secondary infection. There is usually a prompt response to oral metronidazole.

Bacterial pyogenic abscess is much more serious and carries a considerable mortality. Bacterial liver abscesses are usually multiple. There may be a clear history of intrabdominal sepsis, but quite frequently (particularly with abscesses due to microaerophilic *Streptococcus milleri*) there is not. Needle aspiration under ultrasound control should be performed both as therapy and to obtain samples for culture and antibiotic sensitivity.

Is there metastatic carcinoma?

A nodular feel to the liver suggests metastatic carcinoma. It may be tender and an inspiratory rub may be heard on auscultation over the liver.

If there is no previous history of tumour elsewhere malignant melanoma of skin or eye should be considered as a possible primary site.

Histology should always be obtained even when the scan is highly suggestive of tumour (**Figs 14.4 –14.6**. Liver abscesses may resemble tumour on scanning, and some tumours (e.g. carcinoid) may be amenable to chemotherapy or even resection. This should generally be obtained by ultrasound guided needle biopsy to give the best chance of successful biopsy.

Is there a mucocoele or empyema of the gallbladder?

The normal gallbladder lies deep and is not palpable. As it enlarges, the fundus is displaced anteriorly, inferiorly and medially and is felt as a rounded fluid sac, which is often mobile. A mucocoele or empyema of the gallbladder may be felt as tender enlargement, and in the case of the latter, the patient will also have signs of sepsis.

The enlarged gallbladder is usually soft and may be easier to see than to feel. The abdomen should be inspected while the patient breathes deeply and the impression of the gallbladder on the anterior abdominal wall will then be seen moving with respiration. In a jaundiced patient the presence

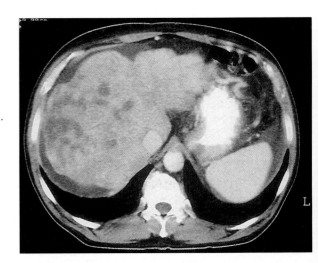

Fig. 14.4 CT scan showing multifocal hepatocellular carcinoma in a patient with hepatitis B-related cirrhosis.

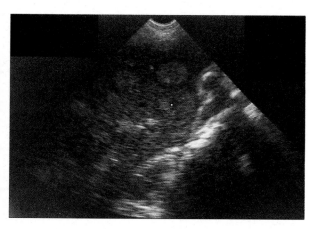

Fig. 14.5 Ultrasound scan showing metastatic carcinoma in the liver. Although these appearances are typical, they should never be regarded as absolutely diagnostic without histological proof since abscesses may give similar appearances.

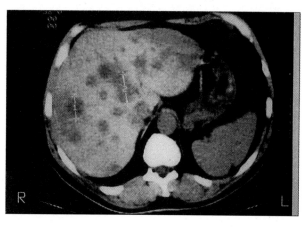

Fig. 14.6 CT scan of metastatic carcinoma. Courtesy of Dr C Garvey.

of a palpable gallbladder indicates that the jaundice is unlikely to be caused by gallstones (Courvoisier's Law), however, the absence of a palpable gallbladder does not necessarily indicate non-malignant obstruction.

Scanning in hepatomegaly

An abdominal ultrasound scan is the most useful investigation of hepatic or gallbladder enlargement. The presence of dilated hepatic veins suggests right heart failure. Sometimes clots in the hepatic veins may be visible, but Doppler ultrasound is a better tool for assessing hepatic venous flow. Metastases larger than 1 cm are readily detected by ultrasonography.

CT scanning sometimes detects lesions of 0.5 cm diameter, but may also miss some metastases, which are radiologically isodense. CT scanning with intravenous contrast improves sensitivity. Ultrasound may also detect parenchymal fatty infiltration or cirrhosis, but this requires biopsy confirmation. CT is superior in the diagnosis of fatty liver as it is possible to quantify the radiodensity of the liver (Hounsfield's numbers). Magnetic resonance scanning has not yet proved any advantage over CT scanning, but research is continuing into new methods for tumour enhancement, which may give it a greater role in the future.

Splenomegaly

A palpable spleen is at least twice its normal size, and is always pathological. The splenic tip as it becomes palpable emerges from the costal margin at the anterior axillary line and is commonly missed because of failure to palpate sufficiently laterally. As the spleen enlarges, the tip moves inferiorly and to the right below the umbilicus and in extreme enlargement towards the right illiac fossa. Hence it

is important to start palpation from the right iliac fossa if a grossly enlarged spleen is not to be missed.

The presence of certain signs may suggest the cause:

- Anaemia and purpura suggest a haematological cause.
- Stigmata of chronic liver disease suggest portal hypertension.
- Lymphadenopathy suggests a reticulosis or infection.

In the absence of any such clues, initial investigation should include full blood count and blood film, chest radiograph and 'liver function tests.' If all these tests are normal an ultrasound scan to exclude splenic vein thrombosis may be helpful. If this is normal referral for further haematological investigation should be sought. If this proves normal then endoscopy or barium swallow to look for oesophageal varices should be performed as cirrhosis may be present without any obvious clinical signs and even with normal biochemical tests.

A renal mass

The kidneys should be palpated bimanually in the flanks. The ability to feel above the mass rules out the liver or the spleen. Unilateral renal masses may be due to tumour or hydronephrosis. Polycystic disease gives bilateral enlarged kidneys. There may be associated haematuria. Renal ultrasound is usually diagnostic.

Other localised masses

A central abdominal mass

A central abdominal mass may be due to stomach, pancreas, abdominal aorta or tumour of lymph nodes or mesentery. A distended stomach is readily seen, but often difficult to feel.

A succussion splash may be elicited by rocking the abdomen sideways. A hard mass in the epigastrium suggests carcinoma of the stomach (or tumour of the left lobe of the liver). Palpable stomach cancer is rarely resectable.

A pancreatic lesion

Pancreatic lesions may be felt in the epigastrium. Pancreatic neoplasms are only palpable when very large and palpable pancreatic masses are more commonly due to post-pancreatitis pseudocysts or inflammatory masses. The pancreas lies anterior to the abdominal aorta and aortic pulsation is often transmitted.

Abdominal lymph nodes

Abdominal lymph nodes may be massively enlarged by lymphoma or abdominal tuberculosis and present as a periumbilical mass.

An abdominal aortic aneurysm

An abdominal aortic aneurysm is palpable as a central abdominal pulsating mass. This is often mimicked in the elderly by a tortuous aorta or merely by transmitted pulsations. To demonstrate an aneurysm, the mass should be expansile (i.e. pulsating in all directions and not merely anteriorly. The presence of a flow murmur supports an aneurysm because they are often clot-laden. A tender aneurysm is an ominous sign because it suggests leakage or impending perforation and must be palpated extremely gently.

A suprapubic mass

A suprapubic mass in a female could represent pregnancy, uterine fibroids or an ovarian lesion. In the male, it is usually due to a full bladder. In chronic bladder neck obstruction, this can be extremely large and surprisingly non-tender.

A right iliac fossa mass

A right iliac fossa mass could represent an appendix abscess, where it follows a history of acute appendicitis. A more chronic tender mass is suggestive of Crohn's disease. A history of chronic abdominal pain, diarrhoea or obstructive symptoms in a younger patient will suggest this diagnosis. Normal small intestine can often be felt in the right iliac fossa and although it should be non tender this is a common cause of confusion. A large caecal carcinoma may be palpable in a thin patient Carcinoid tumours may arise from the ileum, or appendix and may enlarge to a great size. Other accompanying signs (carcinoid syndrome) may provide the diagnostic clue.

The terminal ileum and caecum are the commonest sites for abdominal tuberculosis and this diagnosis must be considered in patients with unexplained pyrexia or anyone from endemic areas.

A left iliac fossa mass

It is not uncommon to be able to feel the sigmoid colon in the left iliac fossa in a thin individual. It may be tender in patients with irritable bowel or diverticular disease. A tender mass in this region can also be due to an abscess, which could be diverticular in origin or due to Crohn's disease.

CONDITIONS CAUSING ABDOMINAL MASSES OR SWELLINGS: NATURAL HISTORY AND MANAGEMENT

Liver tumours

Hepatic tumours may be benign, when they are often of little clinical significance, or malignant. In European populations 90% of malignant tumours of the liver are metastatic, but in parts of East Africa and the Far East, primary hepatocellular carcinoma is a very common cancer.

Hepatocellular carcinoma

Presentation of hepatoma may be insidious and a high degree of clinical suspicion is necessary. In a patient with known cirrhosis with any unexplained clinical deterioration, hepatocellular carcinoma must be suspected. Increasing ascites or jaundice, a palpable local lump over the liver or worsening of chronic encephalopathy are possible pointers to the development of the tumour.

Weight loss, abdominal distension with pain and a low-grade pyrexia are common findings. An irregular hepatic mass may be felt and is often tender. A friction rub due to perihepatitis and an arterial bruit are sometimes heard. Rarely, a patient may present with an acute abdomen with massive intraperitoneal haemorrhage from a ruptured vessel.

INVESTIGATION

Serum alphafetoprotein is raised in 80% of patients. It is a useful screening test for monitoring patients with known cirrhosis. There are a few other causes of a raised alphafetoprotein such as testicular, pancreatic and ovarian tumours and hydatidiform mole, but they are rare causes. Ascites is often blood-stained and high in protein content.

Enhanced CT scanning is often needed to localise the tumour clearly to allow assessment of resectability. If tumour is multifocal or present in both lobes of the liver, then it is deemed inoperable.

Should surgery be contemplated, then angiography is performed, partly to exclude tumour invasion of hepatic or portal veins, but also to delineate the anatomy to allow the surgeon to plan the resection.

A liver biopsy is necessary to make a definitive diagnosis and should be performed under ultrasound control.

EPIDEMIOLOGY

Primary hepatocellular carcinoma (hepatoma) is the second commonest cancer in South East Asia and among East African Bantu populations where it is found in 80% of autopsies. In Caucasians dying of cirrhosis, hepatoma is found in about 50% at post-mortem examination.

AETIOLOGY AND PATHOGENESIS

The main aetiological factors are hepatitis B and cirrhosis from all causes. In the tropics, the carcinogenic aflatoxin from the *Aspergillus flavus* mold, which contaminates the food, is another factor and may act as a co-carcinogen in patients with hepatitis B. The likelihood of hepatocellular carcinoma is increased 100-fold in people infected with the hepatitis B virus and 30% of people with hepatitis B-associated hepatoma are not cirrhotic.

Hepatocellular carcinoma may arise from cirrhosis of any cause, but in areas where hepatitis B is less common the commonest causes are alcoholic liver disease and haemochromatosis. There is a significant male preponderance with a male:female ratio of 4–6:1. Metastatic tumour is uncommon in cirrhotic livers. Hepatocellular carcinoma must be suspected in any patient with known cirrhosis in whom there is clinical deterioration or resistant ascites.

PATHOLOGY

The tumour may be solitary or multifocal and nodular. The malignant cells resemble normal hepatocytes but are somewhat smaller with hyperchromatic nuclei (**Fig. 14.7**). An important variant is the fibrolamellar tumour where fibrosis occurs around sheets of tumour cells (**Fig. 14.8**). This occurs mainly in younger patients and the prognosis is considerably better.

MANAGEMENT

Liver resection offers the only hope of cure. However, for tumours to be resectable, they must be confined to a single lobe of the liver, with no extrahepatic metastases. The presence of cirrhosis itself is not a contraindication provided the hepatic reserve is reasonable. In spite of great technical improvement in recent years, no more than 20% of hepatocellular tumours are resectable. The best results are with younger patients with a fibrolamellar histology.

There is generally an unacceptably high recurrence rate after liver transplantation, which is not indicated except in patients with the fibrolamellar tumour.

Chemotherapy with adriamycin or mitozantrone either as single agents or combination chemotherapy have been used with variable results. They produce tumour shrinkage in just over 50% of patients, but only prolong life by about three months. Palliative measures such as embolisation with gelfoam, alcohol injection and radiotherapy may be considered for bulky painful tumours.

PROGNOSIS

The prognosis is very poor in non-resectable disease with a median survival of 3–4 months after diagnosis. Patients who have their tumours successfully resected have a five-year survival of about 15%.

▶ **Hepatocellular carcinoma in cirrhosis**

- 50% of cirrhotics have hepatoma at postmortem
- α-fetoprotein elevated in 80%
- Hepatitis B an additional risk factor
- 20% resectable with five-year survival of 15%, otherwise very poor prognosis

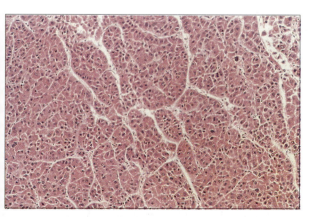

Fig. 14.7 Histology of hepatocellular carcinoma showing sheets of abnormal hepatocytes with dense nuclei and with no recognisable organisation (i.e. no central veins or portal tracts).

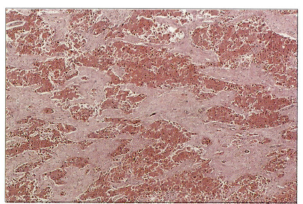

Fig. 14.8 The fibrolamellar variant of hepatocellular carcinoma. Sheets of malignant hepatocytes alternate with fibrous tissue. This usually occurs in younger patients and the prognosis is slightly better.

Other hepatic tumours

HAEMANGIOMA

The commonest benign liver tumour is the haemangioma, which is usually small and single, but occasionally multiple or large. They are mostly of the cavernous variety with true capillary haemangiomas being rare.

Haemangiomas are found in about 5% of autopsies and are increasingly recognised in asymptomatic subjects who undergo abdominal ultrasound or CT examination for other indications. This may cause unnecessary anxiety as haemangiomas may be indistinguishable radiologically from a primary or secondary carcinoma. Attempts at biopsying these lesions occasionally lead to profuse haemorrhage. Enhanced CT scanning usually helps to differentiate these vascular lesions from carcinoma.

In an asymptomatic patient with no history of cirrhosis or other cancers the best approach is usually to perform a follow-up scan a few months later and then discharge with reassurance if no change is seen.

BENIGN ADENOMA

Other primary hepatic tumours are very rare. A benign adenoma may occur in association with the oral contraceptive pill or pregnancy. It will often regress spontaneously with cessation of the oral contraceptive, but occasionally requires resection if causing pain or intraabdominal bleeding. It may coexist with **peliosis hepatis**. This condition is also associated with use of oral contraceptives or anabolic steroids. It consists of blood-filled spaces, which may or may not be lined by endothelial cells. The spaces may range from 1 mm to several cm in diameter and may cause spontaneous bleeding into the liver.

FOCAL NODULAR HYPERPLASIA

Focal nodular hyperplasia may also occur as a result of oral contraceptive usage. Histologically it can be indistinguishable from cirrhosis, but the surrounding liver is normal. The lesions are usually central and are often found by chance on liver scanning, but occasionally rupture with massive bleeding, and are sometimes painful. Regression is common after stopping oral contraceptives and surgery is rarely necessary.

▶ **Oral contraceptive-associated liver lesions**

- Cholestasis
- Peliosis hepatis (blood filled 'lakes' identifiable on histology)
- Adenoma
- Focal nodular hyperplasia

MALIGNANT HAEMANGIOSARCOMA

Malignant haemangiosarcoma is very rare and may be associated with exposure to vinyl chloride, arsenic and anabolic steroids.

PRIMARY SARCOMA

Primary sarcoma is rare, but **Kaposi's sarcoma** occurs in people with human immunodeficiency virus (HIV) infection, where the liver is a common site for the tumour. Antemortem diagnosis is often difficult in these patients.

METASTATIC TUMOUR

The liver is the commonest site of blood-borne metastases. The common primary tumours are colorectal, lung, stomach, breast and pancreas. In European populations it accounts for more than 90% of all malignant liver tumours. Prognosis is poor with the exception of resectable colorectal metastases where five-year survivals of 50% have been reported.

Benign liver infiltration

Glycogen

Hepatomegaly due to massive accumulation of glycogen may occur either as a consequence of diabetes or as a result of an inherited glycogen storage disorder.

Hepatic glycogen accumulation in **diabetes** is commoner in children with newly-diagnosed or poorly-controlled diabetes where its association with hypercholesterolaemia and obesity is known as Mauriac syndrome.

There are at least ten different forms of inherited glycogen storage disorder, each being due to a different enzyme defect in the pathways of glycogen metabolism. Most present in childhood, but patients with milder forms of the following may survive into adult life (or even present in adult life) with few problems except hepatomegaly and short stature:

- Type I (von Gierke's disease) due to glucose-6-phosphatase deficiency.
- Type III (Cori's disease) due to absence of the debranching enzyme amylo-1-6-glucosidase.
- Type VI (Hers' disease) due to phosphorylase deficiency.
- Type IX (phosphorylase kinase deficiency).

Diagnosis of these conditions cannot be made by liver histology alone and requires referral to a centre where the appropriate enzyme assays can be performed.

Fat

Fat in the liver may be either macrovesicular or microvesicular.

MICROVESICULAR FATTY LIVER

Microvesicular fatty liver has a small number of specific causes. Drugs are the commonest cause and include aspirin and valproate. In its severest form (Reye's syndrome), there is severe encephalopathy, hypoglycaemia and coagulopathy. Microvesicular fat is also a feature of hepatitis C.

MACROVESICULAR FATTY LIVER

Macrovesicular fatty liver is commoner, partly because it is most often due to excessive alcohol intake. Fatty liver in the absence of alcoholic hepatitis has a relatively good prognosis, but long-term follow-up studies show a low, but definite risk of cirrhosis. It is commonly associated with mild elevation of serum transaminases. Similar degrees of fatty liver are also seen in severe obesity where other features usually seen in alcoholic liver disease (Mallory's hyaline and neutrophil infiltration) may more rarely occur.

LIPIDOSES

Lipidoses such as **Gaucher's disease** (accumulation of gluco-cerebroside due to β-glucocerebrosidase deficiency) and **Niemann–Pick disease** (accumulation of sphingomyelin due to deficiency of sphingomyelinase) cause hepatosplenomegaly due to infiltration with swollen reticulo-endothelial cells. Similar infiltration with abnormal reticulo-endothelial cells also occurs in the histiocytoses. In the mild form of **Gaucher's disease** seen in adults clinical features include:

- Bone cysts, which may result in pathological fracture.
- Anaemia.
- Massive splenomegaly.
- Yellow thickenings ('pingueculae') on either side of the pupils.
- Massive splenomegaly, sometimes with portal hypertension and ascites.

Milder forms of **Niemann–Pick disease** may present in adolescence with neurological disorders and a diagnostic 'cherry spot' on the macula.

Mucopolysaccharide

The mucopolysaccharidoses are another group of lysosomal storage disorders in which lysosomal enzyme defects result in accumulation of glycosaminoglycans within reticulo-endothelial cells, but also within hepatocytes and fibroblasts. They present in childhood and associated features include abnormal facies and mental retardation.

Amyloid

Amyloid is a mesh of protein with β-pleated sheet structure, either immunoglobulin light chain ('primary amyloid') or acute phase protein (usually amyloid A protein). The β-pleated structure makes it resistant to naturally occurring proteases. Hepatosplenomegaly may occur, but the prognosis depends largely on the effects of amyloid on the heart and kidneys. Cholestasis may occasionally occur (particularly in light chain amyloid) and carries a poor prognosis as does portal hypertension, which is also a rare complication.

Alpha-1-antitrypsin

Alpha-1-antitrypsin is the major alpha-1 serum globulin synthesised in the liver. In the inherited deficiency there is a failure of its transport from the rough endoplasmic reticulum to the Golgi apparatus as a result of which it accumulates in hepatocytes. Three hepatic syndromes may result:

- Neonatal hepatitis, usually followed by compensated cirrhosis with hepatomegaly.
- Cirrhosis, presenting at any stage in later life.
- An increased susceptibility to alcohol-mediated liver damage.

Heterozygotes possibly also have an increased risk of developing alcoholic liver disease. Homozygotes are prone to develop emphysema, particularly if they smoke.

Granulomas

Hepatic enlargement due to granulomatous infiltration occurs in about 20% of patients with **sarcoidosis** and may occasionally be complicated by significant cholestasis and even liver failure. Differential diagnoses of hepatic granulomas are numerous. It is particularly important:

- To diagnose treatable infectious causes such as **mycobacterial infection** and **brucellosis**.
- To recognise occupational exposure (e.g. to **beryllium**) and possible **drug toxicity**.

If these have been excluded and antimitochondrial antibody and chest radiograph are normal, the aetiology is likely to remain unknown.

Hepatic cysts and abscesses

Hepatic cysts

Cystic lesions are increasingly recognised as scanning techniques become more widely applied. They range from small solitary asymptomatic cysts to multiple large cysts, which may be part of adult fibrocystic disease. They are usually asymptomatic, picked up by ultrasound examination and of little clinical significance. However, some patients, particularly in the fourth and fifth decade, may experience abdominal distension and pain when these cysts enlarge. They may cause biliary obstruction with jaundice or rupture.

MANAGEMENT

When symptomatic, the large cysts may be drained percutaneously. Instillation of absolute alcohol may delay their recurrence, but is rarely necessary and must only be done when it has been ascertained that there is no communication between the cyst and the biliary tree otherwise severe damage to the bile ducts may occur. Only in exceptional circumstances is surgery required.

Hydatid cysts

NATURAL HISTORY

Hydatid disease is caused by the cyst of the tapeworm *Echinococcus granulosus*. The disease is endemic in sheep-rearing countries in the Eastern Mediterranean, Middle East, Africa, South Australia and New Zealand. The incidence of new cases in Wales is 1.5/million/year.

Hydatid disease is a zoonosis with the dog as primary host and man, sheep and cattle acting as intermediate hosts. Man is infected by ingesting the ova, which are picked up when handling dogs or their excreta. The ovum hatches into an embryo, which passes through the intestinal wall and is delivered to the liver in the portal flow. The liver is the main infected organ with lungs the next most commonly affected site. Spleen, bone and brain may rarely be affected. Once in the liver, host cellular responses produce a thick ectocyst, which may calcify. These cysts may be single or multiple and usually affect the inferior of the right lobe of liver.

The cysts themselves are usually asymptomatic although the larger ones cause abdominal distension and discomfort. Cysts may occasionally rupture intraperitoneally resulting in ascites or into the bile ducts causing jaundice. Occasionally secondary infection with pyogenic organisms occurs. The cyst fluid is antigenic, and as the host is sensitised, leakage of the fluid may lead to anaphylaxis.

MANAGEMENT

Small asymptomatic cysts are best left alone. Aspiration or biopsy is absolutely contraindicated because of risk of anaphylaxis and dissemination. Large solitary cysts may be surgically removed with care to shell out the entire cyst without spilling. Medical treatment with mebendazole or the less toxic albendazole should be given before surgery, but it is not yet clear how effective this is.

Pyogenic abscess

Pyogenic liver abscesses may result from the following:

- Portal spread of infection from intra-abdominal sepsis (e.g. appendix abscess).
- Direct spread from an adjacent infective focus.
- Penetrating wounds or biliary infections.

The latter route is increasingly common, especially in the elderly and people with HIV (see Chapter 17) In about 50% of patients, particularly in elderly patients, there may be no obvious source of infection. The commonest infecting organisms are Gram-negative cocci, *Escherichia coli*, *Streptococcus faecalis* and *S. milleri*. Staphylococci and anaerobic bacteria are increasingly encountered. *Salmonella typhi* causes a relapsing cholangitis.

MANAGEMENT

Antibiotic therapy should be guided by bacteriology. If the abscess is culture-negative, a combination of a broad-spectrum antibiotic with Gram-negative activity such as a cephalosporin and metronidazole should be used. If there is no obvious primary focus of infection *S. milleri* is likely and benzylpenicillin should be given in addition.

Antibiotics alone are rarely sufficient and a drainage procedure should be attempted under ultrasound or CT control. This may not be feasible if the abscesses are small and numerous. Any biliary obstruction must be relieved by endoscopic sphincterotomy and stone removal or stent insertion.

Amoebic abscess

NATURAL HISTORY

Patients present with fever and right upper quadrant pain. The systemic features of an amoebic liver abscess are usually less marked than with pyogenic abscesses. Alcohol is said to exacerbate the pain. A tender liver is usual and the swelling may be visible in the epigastrium. Abscesses near the diaphragmatic surface may present with shoulder-tip pain and pleural effusion.

AETIOLOGY AND PATHOGENESIS

Amoebiasis is a disease of the sub-tropics and tropics. It is rare in European populations except those who have visited endemic areas. It may present many years after exposure. The organism *Entamoeba histolytica* exists in a free-living cystic form outside the host and when ingested, passes through to the colon where it invades the mucosa causing typical flask-shaped ulcers. From there the amoebae invade the portal system and pass into the liver.

MANAGEMENT

Metronidazole, 800 mg three times a day for ten days, is the standard therapy and drainage should be avoided because of the risk of introducing secondary infection. This should followed by oral diloxanide, 500 mg three times daily for 10 days, which eliminates amoebae from the gut and prevents relapse.

Peritoneal disease

Malignant ascites

Malignant ascites may present late in the course of malignant disease, but is quite commonly the presenting complaint. The primary tumour may be asymptomatic and therefore very difficult to identify.

The most important aspect of diagnosis is the certainty of distinction from infection, particularly tuberculosis, and lymphoma. Distinction from lymphoma may require expert assessment of cell surface markers as well as morphology. If ascites is due to a malignant lymphoma the prognosis may be reasonable with aggressive chemotherapy whereas it is uniformly poor for ascites due to carcinoma. The presence of mucus is diagnostic of a mucin-secreting adenocarcinoma or adenoma, usually ovarian ('pseudomyxoma peritonei').

MANAGEMENT

Gynaecological tumours are worth searching for by scanning because they stand a slightly better chance of response to chemotherapy. For most patients with ascites due to adenocarcinoma, however, there is little that can be usefully offered other than repeated aspiration as necessary to relieve discomfort.

If fluid re-accumulates rapidly insertion of a peritoneo-jugular shunt may have to be considered although this carries some risk of inducing disseminated intravascular coagulation.

Peritoneal mesothelioma

BENIGN MESOTHELIOMAS

Benign mesotheliomas, which may be cystic, are rare tumours that usually occur in women of childbearing age and present with abdominal pain or distension. CT and ultrasound scanning show a multiseptate cystic mass. Prognosis after resection is excellent although recurrence may occur.

MALIGNANT MESOTHELIOMAS

Malignant mesotheliomas are usually a response to asbestos exposure, often 30-40 years previously. About 50% of patients have evidence of pulmonary asbestosis in addition. There is no effective treatment and prognosis is poor.

Vasculitis

Ascites may occur as a rare complication of vasculitis, usually in systemic lupus erythematosus (SLE). It may be painless and the diagnosis is usually made by exclusion of infection in a patient with positive serological markers for SLE. There is usually a good response to corticosteroids.

Sclerosing peritonitis

Sclerosing peritonitis is an unusual clinical syndrome, best recognised as a complication of the beta blocker practolol, but can also occur as a result of intrabdominal sepsis or as a consequence of chronic peritoneal dialysis. The peritoneum becomes thickened with intense fibrosis and patients may initially present with abdominal pain, obstruction or an abdominal mass.

Disease of the mesentery

Mesenteric panniculitis

Mesenteric panniculitis is a curious condition in which spontaneous fat necrosis in the mesentery is followed by a granulomatous reaction. It presents as recurrent episodes of abdominal pain, which may be localised or generalised associated with weight loss, low-grade fever and vomiting. It is often found as an incidental finding at laparotomy. Barium studies may show distorted and separated loops of small intestine.

MANAGEMENT

Regression usually occurs spontaneously over about two years, but there may be a prompt response to corticosteroid therapy. Lymphoma is an occasional complication.

Mesenteric fibromatosis (desmoid)

Desmoids are benign lesions that occur either in isolation or as part of the adenomatous polyposis (Gardner's) syndrome.

Treatment is often unnecessary once histological diagnosis has been made by biopsy, but local compression of vital structures may necessitate surgical resection.

Mesenteric and omental cysts and tumours

Mesenteric cysts are either lined by mesothelial cells or less commonly by endothelial cells (cystic lymphangioma). They may present with abdominal pain, and are only moveable longitudinally on abdominal palpation. Omental cysts, which are more common in childhood, are mobile in all directions. Surgical resection or enucleation should be performed.

Primary tumours of the mesentery and omentum are rarer than secondary tumours. They include fibromas, leiomyomas, lipomas and histiocytomas as well as malignant leiomyosarcomas and are treated by surgical resection.

FURTHER READING

Hepatoma

Colombo M. Hepatocellular carcinoma. *J Hepat* 1992: **15**: 225–236.

Farmer DG, Rosove MH, Shaked A, Busutilli RW Current treatment modalities for hepatocellular carcinoma. *Ann Surg* 1994; **219**: 236–47.

Hobbs KE, Dusheiko GM. Management of hepatocellular carcinoma. *J Hepatol* 1992; **15**(3): 281–3.

Luporini G, Labianca R, Pancera G. Medical treatment of hepatocellular carcinoma. *J Surg Oncol* Suppl. 1993; **3**: 115–18.

Moore D Jr, Pazdur R. Systemic therapies for unresectable primary hepatic tumors. *J Surg Oncol* Suppl. 1993; **3**: 112–14.

Pichlmayer R. Liver transplantation in primary hepatocellular carcinoma. *J Hepatol* 1993; **18**: 151–153.

Ravoet C, Bleiberg H, Gerard B. Non-surgical treatment of hepatocarcinoma. *J Surg Oncol* Suppl. 1993; **3**: 104–11.

Robinson WS. The role of hepatitis B virus in the development of primary hepatocellular carcinoma: Part I. *J Gastroenterol Hepatol* 1992; **7**(6): 622–38.

Robinson WS. The role of hepatitis B virus in development of primary hepatocellular carcinoma: Part II. *J Gastroenterol Hepatol* 1993; **8**(1): 95–106.

Sherlock S Viruses and hepatocellular carcinoma. *Gut* 1994; **35**:828–32.

Wanebo HJ, Vezeridis MP. Hepatoma. *J Surg Oncol* Suppl. 1993; **3**: 40–5.Okuda K. Hepatocellular carcinoma: Recent progress. *Hepatology* 1992; **15**: 948–63.

Cystic diseases of the liver and biliary tree

Cuschieri A, Byrne D. Cystic disease of the biliary tract. *Ann Chir Gynaecol* 1989; **78**(4): 259–66.

Forbes A, Murray Lyon IM. Cystic disease of the liver and biliary tract. *Gut* 1991; Suppl.: S116–22.

Karrer FM, Hall RJ, Stewart BA, Lilly JR. Congenital biliary tract disease. *Surg Clin North Am* 1990; **70**(6): 1403–18.

Lindberg MC. Hepatobiliary complications of oral contraceptives. *J Gen Intern Med* 1992; **7**(2): 199–209.

Vauthey JN, Maddern GJ, Blumgart LH. Adult polycystic disease of the liver. *Br J Surg* 1991; **78**(5): 524–7.

Hydatid disease

al Karawi MA, el Shiekh Mohamed AR, Yasawy MI. Advances in diagnosis and management of hydatid disease. *Hepatogastroenterology* 1990; **37**(3): 327–31.

Farmer PM, Chatterley S, Spier N Echinococcal cyst of the liver: diagnosis and surgical management. *Ann Clin Lab Sci* 1990; **20**(6): 385–91.

Munzer D. New perspectives in the diagnosis of Echinococcal disease. *J Clin Gastroenterol* 1991; **13**(4): 415–23.

Other tumours

Hidvegi J, Schneider F, Rohonyi B, Flautner L, Szlavik L. Peritoneal benign cystic mesothelioma. (Review.) *Path Res Pract* 1991; **187**(1):103–6; discussion 106–8.

Kittur DS, Korpe SW, Raytch RE, Smith GW. Surgical aspects of sclerosing encapsulating peritonitis. (Review.) *Arch Surg* 1990 Dec; **125**(12). 1626–8.Ros PR, Li KC. Benign liver tumors. *Curr Probl Diagn Radiol* 1989; **18**(3): 125–55.

15
LIVER FAILURE

REACHING A DIAGNOSIS AND MANAGEMENT

There are two different clinical syndromes of liver failure :

- Acute (fulminant) failure.
- Chronic (or acute on chronic) failure.

There is considerable overlap between the syndromes, but:

- **Acute (fulminant) liver failure** is typified by cerebral oedema, severe hypoglycaemia, severe coagulopathy and the potential for rapid improvement if the underlying liver disease is reversible. It is usually due to an acute illness or insult such as acute viral hepatitis, poisoning (paracetamol or mushroom), drug reaction (halothane or isoniazid), fatty liver of pregnancy. It may occasionally be an acute presentation of chronic liver disease (particularly chronic active hepatitis or Wilson's disease).
- **Chronic or acute on chronic liver failure** is characterised by ascites, portal–systemic encephalopathy (PSE) and variceal bleeding, which is a consequence of portal hypertension rather than liver failure, but is nevertheless common in this group of patients. There is usually underlying cirrhosis (or alcoholic hepatitis) and deterioration is often precipitated by variceal bleeding, sepsis or overvigorous use of diuretics.

Both acute and chronic liver failure are frequently complicated by renal failure and sepsis.

Acute (fulminant) liver failure

Acute liver failure usually occurs in patients with previously normal livers. It is important to distinguish this group of patients from those who have an acute-on-chronic liver disease. In acute liver disease, there is potential for complete recovery of the liver and even in patients with chronic active hepatitis or Wilson's disease there is potential for recovery with appropriate treatment of the underlying liver disease.

Acute fulminant hepatic failure is defined as the onset of hepatic encephalopathy within six weeks of the onset of symptoms. A further group is recognised in which

▶ **Is it acute rather than acute-on-chronic liver disease?**

Acute liver disease more likely

- Short history
- Small liver
- No spider naevi
- Well nourished
- Ascites late
- Early encephalopathy
- Small or absent varices
- No identifiable precipitating event

Acute-on-chronic liver disease more likely

- Long history of known liver disease
- Large liver
- Enlarged spleen
- Spider naevi present
- Poor nutritional state
- Ascites early
- Late encephalopathy
- Varices present
- Gastrointestinal bleed, infection, drugs as precipitant

encephalopathy sets in after six weeks from the onset of symptoms, but before six months. This is sometimes referred to as **subacute fulminant hepatic failure** or late-onset acute liver failure. This is quite an important clinical distinction because the mortality is considerably higher in the subacute group, with coma carrying a mortality of 80–90% and being an indication for immediate transfer to a transplant centre. Coma in acute fulminant hepatic failure carries a mortality of approximately 50% (lower in paracetamol injury than viral hepatitis).

Fulminant hepatic failure is a medical emergency. Suspected patients must be admitted immediately.

There are several questions that need to be answered urgently:

- Is the diagnosis correct?
- What is the aetiology?
- Are there complicating medical problems?
- Is the patient to be considered for urgent liver transplantation?

Is the diagnosis correct?

Encephalopathy may initially manifest as subtle behavioural changes. The patient may be antisocial and aggressive and signs of disinhibition, mania and delirium may follow. This is because inhibitory pathways are affected first, but in the latter stages, there is increasing drowsiness leading, as cerebral oedema worsens, to decerebrate rigidity. At this stage there may be spasticity, extension and hyperpronation of limbs and dysconjugate eye movements, but plantar responses remain flexor till very late.

It is important to realise that the degree of neuro-psychiatric disturbance (and hence the risk of death from coning and respiratory arrest) does not correlate well with the degree of jaundice.

Other neuropsychiatric disorders presenting in a patient with co-existing liver disease (particularly Wilson's disease) may confuse the picture. If the diagnosis is not clear, an electroencephalogram is often very helpful in differentiating between hepatic coma and other causes.

Coagulation is invariably impaired, serum transaminase is usually markedly elevated (although may fall within a few days if a large proportion of the hepatocytes have already been destroyed), but bilirubin may be only modestly elevated at first (**Figs 15.1–15.4**).

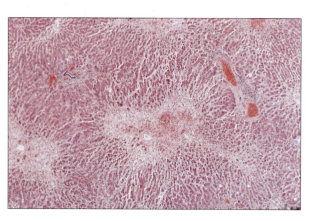

Fig. 15.1 Paracetamol liver injury showing the centrilobular necrosis (i.e. around the central vein) that is typical of acute drug-induced hepatic necrosis.

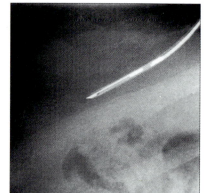

Fig. 15.2 Trans-jugular liver biopsy. This techique can be used to obtain biopsy samples when a diagnosis is urgently required, but coagulation is too poor to allow conventional biopsy (e.g. hepatic failure due to possible Wilson's disease).

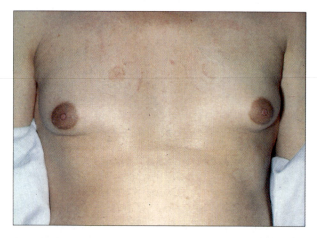

Fig. 15.3 Gynaecomastia. This can be a feature of cirrhosis (due to reduced metabolism of oestrogens), but is more commonly due to spironolactone therapy.

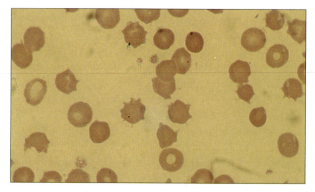

Fig. 15.4 Spur cells. These are an uncommon, but specific feature of end-stage alcoholic liver disease; usually in a patient who has stopped drinking too late and has ended up with a small cirrhotic liver. They are probably due to failure of apolipoprotein synthesis and indicate a poor prognosis, most patients dying within six months unless transplanted. Severe haemolytic anaemia may result.

What is the aetiology?
The main causes of acute fulminant hepatic failure are listed below.

▶ **Causes of fulminant liver failure**

- Viral hepatitis: A (rare), B, C, D, E(rare except in pregnancy), ?F(non-A non-B non-C)
- Other infective hepatitis: yellow fever, leptospirosis
- Paracetamol overdose
- Other drugs: idiosyncratic reactions (halothane, isoniazid, NSAIDs, antidepressants)
- Alcohol
- Wilson's disease
- Budd–Chiari syndrome
- Acute fatty liver of pregnancy
- Metastatic malignancy
- Mushroom poisoning

In Britain, the commonest causes are viral hepatitis and paracetamol (acetaminophen) poisoning. In France, ingestion of the poisonous mushroom *Amanita phalloides* is a major cause in the autumn. The main diagnostic difficulty is the differentiation between acute liver disease and an acute presentation of chronic liver disease. An accurate history, from a relative if necessary, is particularly important. It is important to look for any stigmata of chronic disease such as cutaneous spiders, palmar erythema and more particularly, evidence of portal hypertension such as splenomegaly or distended abdominal wall veins.

VIRAL HEPATITIS
History of contact, foreign travel, drug abuse, homosexuality and blood transfusion should be sought. Hepatitis A is a rare cause of fulminant failure although in the UK it is high compared to many other countries as exposure to the virus later in life gives a higher risk of acute liver failure. Diagnosis is made by serum anti-HAV IgM antibody.

There is a higher risk (approximately 5%) of developing acute liver failure with hepatitis B infection. Females are at particularly high risk. There is evidence that people with human immunodeficiency virus (HIV) infection are less likely to develop fulminant failure, and this is to be expected because the virus itself is not cytotoxic and the hepatocellular damage is the result of the cellular immune response to infected cells.

Diagnosis is made by presence of IgM anti-core antibody because HBsAg (surface antigen) may be absent in up to 50% of patients with acute fulminant failure.

Co-infection or superinfection with hepatitis D (delta agent) also predisposes to acute liver failure. Hepatitis C may be diagnosed by the anti-HCV antibody, but the antibody may not appear in the serum for many weeks.

Hepatitis E (orofaecal non-A non-B hepatitis) is uncommon in the UK and is thought to be a rare cause of acute liver failure except when acquired in pregnancy. In many patients with acute fulminant liver failure viral serology is negative, but no other cause is found and it is likely that further hepatotrophic viruses may be responsible.

PARACETAMOL (ACETAMINOPHEN) POISONING
In the UK deliberate self-poisoning with paracetamol is the commonest cause of acute liver failure. The diagnosis is usually clear if a history can be obtained, but may be more difficult if the patient is admitted late.

The liver metabolises paracetamol, which is not itself toxic, by the cytochrome P450 system into an unstable toxic metabolite. This metabolite is normally rapidly inactivated by glutathione. Ingestion of high doses (usually higher than 20 g of paracetamol) depletes the glutathione and results in toxicity. However even modest doses may result in hepatocellular damage in some individuals including:

- Patients receiving enzyme-inducing agents such as antiepileptic agents whose cytochrome P450 system is stimulated.
- Alcoholics, whose glutathione may be depleted.

DRUG REACTIONS
Halothane hepatitis still occurs. It is an idiosyncratic reaction that probably has an allergic component and patients have usually had a previous exposure. Even subsequent exposure to minute amounts of halothane such as may be found in the piping of the anaesthetic machine may provoke hepatitis in susceptible individuals.

A specific antibody test has been described, but the diagnosis can usually be made from the history and clinical features. Careful examination of the patient's records will often reveal an unexplained pyrexia.

Jaundice usually develops 5–15 days after exposure, the period typically being shorter after second or subsequent exposure. About 75% of patients have an associated fever and 40% have eosinophilia. The prognosis is worse in obese patients, presumably because the drug is lipid-soluble and body stores are greater.

Many other drugs produce idiosyncratic hepatitic reactions. Common current causes include co-amoxyclav, flucloxacillin, isoniazid, ketoconazole and valproate.

RARE CAUSES OF ACUTE PRESENTATIONS OF CHRONIC LIVER DISEASE
Wilson's disease may present acutely and should be suspected in any patient under 40 years of age if there is no clear alternative diagnosis, particularly if there is evidence of haemolysis (see Chapter 13). Very rarely, malignant disease also presents with fulminant hepatic failure.

Are there complicating medical problems?

Intensive supportive therapy and treatment of complications is the mainstay of management of fulminant liver failure. Patients are best managed in an intensive care unit with full monitoring facilities. Improvement in prognosis in recent years have been largely due to better supportive therapy.

IS COAGULATION IMPAIRED?

Coagulation is a good guide to hepatic synthetic function. Following paracetamol overdose a prothrombin ratio of less than twice control at 48 hours implies almost certain survival. Thrombocytopenia may also occur due to mechanisms that are poorly understood.

IS THERE A RESPIRATORY ALKALOSIS? IS THERE A METABOLIC ACIDOSIS?

Respiratory alkalosis associated with hyperventilation is usual until a late stage when metabolic acidosis appears. This is a grave feature because it can rapidly become irreversible despite attempts at correction with dialysis or intravenous bicarbonate. With paracetamol poisoning, when the pH falls to less than 7.3 mortality is higher than 90% without transplantation.

IS THERE RENAL FAILURE?

Renal failure is not as grave a feature in fulminant failure as it is in acute on chronic liver failure, but nevertheless complicates management considerably. It is particularly common following paracetamol overdose, because of the nephrotoxicity of the drug itself (75% incidence in patients with grade 4 encephalopathy following paracetamol compared with 30% due to other causes). Survival figures of 30% for renal failure complicating viral hepatitis and 50% for renal failure complicating paracetamol poisoning have been reported.

HAS THE LIVER SHRUNK IN SIZE?

Liver size is a useful clinical guide. The liver usually shrinks rapidly during the acute injury and its size can be monitored approximately by percussion. Absence of any hepatic dullness is a grave sign.

What is the underlying liver disease?

The nature of the underlying liver disease is probably the most important determinant of survival. Paracetamol injury carries a relatively good prognosis while grade 4 coma associated with Wilson's disease, halothane hepatitis, idiosyncratic drug reactions or non-A, non-B hepatitis all carry mortalities of 80% without transplantation.

Acute or subacute?

The speed of onset is also an important prognostic feature. Coma occurring more than six weeks after the onset of symptoms (subacute hepatic failure) carries a mortality of 80% and is a clear indication for transplantation.

Management

GENERAL PRINCIPLES

Prevent hypoglycaemia

The most important yet simple action that can be taken is the prevention of hypoglycaemia. Considerable amounts of glucose may be required to do this. A sensible approach is to commence with an infusion of 10% dextrose, 1 litre 12-hourly, on admission increasing to 20% dextrose or greater if hypoglycaemia is documented. Blood glucose should be monitored two-hourly aiming to keep the blood glucose above 5 mmol/l. Prevention of hypoglycaemia is much better than reacting after the event. It is also appropriate to follow this course in a patient following a large paracetamol overdose even before any features of liver failure have developed.

Avoid cerebral oedema

In a severe case there may be little that can be done to prevent cerebral oedema, but care should be taken to avoid fluid overload and the patient should be nursed head up providing that perfusion is adequate.

Avoid sedation

Any drugs metabolised by the liver will remain in circulation almost indefinitely and if they impair consciousness will at least make assessment of prognosis (and hence consideration of transplantation) difficult and may precipitate coma. They should therefore be avoided unless absolutely necessary to calm a violently agitated patient (in which case sedation and ventilation may be necessary).

SPECIFIC PROBLEMS

Encephalopathy and cerebral oedema

Cerebral oedema is much more of a problem than PSE in acute liver failure. This presumably reflects the relative lack of portal hypertension and shunting. Conventional treatments for PSE such as lactulose and neomycin, rarely have an impressive effect on mental status. Cerebral oedema occurs in over 75% of fulminant failure patients with grade IV encephalopathy, who may eventually develop decerebrate rigidity, but can occasionally make a full recovery, even from this state.

The patient should be managed in a specialist intensive care unit and some units advocate monitoring of intracranial pressure. Specific treatment with mannitol, 0.3–0.4 mg/kg intravenously by rapid bolus, is given if the cerebral pressure exceeds 25 mmHg (normal < 12 mmHg) or if the mental status is deteriorating. Care should be taken not to give repeated mannitol in the absence of response, particularly if

▶ **Main principles of therapy for acute liver failure**

- Prevent hypoglycaemia
- Avoid sedation
- Avoid fluid overload
- Contact transplant centre early
- Coma occurring more than six weeks after the onset of symptoms carries a mortality of over 90% unless transplanted

▶ **Investigations of acute (fulminant) hepatic failure:**

To establish diagnosis and aetiology

- EEG (not usually necessary)
- Serum liver enzymes
- Virology
    Hepatitis B IgM anti-core
    Hepatitis C,D
    Hepatitis A IgM
- Paracetamol level
- Alcohol level (if relevant)

If diagnosis still in doubt:

- CT scan (acute fatty liver of pregnancy, malignancy)
- Serum caeruloplasmin, copper excretion, slit lamp examination (Wilson's disease)
- Liver biopsy if clotting is acceptable

To assess severity

- Full biochemistry profile (U and Es, albumin, calcium, bilirubin, creatinine)
- Blood glucose
- Full blood count
- Prothrombin time
- Blood gases (especially in paracetamol poisoning)

To monitor for complicating conditions (daily)

- Renal (urine output,creatinine: note, urea is unhelpful)
- Sepsis (microbiological samples, e.g. blood,urine, sputum, ascitic fluid)
- Coagulation (prothrombin time)
- Metabolic(glucose, electrolytes)

the patient is in renal failure, otherwise a hyperosmolar state will result unless the mannitol is removed by haemo-filtration. If mannitol is ineffective, intravenous thiopentone or hyperventilation may be tried. Dexamethasone is ineffective in this situation. Residual brain damage is extremely rare in patients who survive.

Renal failure, hypotension and metabolic acidosis

Vascular and haemodynamic changes may be profound in patients with fulminant failure with hypovolaemia through vasodilation. Renal vascular support may be achieved by intravenous dopamine. Frusemide is ineffective and best avoided. Care should be taken to avoid fluid overload because of the risk of cerebral oedema. Dialysis or haemo-filtration may be required for correction of acidosis or fluid overload at a time when the serum creatinine is only mod-erately increased. It is important to monitor creatinine and not urea because urea synthesis is impaired in liver failure.

Severe acidosis is a bad prognostic sign and does not usually respond to intravenous bicarbonate. If dialysis is required great care needs to be taken to avoid excessive heparinisation of the patient, preferably by strict regional heparinisation of the dialysis equipment. Peritoneal dialysis can be used as a short-term therapy, but is rarely sufficient to correct the severe metabolic problems.

Haemodynamic support may require colloid infusions and noradrenaline infusion, but when a patient requires such inotropic support the prognosis is hopeless except to buy time until a suitable liver homograft is available.

Coagulopathy

As the liver is the source of most clotting factors (except Factor VIII), profound coagulopathy may result in haem-orrhage. Prothrombin time is the most commonly used indicator of severity of liver failure. Factor V has a short half-life and is theoretically a better indicator of deterioration, but assay is not generally available. The commonest source of haemorrhage is the upper gastrointestinal tract from gastric erosions. The prophylactic use of H_2 receptor antagonists reduces this risk. Any blood loss should be replaced by fresh blood or stored blood with fresh frozen plasma and platelet transfusion may be required. Prophylactic infusion of clotting factors has not been shown to reduce morbidity or mortality and is not recommended in the absence of bleeding.

Sepsis

Sepsis is very common in patients with acute fulminant failure. Daily blood culture specimens should be obtained and evidence of infection rigorously treated. There is no clear evidence that prophylactic antibiotics or bowel decontamination are of benefit. Infection should be suspected particularly if coagulation deteriorates while other parameters improve. Fungal sepsis is a common cause of late deterioration.

Treatment of paracetamol poisoning

Treatment with N-acetylcysteine intravenously will protect the liver by increasing the availability of sulphhydryl groups with which the active metabolite can react. It is important to determine as accurately as possible the time of ingestion and blood levels of paracetamol.

If the blood paracetamol level is above the 'treatment line' at 4–16 hours after ingestion, N-acetylcysteine should be administered. However, if the time of ingestion is uncertain, particularly when the patient is under the influence of alcohol or other psychotropics, treatment with N-acetylcysteine should also be commenced. Although there are occasional cases of anaphylaxis, N-acetylcysteine is generally non-toxic. There is accumulating evidence that administration of N-acetylcysteine given more than 16 hours after ingestion may also be beneficial. 'If in doubt, treat' is a good policy.

Experimental evidence suggests that the earlier after ingestion the prophylaxis is given the better, even during the first 12 hours after overdose. It is therefore important to avoid lengthy delays between patient admission and treatment. Such delays sometimes result while paracetamol assays are being performed. In order to avoid this problem rapid assay kits can be kept in the emergency department or alternatively a policy can be adopted of giving all patients immediate oral methionine 2.5 g (an alternative, safe and cheap glutathione precursor) while awaiting drug levels. It is probably safest to follow this with N-acetylcysteine rather than further methionine if levels are high because vomiting or ileus may make absorption unreliable.

INDICATIONS FOR TRANSPLANTATION

Liver transplantation is a well-established treatment option for patients with fulminant failure. However, in patients with paracetamol poisoning or acute viral hepatitis A or B, the liver may completely recover if the patient survives the acute episode. Hence the decision to transplant must be made on the basis of accurate measurement of prognosis.

Survival rates after transplantation for acute liver failure are 60–75%. The adjacent table shows the criteria used by the King's College Hospital Liver Unit, London, for deciding whether to transplant. It is important to discuss any patient with fulminant hepatic failure with a transplant unit

▶ **King's College Hospital criteria for selection of patients with fulminant hepatic failure for transplantation**

Paracetamol-induced

- pH < 7.3 (irrespective of grade of encephalopathy)

or

- Prothrombin time > 100 secs and serum creatinine > 300 µmol/l in patients with grade III or IV encephalopathy (see page 232)

Other causes

- Prothrombin time > 100secs (irrespective of grade of encephalopathy)

or

- Any three of the following variables (irrespective of grade of encephalopathy):
  - Age < 10 years or > 40 years
  - Aetiology: non A, non B hepatitis, halothane hepatitis, idiosyncratic drug reaction
  - Duration of jaundice before onset of encephalopathy > 7days
  - Prothrombin time > 50 secs
  - Serum bilirubin > 300 µmol/l

at an early stage as there may only be a very narrow 'window of opportunity' for transplantation once the decision has been made.

Chronic (or acute on chronic) liver failure

Chronic (or acute on chronic) liver failure differs from acute liver failure in that:

- Coma is usually due to portal-systemic encephalopathy (PSE) rather than cerebral oedema and is usually reversible.
- Bleeding is more commonly due to oesophageal varices or some other consequence of portal hypertension than to gastric erosions.
- Renal failure carries a very grave prognosis.
- The underlying liver disease is likely to be irreversible (with the exception of autoimmune chronic active hepatitis and some cases of alcoholic hepatitis).

Chronic liver failure is a clinical syndrome with multisystem involvement. It may result from almost any form of liver disease.

- The failure of the liver to excrete bilirubin results in **jaundice**.
- The failure of synthesis of coagulation factors and other proteins results in **coagulopathy** and **muscle wasting**.
- The almost invariable alteration in liver architecture (cirrhosis) results in **portal hypertension**.

▶ **Characteristic features of acute and chronic liver failure**

Acute	Chronic
Coma due to cerebral oedema	Coma due to portal-systemic encephalopathy
Hypoglycaemia often severe	Hypoglycaemia less common
GI bleeding usually due to erosions	GI bleeding usually due to varices
Renal failure commonly reversible	Renal failure usually irreversible
Occasional sepsis	Sepsis frequent

- **Ascites** results from a combination of factors, which include renal dysfunction (salt retention and failure to excrete a water load), hypoproteinaemia and raised portal pressure.
- Shunting of portal blood past the liver and alterations in amino acid balance result in the passage of nitrogenous compounds across the blood–brain barrier leading to **hepatic encephalopathy**.
- Vascular vasodilatation due to factors that probably include nitric oxide leads to a **hyperdynamic circulation**.
- The patient is anorexic, weak and listless.

Coagulation disorders and bleeding

The liver is the source of most of the clotting factors (with the exception of Factor VIII). In hepatocellular failure, there is therefore abnormal clotting. The prothrombin time is a reliable indicator of hepatic dysfunction. With portal hypertension and hypersplenism, the platelet count may also below.

Portal hypertension leads to varices in the oesophagus, stomach and rectum at sites of portosystemic anastomoses. When bleeding occurs it is often catastrophic. Portal hypertensive gastropathy and colopathy are also not uncommon, and may also lead to bleeding and anaemia. These are discussed in more detail in Chapter 6.

Ascites

Ascites is the presence of free fluid in the peritoneal cavity, of at least two litres before it is clinically detected. It often presents insidiously as increasing abdominal girth in a patient with stigmata of chronic liver disease, but may occur suddenly if there is an accompanying decompensating event such as sepsis or haemorrhage. Diagnosis is discussed in Chapter 14.

The pathogenesis of ascites is complex, but the earliest pathological event is probably peripheral arterial vasodilation, probably due to an accumulation of nitric oxide (endothelium relaxant factor). This results in 'underfilling' of the intravascular space and stimulation of the renin–angiotensin system, vasopressin release and increased sympathetic acivity, all resulting in water and sodium retention. The avid sodium and water retention spills over into the peritoneal space, encouraged by a high portal pressure and a low serum oncotic pressure due to hypoalbuminaemia.

MANAGEMENT
Apart from the usual blood biochemistry:

- Serum α-fetoprotein should be measured to look for occult hepatoma.
- It is important to perform a diagnostic tap. Samples should be sent for bacteriology, biochemistry and cytology. The protein content of ascitic fluid complicating cirrhosis rarely exceeds 15 g/litre, and higher values may suggest infection, venous obstruction or malignancy. A high amylase indicates pancreatic ascites.

Spontaneous bacterial peritonitis is extremely common in cirrhosis, and culture is particularly important. The chance of culturing pathogens is increased if the samples are inoculated into blood culture bottles before transit to the laboratory. *Escherichia coli* and streptococci spp. are the most frequently encountered pathogens.

Before the culture result is obtained the white blood cell (WBC) count of the ascitic fluid is the single most useful indicator of the presence of infection. A total WBC count in excess of 500/mm^3 or neutrophil count of over 250/mm^3 is indicative of infection, and antibiotic treatment should be started. The antibiotic should be broad-spectrum, such as one of the third generation cephalosporins (e.g. cefotaxime). Minor ascites may not warrant treatment and inappropriate use of powerful loop diuretics may precipitate renal failure.

▶ **Principles of treatment of ascites**

- Do not aim for more than 0.5 kg weight loss per day
- Avoid loop diuretics
- Avoid precipitation of hyponatraemia, hypokalaemia or hypovolaemia and therefore avoid precipitating renal failure
- Aim to make the patient comfortable rather than necessarily aiming for complete eradication of ascites (which may result in hypovolaemia)

As a rule, treatment aims to relieve patient discomfort without compromising renal function or causing postural hypotension. Overdiuresis may cause fatal hepatorenal syndrome.

The patient should be rested in bed, and weight, serum electrolytes and creatinine and urine output monitored daily. Weight loss should not exceed 0.5 kg/day, which is about the limit of ascitic fluid transfer into the intravascular compartment. Fluid restriction (1.5 litres is usual), salt restriction (40 mmol/day is adequate without making food too unpalatable), and spironolactone, are the mainstay of therapy. A dose of 200 mg of spironolactone is usually necessary, and may be increased if there is no significant response after three days. Urinary electrolytes should be monitored twice a week when on spironolactone, aiming for a sodium:potassium ratio higher than 1. Xipamide, 20 mg daily, may be added if there is no response after a week on the above regimen, keeping a close eye on the electrolytes and renal function.

Paracentesis can be safely carried out with concomitant infusion of 6–8 g of albumin for every litre of fluid removed. A large bore or indwelling catheter should not be used because it may cause persistent leakage and has an increased risk of bacterial contamination. A modified Kuss needle (with additional side-holes) under low-grade suction is preferred. Paracentesis is effective, and the high cost of the albumin may be offset by the shorter hospital stay.

Renal failure

Hepatorenal syndrome is a functional renal failure that results partly as a result of poorly understood changes in regional renal perfusion, and partly from fluid shifts due to over-diuresis or diarrhoea in patients with severe liver disease. It may occur spontaneously. It is described as 'functional' because renal histology is normal and when patients are transplanted, the kidney function returns.

Once renal failure is established with a high serum creatinine in a patient with chronic liver disease, death is almost inevitable, and dialysis is of no benefit. Only hepatic transplantation may save the patient.

It is important to exclude iatrogenic causes including overdiuresis, diarrhoea from over-enthusiastic use of lactulose, and non-steroidal anti-inflammatory drugs.

Encephalopathy

Hepatic encephalopathy may present with a wide variety of manifestations, from agression through delirium to coma. It may fluctuate and often passes through a disinhibited phase that may prompt administration of a sedative which may be fatal. Often alcoholic patients are assumed to be withdrawing from alcohol and given high doses of chlormethiazole, which is dangerous if there is established liver failure.

In the early stages of encephalopathy there may be an associated:

- Flapping tremor (asterixis).
- Slurred speech.
- Constructional apraxia.
- Inversion of normal sleep pattern.
- Deterioration of intellectual function.
- Hepatic foetor, a sweet, faecal breath may be detected.

In later stages, coma, increased muscle rigidity and hyperventilation occurs. Two clinical types of encephalopathy are recognised in patients with chronic liver disease:

▶ **Grade of encephalopathy**

I

Mild or episodic drowsiness, intellectual impairment, but rousable and coherent

II

Increased drowsiness with confusion and disorientation, but rousable

III

Very drowsy, disorientated, often agitated

IV

Comatose, unresponsive or responding only to pain, may be complicated by evidence of cerebral oedema

▶ **Assessment of severity**

There are seven main determinants of severity and prognosis
• Mental state
• Coagulation
• Acid/base balance
• Renal function
• Liver size: small is associated with a poor prognosis
• The nature of the underlying liver disease
• The speed of onset: (over six weeks is associated with a poor prognosis)

- Acute-on-chronic encephalopathy seen in patients with decompensated cirrhosis in which a precipitant is usually identified (e.g. drugs, gastrointestinal bleed, electrolyte disturbance; see list on page 233).
- Chronic encephalopathy in patients with portosystemic shunting, but relatively preserved liver function.

The exact factors responsible for the encephalopathy are unknown, but a recent demonstration that coma can occasionally be reversed by specific benzodiazepine antagonists suggests that at least part of the problem is due to false neurotransmitters crossing the blood–brain barrier and interacting with gamma-aminobenzoic acid (GABA) (i.e. benzodiazepine) receptors. In all cases it can be demonstrated that there is:

- Substantial portal-systemic shunting.
- A high protein load in the intestine, either due to diet or bleeding.

MANAGEMENT
Treatment of encephalopathy is with lactulose (or lactitol) and removal of the precipitant. The dosage should be increased until diarrhoea occurs (e.g. 20 ml three times per day) and then reduced until the stool starts to form.

Addition of neomycin usually has relatively little additional effect and care should be taken if it is used long term because small amounts of the drug can get absorbed and cause ototoxicity.

Magnesium sulphate enemas should be used in the acute situation, particularly if there is constipation or melaena.

Patients with chronic encephalopathy need to be advised to take a very low intake of animal protein. A single hamburger 'binge' may be sufficient to precipitate coma in some patients. A high vegetable protein diet often seems to be successful, allowing maintenance of serum albumin and muscle bulk without precipitation of encephalopathy.

Look for the following as possible **precipitants of acute-on-chronic encephalopathy**:

- Constipation.
- Gastrointestinal bleeding.
- Infection.
- Alcohol.
- Sedative drugs (e.g. barbiturates, benzodiazepines).
- Opiates.
- Overdiuresis.
- Hypokalemia.
- Protein excess.
- Metabolic alkalosis.
- Paracentesis without adequate albumin reinfusion.
- Renal failure.
- Acute on chronic liver disease.

▶ **Child's grading (modified by Pugh scoring method)**

Parameter	Score 1	Score 2	Score 3
Albumin	> 35 g/l	30–35 g/l	< 35 g/l
Bilirubin	< 34	34–51	> 51
Prothrombin time	< 4 secs prolonged	4-6 secs prolonged	> 6 secs prolonged
Ascites	Nil	Moderate	Severe
Encephalopathy	Nil	Moderate	Severe

Child's score

Grade A, total score 5–6; Grade B, total score 7–9; Grade C, total score > 9

FURTHER READING

Blei AT. Cerebral oedema and intracranial hypertention in acute liver failure: distinct aspects of the same problem. *Hepatology* 1991; **13**: 376–379

Conn HO. Transjugular intrahepatic Portal-systemic shunts: the state of the art. *Hepatology* 1993; **17**: 148–155.

Donovan JP, Shaw BW, Langnas AN, Sorrel MF. Brain water and acute liver failure: The emerging role of intracranial pressure monitoring. *Hepatology* 1992; **16**: 267–268.

Fagan EA. Acute liver failure and unknown pathogenesis: the hidden agenda. Hepatology 1994; 19:1307.

Fingerote RJ, Bain VG. Fulminant hepatic failure. *Am J Gastroenterol* 1993; **88**: 1000–1010.

Grose RD, Hayes PC. Review article: the pathophysiology and pharmacological treatment of portal hypertension. *Aliment Pharmacol Ther* 1992; **6**(5): 521-40.

Jimenez W, Arroyo V. Pathogenesis of sodium retention in cirrhosis. *J Hepatol* 1993; **18**: 147–150.

Lee WM. Acute liver failure. *Am J Med* 1994; **96**: 35–95.

Runyon BA. Bacterial infections in patients with cirrhosis. *J Hepatol*; **18**: 271–272.

Salerno F. Large-volume paracentesis and re-expansion: can synthetic plasma expanders safely replace albumin? *J Hepatol* 1992; **14**: 143–145.

Shafirstein R, Levitt MF. A hepatorenal depressor reflex: A possible clue to the pathogenesis of hepatorenal syndrome. *Hepatology* 1991; **14**: 734–735.

Triger DR. Endotoxemia in liver disease-time for reappraisal? *J Hepatol* 1991; **12**: 136–137.

van der Rijt CCD, Schalm SW. Quantitative EEG analysis and evoked potentials to measure (latent) hepatic encephalopathy. *J Hepatol* 1992; **14**: 141–142.

Warner L, Skorecki K, Blendis L, Epstein M. Atrial natriuretic factor and liver disease. *Hepatology* 1993; **17**: 500–513.

Whittle JR, Moncada S. Nitric oxide: The elusive mediator of the hyperdynamic circulation of cirrhosis? *Hepatology* 1992; **16**: 1089–1092.

16
ABNORMAL LIVER BIOCHEMISTRY

TESTING LIVER FUNCTION

The use of screening tests, including multichannel biochemical analysis, in asymptomatic people or in patients attending general clinics, is now widespread. This practice often reveals an unexpected abnormality in liver biochemistry, which itself becomes a clinical problem requiring solution. Considerable clinical skill is needed to know when to investigate further and when to avoid potentially hazardous investigations (e.g. liver biopsy, ERCP) in patients who are unlikely to benefit from them.

The serum enzymes alanine transaminase, aspartate transaminase, alkaline phosphatase (ALP) and gamma-glutamyltranspeptidase (γGT) are often erroneously referred to as 'liver function tests.' This is a misnomer on two counts:

- The enzymes (except γGT) are not exclusively hepatic in origin.
- They do not reflect the function of the liver.

In fact, in advanced cirrhosis, the liver enzymes may even be normal. Better indicators of hepatic synthetic activity include serum albumin and coagulation studies. Amino-pyrine breath testing is sometimes performed as a research procedure, but there is no very satisfactory readily available and sensitive test of liver function.

REACHING A DIAGNOSIS

Raised alkaline phosphatase (ALP) as the sole abnormality

The first step is to determine whether the ALP is of hepatic or other origin. Sole elevation of ALP is more commonly due to a bony origin and may very rarely be intestinal or renal. There are two ways of assessing this.

- Measurement of ALP isoenzymes. ALP from different sources have different isoelectric points and this can be used to identify and quantify the contribution of the different isoenzymes to an elevated ALP. This is the most logical approach, but is relatively complicated and sometimes produces an equivocal result. Sometimes an unusual isoenzyme is found and is taken to be suggestive of

▶ Patterns of serum biochemical changes (+, may be raised or normal; ++, moderately raised; +++, greatly raised)

	ALP	γGT	AST	ALT
Primarily cholestatic				
Intrahepatic cholestasis	+++	+++	N	N
Extrahepatic obstruction	+++	++	+	+
Primary biliary cirrhosis	+++	++	+	+
Primarily hepatitic				
Acute hepatitis	+	++	+++	+++
Drug hepatitis	+	++	++	++
Chronic active hepatitis	+	++	++	++
Alcoholic hepatitis	+	+++	++	+
Others				
Metastatic disease	++	+	+	+
Cirrhosis	+	++	+	+

underlying malignancy, but the specificity of this finding is not sufficient to make it a reliable test.

- The alternative is to quantify another enzyme that is more liver specific such as γGT or 5-nucleotidase. It is very rare for a hepatic cause of raised ALP not to be associated also with raised γGT or 5-nucleotidase.

Raised ALP of bony origin
Further investigation tends to be unrewarding in the asymptomatic patient. Serum calcium and phosphate and proximal muscle strength should be checked with osteomalacia in mind. A limited bony X-ray screen (e.g. chest, pelvis and skull) can be performed as a search for malignant disease or Paget's disease. A raised bony ALP is normal in adolescence.

Raised ALP of hepatic origin
The significant liver diseases that are most likely to present in an asymptomatic patient with lone elevation of serum ALP are primary biliary cirrhosis, sclerosing cholangitis, infiltrative conditions such as carcinoma, granulomatous diseases such as sarcoidosis, drug reactions and inactive cirrhosis. However the majority of patients have no sinister disease or any condition requiring treatment. Investigation therefore tends to be unrewarding.

If the patient is asymptomatic, is not taking any potentially hepatotoxic drugs, no abnormality has been found on general examination and there is no other biochemical abnormality a reasonable plan would include ultrasound examination of the liver, chest X-ray, a blood screen for chronic liver diseases (hepatitis BsAg and core Ab, hepatitis C Ab, antimitochondrial antibody, ferritin, alphafetoprotein). If the patient has underlying inflammatory bowel disease sclerosing cholangitis may need to be excluded even if ultrasound is normal. If all these tests are normal the most sensible course is usually just to keep the patient under intermittent review combined with reassurance that there is very unlikely to be any serious underlying disease. Liver biopsy is hard to justify in this situation since it is very unlikely to lead to any change in management and at best may just yield a granuloma of unknown cause.

▶ **Sole elevation of serum alkaline phosphatase (ALP)**

- Check gamma GT, 5-nucleotidase or alkaline phosphatase isoenzymes
- **If bony**: check calcium, phosphate, X-ray pelvis, chest and skull
- **If hepatic**: check antimitochondrial antibody, ferritin, alphafetoprotein, liver ultrasound scan
- **If these tests are normal**: liver biopsy is unlikely to be rewarding

Raised gamma-glutamyltranspeptidase (γGT)
The serum γGT is a very sensitive indicator of hepatic disease and is rarely normal in established liver disease. It is an inducible enzyme and many drugs including alcohol can cause an isolated raised γGT in the absence of liver disease.

A raised γGT is useful in verifying that the abnormal serum ALP or transaminases are of hepatic origin.

A raised γGT in the absence of any other biochemical abnormality is most commonly due to alcohol. It usually implies excessive alcohol consumption, but does not necessarily imply significant liver damage and should not be taken as an indication for liver biopsy. The correlation between quantity of alcohol consumed and height of γGT is poor, but it is useful for monitoring abstinence. Other drugs that induce γGT include anticonvulsants, barbiturates, tricyclic antidepressants, lipid lowering drugs and oral contraceptives. It is not necessary to stop the use of these drugs if they are clinically indicated unless there are other reasons to suspect hepatotoxicity.

▶ **Sole elevation of serum gamma-glutamyltranspeptidase (γGT)**

- Check history for alcohol and drugs
- No further action usually needed if other tests normal

Raised transaminases
The two commonly measured transaminases, aspartate aminotransferase (AST) and alanine aminotransferase (ALT), are sensitive indicators of hepatocellular damage. Most laboratories tend to offer one or the other rather than both. ALT is somewhat more specific for liver damage because AST is also released in muscle damage (e.g. myocardial infarction and rhabdomyolysis), haemolysis and hypothyroidism.

Sole elevation of aspartate aminotransferase (AST)
Causes include liver disease, myocardial infarction, pulmonary embolism, haemolysis, pernicious anaemia, leukaemia, rhabdomyolysis and hypothyroidism. Many of these conditions usually give rise to obvious symptoms, but some may be asymptomatic, in particular hypothyroidism and pernicious anaemia. Blood count, vitamin B_{12} and thyroid function tests should therefore be performed before assuming that the AST is hepatic.

Liver diseases that cause sole elevation of AST include acute and chronic viral hepatitis, alcoholic liver disease, autoimmune chronic active hepatitis, haemochromatosis, hepatic congestion due to heart failure and occasionally fatty infiltration in obesity.

▶ **Sole elevation of serum aspartate aminotransferase (AST)**

> - Exclude non-hepatic cause
> - Check B12, thyroid function, full blood count, film
> - Then proceed as for an elevated ALT

Sole elevation of alanine aminotransferase (ALT)

ALT is much more liver-specific than AST. Elevation of ALT will nearly always be associated with elevation of AST, but most laboratories perform one or other test, but not both.

Blood tests should be performed to help exclude significant liver disease. These should include tests for hepatitis A, B and C, autoantibodies (particularly antinuclear factor), ferritin and caeruloplasmin (if under 40 years of age). If all these tests are normal and the patient remains asymptomatic it is sensible to advise avoidance of alcohol and repeat the tests within one month.

▶ **Sole elevation of serum alanine aminotransferase (ALT)**

> - Liver-specific, but sensitive
> - Check blood tests for chronic liver disease (antinuclear antibody, ferritin, caeruloplasmin) and hepatitis A, B, C serology
> - If markedly (> 100 iu/l) and persistently raised (longer than six weeks) and no obvious clinical diagnosis (e.g. alcohol), biopsy liver

Is liver biopsy indicated?

If the ALT remains elevated a difficult decision may have to be made about liver biopsy. Biopsy in this situation is more likely to alter clinical management than biopsy for sole elevation of ALP, but the urgency depends to some extent on the degree of enzyme elevation. Persistent elevation above 100 iu/l should probably be taken as an indication to biopsy whereas a more modest elevation may reasonably be monitored for a few months if the patient remains well. The height of the elevated ALT may give a clue to the diagnosis.

- In alcoholic hepatitis, the ALT rarely exceeds 200 iu/l. Here, the AST rise is often more pronounced and the ratio of AST to ALT usually exceeds 2.
- In acute viral hepatitis, ALT typically rises 20 times or more above normal.
- Drug-induced hepatitis results in very high transaminases.
- In conditions where there is massive hepatic necrosis, as in severe paracetamol poisoning or from mushroom toxin, the transaminases may rise to many thousands of iu/l, but fall quickly over the next few days even when fatal liver damage has already occurred.

- Transaminases may be raised, sometimes dramatically, in patients with hepatic congestion from heart failure or reduced perfusion.

Serum albumin, prothrombin time and bilirubin

Serum albumin, prothrombin time and bilirubin are important indicators of hepatic function. The first two are indicators of synthetic function and bilirubin of excretory function. They are used in many indices of hepatic dysfunction, the most widely used for chronic liver disease being the Child–Pugh grading (see Chapter 15). Other indices have been devised specifically for timing of transplantation for patients with chronic liver diseases like primary biliary cirrhosis and primary sclerosing cholangitis, but all have limitations. There are also schemes adapted for use in acute liver failure for prognostication and timing of liver transplantation (e.g. for paracetamol poisoning).

A low serum albumin

A low serum albumin in the context of liver disease indicates poor hepatic synthetic function. However, low albumin may be also be caused by poor nutritional status, severe catabolic states and protein-losing enteropathy.

Any event such as sepsis that causes an acute phase response will result in a marked decrease in hepatic albumin synthesis that reciprocates with the increased synthesis of hepatic globulins.

Coagulation studies

Coagulation studies are useful in assessing severity and prognosis in patients with liver disease. However in patients with a cholestatic element to the liver pathology, the prolongation of the prothrombin time may in part be contributed by vitamin K malabsorption and a parenteral administration of 10 mg of vitamin K should be given to check for reversibility. Some units therefore use quantification of Factor V levels to give a vitamin K-independent measure of hepatic synthetic function.

A low serum urea

A low serum urea is typical in advanced liver insufficiency and reflects reduced hepatic synthesis. Thus serum creatinine is a better indicator of renal failure in the presence of hepatic disease. A rise in serum urea while the serum creatinine remains stable is suggestive of upper gastro-intestinal bleeding.

Raised serum bilirubin

The approach to sole elevation of serum bilirubin is discussed in Chapter 13, pages 181–182.

FURTHER READING

Liver enzymology

Herrera JL. Abnormal liver enzyme levels. The spectrum of causes. *Postgrad Med* 1993; **93**(2): 113–6.

Narayanan S. Serum alkaline phosphatase isoenzymes as markers of liver disease. *Ann Clin Lab Sci* 1991; **21**(1): 12–8.

King PD. Abnormal liver enzyme levels. Evaluation in asymptomatic patients. *Postgrad Med* 1991; **89**(4): 137–41.

Griffiths J. Alkaline phosphatases. Newer concepts in isoenzymes and clinical applications. *Clin Lab Med* 1989; **9**(4): 717–30.

17
GASTROINTESTINAL PROBLEMS IN PATIENTS WITH HIV

REACHING A DIAGNOSIS AND MANAGEMENT

People with human immunodeficiency virus (HIV) infection may present with a wide variety of gastrointestinal symptoms. Many of the problems result from opportunistic infections in the gastrointestinal tract and hepatobiliary system, but many people with HIV are also at risk of other sexually acquired gastrointestinal problems like hepatitis B and C and gonococcal proctitis. The gut may be the site of HIV-associated tumours and HIV itself affects the gatrointestinal mucosa.

Gastrointestinal problems associated with HIV are often debilitating and, as effective treatment is often available, a diagnosis should be vigorously sought. Presence of gastrointestinal symptoms may also herald the onset of full-blown acquired immune deficiency syndrome (AIDS).

Oral lesions
Painful lesions of the mouth are common in people with HIV.

Oral candidiasis
The most common problem is oral candidiasis and a simple examination of the fauces is usually sufficient to make a diagnosis. The infection is often extensive. This can be treated with local nystatin, but a systemic antifungal agent such as ketoconazole, fluconazole or itraconazole is often required.

Oral fluconazole is probably the drug of choice. Recurrence is very common and maintenance therapy is recommended in recurrent oral candidiasis. Almost 50% of people with HIV and oral candidiasis will develop AIDS within a year.

Herpes simplex infection
Herpes simplex infection usually presents as cold sores, but may also affect gums and palate. Treatment is with oral acyclovir, but as with candidiasis recurrence is common and necessitates maintenance treatment.

Aphthous mouth ulceration
Aphthous mouth ulcers may occur and are treated symtomatically, but the occasional patient with large painful ulcers may respond to thalidomide.

Hairy leukoplakia
Hairy leukoplakia (see page 178) is a characteristic lesion of HIV infection, affecting the side of the tongue. It is usually asymptomatic, but may herald progression to AIDS. It is probably caused by Epstein–Barr virus infection.

Kaposi's sarcoma
Kaposi's sarcoma is a very rare tumour among people without HIV, but may affect any part of the gastrointestinal tract in HIV-seropositive patients. In the mouth it tends to affect the gums and palate. Radiotherapy is effective if lesion is localised. Cytotoxic chemotherapy is sometimes effective if lesions are more widespread.

Dysphagia
Dysphagia and odynophagia are common in people with HIV. Patients with any symptoms of oesophageal disease should have upper gastrointestinal endoscopy because barium examination has a low diagnostic yield (**Fig. 17.1**).

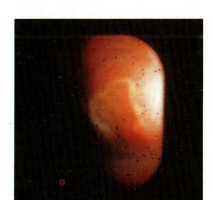

Fig. 17.1 Primary herpetic ulcer in the oesophagus. This can be seen in patients without immune deficiency and causes intense pain on swallowing.

Provided adequate care is taken the procedure is safe to both operator and patient and the HIV organism is readily killed with routine endoscopic sterilisation (care being taken as always to ensure particulate material has been cleared from endoscope channels before washing).

Endoscopy is particularly helpful because biopsy specimens can be obtained and are vital in diagnosing cytomegalovirus (CMV) infection and Kaposi's sarcoma. Patients with HIV are commonly hypochlorhydric and have reduced pepsin secretion, and are less likely to suffer from acid-related disorders.

Oesophageal candidiasis

Oesophageal candidiasis is the commonest oesophageal lesion (**Figs 17.2** and **17.3**). Although it may be asymptomatic, patients may complain of odynophagia, particularly with hot liquids. It is readily diagnosed by characteristic endoscopic appearances of raised white plaques often appearing as vertical columns particularly in the lower oesophagus. In more severe infection, the plaques become confluent. Since other lesions (particularly leukoplakia) may mimic candidiasis a biopsy specimen should be taken if there is doubt. Cytology of brushings may also be helpful. Systemic antifungals are recommended for patients with HIV, and fluconazole is probably superior to ketoconazole.

Cytomegalovirus infection

CMV infection of the oesophagus is more likely to present as dysphagia, which is often painful. Diagnosis is by endoscopy and biopsy. The endoscopic lesions may mimic oesophageal carcinoma because CMV infection classically produces discrete ulcers with raised edges. Histology may show CMV inclusion bodies, but repeated biopsies may be required to confirm the diagnosis. If immunohistochemistry is available, CMV antigens may be visualised in infected cells. Treatment is with ganciclovir or foscarnet intravenously. Ganciclovir is toxic and may cause neutropenia.

Other types of infection

Other infections of the oesophagus include herpes simplex virus, *Cryptosporidium* and *Mycobacterium avium intracellulare*. Herpes simplex (Type I) usually produces vesicular lesions, or less commonly, a diffuse oesophagitis. Epstein–Barr virus has also been implicated in oesophageal ulceration. Diagnosis is by biopsy and culture.

Kaposi's sarcoma

Kaposi's sarcoma of the oesophagus may present as dysphagia. Its presence fulfils the criteria for diagnosing AIDS. Oesophageal lymphoma is exceedingly rare in the immune competent, but has also been reported in those patients with AIDS. The presence of oesophageal disease is a bad prognostic indicator with a majority of patients surviving less than 12 months.

Diarrhoea

Diarrhoea is a common and often incapacitating syptom in patients with HIV. More than 50% of all patients with HIV will suffer from diarrhoea at some stage of their illness. In Africans with AIDS, more than 90% have debilitating diarrhoea. A large number of pathogens have been identified presenting a considerable diagnostic challenge

The key to diagnosis is repeated stool cultures and rectal biopsy (**Fig. 17.4**). Direct microscopy of stool specimens must be carried out. Even after exhaustive microbiological examination, a pathogen may not be isolated from more

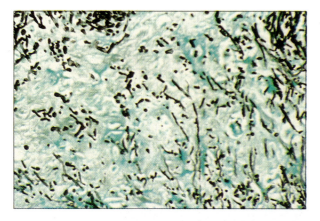

Fig. 17.2 *Candida* oesophagitis showing numerous fungal hyphae in surface slough.

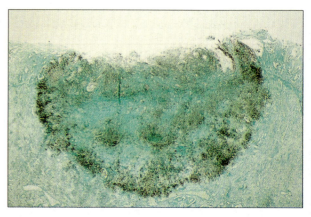

Fig. 17.3 Invasive candidal infection of the oesophagus in a patient with acquired immune deficiency syndrome (AIDS).

than 50% of patients. In these patients measurements of stool volumes, sigmoidoscopy and biopsy, hydrogen breath tests and Schilling test may be helpful. If stool volumes exceed 500 ml/day, or if the rectal mucosa looks abnormal, persistence with the microbiological search for a pathogen should be maintained. However, if stool volume is less than 500 ml/day, further search for a pathogen is less likely to be rewarding in these patients.

A Schilling test demonstrating malabsorption of vitamin B_{12} suggests *Cryptosporidium* or *Isospora* infection, but HIV itself may cause B_{12} malabsorption. It has been demonstrated that HIV infects the mucosa of the gastrointestinal tract and it is likely that in some patients, diarrhoea is a result of HIV infection rather than any superinfection.

Diarrhoea may be the presenting symptom of seroconversion illness where it is associated with fever, rash and lymphadenopathy. Diarrhoea may also herald the onset of full-blown AIDS, especially in Africans when it is associated with weight loss and wasting (slim disease).

▶ **Pathogens causing diarrhoea in association with HIV**

Protozoa

Cryptosporidium
Isospora belli
Giardia lamblia
Entamoeba histolytica

Bacteria

Campylobacter jejuni
Salmonella typhimurium
Mycoplasma avium intracellulare
Shigella flexneri

Viruses

Cytomegalovirus
Adenovirus
Herpes simplex
HIV

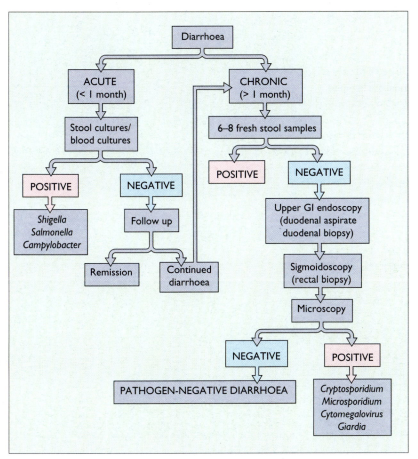

Fig. 17.4 Algorithm for the diagnosis of diarrhoea in patients with HIV.

Symptoms

The pattern of diarrhoea, nausea and vomiting is common to all the enteric pathogens. Voluminous prolonged diarrhoea is seen in *Cryptosporidium* and *Isospora* infection, often associated with abdominal pain. Bloody diarrhoea with abdominal pain usually indicates severe CMV colitis or *Shigella flexneri* infection.

'Gay bowel' syndrome

As homosexual males with HIV may acquire infections as a result of their life-style, gonococcal proctitis, perianal herpes simplex and chlamydial infections should also be sought. Other pathogens of 'gay bowel' syndrome include *Giardia lamblia* and *Entamoeba histolytica*, which are not uncommon as sexually-acquired pathogens among homosexuals.

Giardiasis behaves similarly in HIV patients and non-HIV individuals. Microscopy of a freshly-voided stool sample should allow identification of amoebiasis, but giardia may be difficult to identify or be absent from stool samples even when there is significant small bowel infestation.

Treatment with metronidazole is effective for both organisms. Endoscopic duodenal biopsy and aspiration may assist in diagnosis, but a trial of metronidazole is a reasonable course if suspicion of giardiasis is high.

Cryptosporidiosis

Infection with *Cryptosporidium* is the commonest opportunistic bowel infection and the commonest cause of diarrhoea in HIV patients. It is an intracellular parasite. It causes a chronic high-output diarrhoea associated with abdominal pain, fever and electrolyte disturbances.

Diagnosis is made by smears of freshly voided stool samples, staining of which with a modified Ziehl–Neelsen stain demonstrates *Cryptosporidium* oocytes. The organism may also be seen in duodenal and rectal biopsies (**Fig. 17.5**). As secretion of the parasite is intermittent, repeated stool examination is often required.

There is no specific treatment. Management consists of antidiarrhoeal drugs, rehydration and salt replacement. Intravenous fluid and electrolytes may be necessary. Simple antidiarrhoeals such as codeine phosphate and loperamide may be tried, but relief is often temporary. Oral morphine or even subcutaneous diamorphine may be required.

Isospora

Isospora belli causes a similar illness to *Cryptosporidium* infection. It is a more common pathogen in African AIDS than in the West, where it accounts for less than 1% of diarrhoeas.

Cytomegalovirus

CMV colitis is often a severe illness with bloody diarrhoea and abdominal pain with signs of peritonism. An abdominal radiograph may show large bowel dilatation and colonic perforation is not uncommon. Diagnosis is made by simoidoscopic examination, which usually show a severe mucosal inflammation with ulceration. Biopsy may show CMV inclusion bodies (**Figs 17.6** and **17.7**). Treatment is with ganciclovir or foscarnet, but response is variable and prognosis is poor.

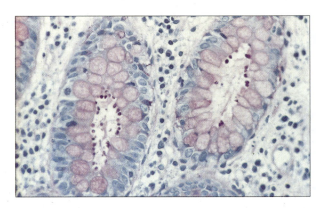

Fig. 17.5 Cryptosporidial infestation of the colon (Giemsa stain).

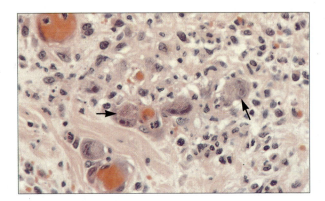

Fig. 17.6 Cytomegaloviral inclusions (arrowed) in cytomegalovirus colitis.

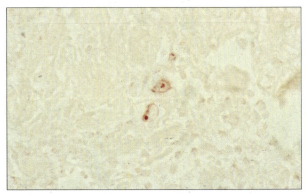

Fig. 17.7 Cytomegalovirus demonstrated by *in situ* hybridisation.

Mycobacterium avium intracellulare

Mycobacterium avium intracellulare (MAI) is a cause of abdominal pain, fever and diarrhoea in patients with HIV, who usually have infection in other sites such as lung, liver and bone marrow. Diagnosis is made by finding acid-fast bacilli in faecal smears or duodenal biopsy. Characteristic white nodules in the duodenal mucosa have been described. When biopsied, these duodenal lesions show foamy macrophages filled with acid fast bacilli, histologically indistinguishable from Whipple's disease. There is no effective treatment for MAI infections.

Campylobacter, Shigella, Salmonella

Campylobacter jejuni causes a watery diarrhoea with abdominal pain in seropositive individuals similar to that in non-HIV patients, but may run a prolonged course.

In HIV-positive patients, *Shigella flexneri* causes a more severe disease, with bloody diarrhoea, fever and abdominal pain. Both *Shigella and Salmonella* infections are often invasive with resulting bacteraemia. Stool and blood cultures may identify the organism and treatment of choice is ciprofloxacin, which may need to be given intravenously.

Abdominal pain

Abdominal pain in patients with HIV requires careful clinical assessment. If associated with diarrhoea, an infective aetiology should be sought. If the patient has signs of intestinal obstruction and weight loss, **lymphoma** and **Kaposi's sarcoma** of the bowel should be considered and small bowel barium studies should be performed. Common causes of an acute abdomen such as appendicitis, cholecystitis, pancreatitis and perforated viscus will also have to be excluded.

Right upper quadrant pain in a person with HIV may be due to:

- **Acalculous cholecystitis** caused by **CMV** or *Campylobacter fetus*.
- A well-recognised syndrome of **ascending cholangitis** with fever, right upper quadrant pain and less commonly jaundice with cholangiographic appearance similar to sclerosing cholangitis. ERCP is necessary for diagnosis (see page 244).

Kaposi's sarcoma

Kaposi's sarcoma commonly affects the gastrointestinal tract and is found at postmortem in about 70% of patients dying from AIDS. It is often asymptomatic. Bleeding, obstruction and perforation may occur and occasionally, a protein-losing enteropathy. The tumour may be visualised radiologically by barium enema or small bowel radiology. Endoscopically, it appears as raised purple nodules with or without haemorrhage, but may also appear polypoid or as confluent flat haemorrhagic plaques (**Figs 17.8** and **17.9**). Endoscopic biopsies are often negative as the lesion is submucosal.

In the absence of symptoms, Kaposi's sarcoma does not require treatment. Symptomatic lesions may be treated with radiotherapy for localised accessible lesions or single-agent chemotherapy. Chemotherapy carries a risk of further immunocompromising these patients, but may nevertheless be effective in some patients with disseminated Kaposi's sarcoma.

Non-Hodgkin's lymphoma

Patients with HIV may develop a high-grade and widespread non-Hodgkin's lymphoma. The gastrointestinal tract

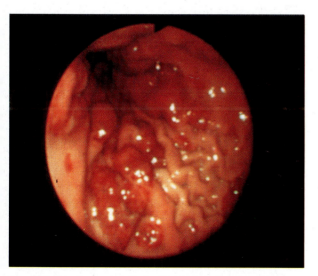

Fig. 17.8 Kaposi's sarcoma affecting the stomach. Courtesy of Dr J Smithson.

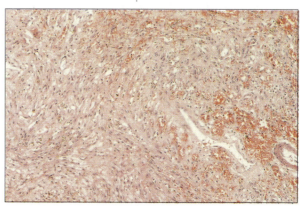

Fig. 17.9 Kaposi's sarcoma affecting the stomach. Whorls of malignant endothelial cells are seen.

is the commonest extranodal site and the majority are B-cell lymphomas. It may present with abdominal pain, weight loss, perforation or obstruction. Chemotherapy is indicated, but prognosis is poor.

Jaundice and abnormal liver function tests

Abnormalities of hepatic enzymes ('liver function tests') are very common in patients with HIV. They reflect the susceptibility of the liver to the wide variety of infections that these patients encounter.

The drugs used to treat these patients including keto-conazole, antituberculous therapy and cotrimoxazole may also cause significant hepatotoxicity or elevation of gamma-glutamyltransferase and transaminases. The risk factors for acquiring HIV infection are the same as those for blood-borne hepatitis viruses B, C, and D. Hepatic involvement with HIV-associated tumours may also occur.

Infectious hepatitis

- Hepatitis A is common in homosexuals and the course of illness is no different from that in people without HIV.
- Hepatitis B tends to run a more chronic course with high viral replication and relatively little hepatocellular damage because of the host's compromised immunocompetence.
- Hepatitis C similarly runs a prolonged course.
- Hepatitis D is uncommon in the UK.

Management of viral hepatitis in patients with HIV does not differ from that for patients without HIV. HIV patients seronegative for hepatitis B should be offered immunisation, although the conversion rate is likely to be low.

Other infections of the liver include CMV hepatitis, which usually presents as part of a disseminated infectious process with fever, weight loss and malaise. Jaundice is unusual. Diagnosis is made by histological demonstration of inclusion bodies and treatment is with gancyclovir or foscarnet. The liver is often involved in the opportunistic infections of the gut, notably with *Cryptococcus neoformans* and MAI. Fungal infections may present as hepatic abcesses.

Hepatomegaly

An enlarged liver is common in patients with HIV, and is usually asymptomatic. About 85% of people with AIDS have a large liver at postmortem. Patients should be investigated if symptomatic, jaundiced or if serum transaminases are markedly elevated: hepatitis serology should be checked and the liver scanned by ultrasound or CT scan. Liver biopsy is usually inappropriate in the asymptomatic patient because few therapeutic options are likely to be available:

- Hepatic steatosis (fatty infiltration) is common in people with AIDS and probably reflects profound malnutrition.
- Granulomatous disease of the liver is also common, and is usually caused by MAI.
- Kaposi's sarcoma is the commonest tumour to affect the liver, but antemortem diagnosis is difficult because the lesions are often focal and patchy.
- Lymphomatous involvement of the liver may present with hepatosplenomegaly and, typically, a mild jaundice, but markedly raised serum alkaline phosphatase.

Right upper quadrant pain and fever

The patient with HIV may present with biliary symptoms of right upper quadrant pain, with or without jaundice. Biliary problems in these patients are important because the diagnostic approach is different and specific therapy is often available. Two particular syndromes are well recognised:

- Acalculous cholecystitis.
- AIDS-related sclerosing cholangitis.

Abdominal ultrasound is a very helpful in diagnosis of biliary problems.

Acalculous cholecystitis

Acalculous cholecystitis may present as an acute or subacute illness lasting a few weeks presenting with fever, right upper quadrant pain and tenderness and a positive Murphy's sign. Ultrasound scan shows gallbladder wall thickening and an absence of stones. Air in the gallbladder wall is seen in severe disease. CMV infection is the commonest cause, but in the presence of diarrhoea *Cryptosporidium* infection is likely. Treatment is by cholecystectomy.

AIDS-sclerosing cholangitis

AIDS-sclerosing cholangitis is a well-recognised syndrome presenting as a cholangitis with fever, right upper quadrant pain, nausea and vomiting in a patient with AIDS. Typically the serum alkaline phosphatase is raised, but jaundice is rare as biliary obstruction is incomplete. Ultrasound of the abdomen will reveal dilated intra- and extrahepatic ducts. Differential diagnosis includes lymphoma and Kaposi's sarcoma of the biliary tree. This condition is often associated with a cryptosporidial diarrhoea and is believed to be a manifestation of infection of the biliary tree with *Cryptosporidium*. Diagnosis is made by ERCP, which shows ductal dilatation and stricturing similar to that of primary sclerosing cholangitis (**Fig. 17.10**). Associated papillary stenosis is usual. Treatment of cholangitis is by improving biliary drainage with sphincterotomy.

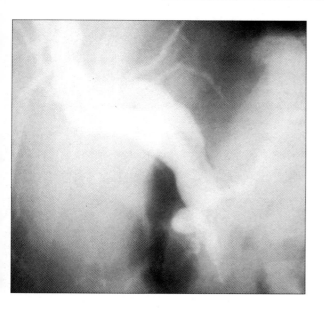

Fig. 17.10 ERCP showing biliary tree dilatation and stricturing in AIDS-sclerosing cholangitis. Sphincterotomy may relieve symptoms in this condition. Courtesy of Dr J Smithson.

FURTHER READING

Gastrointestinal manifestations of HIV infection: general

Anderson M. Gastroenterological aspects of AIDS in the Third World. *Baillières Clin Gastroenterol* 1990; 4(2): 375–83.

Chui DW, Owen RL. AIDS and the gut. *J Gastroenterol Hepatol* 1994; 9: 291–303.

Forsmark CE. AIDS and the gastrointestinal tract. *Postgrad Med* 1993; 93(2): 143–8, 151–2.

Gazzard BG. Practical advice for the gastroenterologist dealing with symptomatic HIV disease (see comments) *Gut* 1990; 31(7): 733–5.

Gazzard BG. Review article: treatment of the gastrointestinal manifestations of AIDS. *Aliment Pharmacol Ther* 1990; 4(4): 317–24.

Tanowitz HB, Simon D, Wittner M. Medical management of AIDS patients. Gastrointestinal manifestations. *Med Clin North Am* 1992; 76(1): 45–62.

Wexner SD. Sexually transmitted diseases of the colon, rectum, and anus. The challenge of the nineties. *Dis Colon Rectum* 1990; 33(12): 1048–62.

Oral lesions

Barr CE. Oral diseases in HIV-1 infection. *Dysphagia* 1992; 7(3): 126–37.

Gillespie GM, Marino R. Oral manifestations of HIV infection: a Panamerican perspective. *J Oral Pathol Med* 1993; 22(1): 2–7.

Greenspan D, Greenspan JS. Oral manifestations of human immunodeficiency virus infection. *Dent Clin North Am* 1993; 37(1): 21–32.

Greenspan D, Greenspan JS. Oral lesions of HIV infection: features and therapy. *AIDS Clin Rev* 1992: 225–39.

Greenspan D; Greenspan JS. Oral manifestations of HIV infection. *Dermatol Clin* 1991; 9(3): 517–22.

Heinic GS, Greenspan D, Greenspan JS. Oral CMV lesions and the HIV infected. Early recognition can help prevent morbidity. *J Am Dent Assoc* 1993; 124(2): 99–105.

Smith GL, Felix DH, Wray D. Current classifications of HIV-associated periodontal diseases. *Br Dent J* 1993; 174(3): 102–5.

Oesophageal lesions

Wilcox CM. Esophageal disease in the acquired immunodeficiency syndrome: etiology, diagnosis, and management. *Am J Med* 1992; 92(4): 412–21.

Diarrhoea

Anthony SJ. HIV enteropathy - a challnege in diagnosis and management. *J Natl Med Assoc* 1994; 86: 347–51.

Bartlett JG, Belitsos PC, Sears CL. AIDS enteropathy. *Clin Infect Dis* 1992; 15(4): 726–35.

Gazzard BG. Diarrhea in human immunodeficiency virus antibody-positive patients. *Semin Liver Dis* 1992; 12(2): 154–66.

Griffin GE. Malabsorption, malnutrition and HIV disease. *Baillières Clin Gastroenterol* 1990; 4(2): 361–73.

Grohmann GS, Glass RI, Pereira HG, et al. Enteric viruses and diarrhea in HIV-infected patients. Enteric Opportunistic Infections Working Group. *N Engl J Med* 1993; 329(1): 14–20.

Rabeneck L. Diagnostic workup strategies for patients with HIV-related chronic diarrhea. What is the end result? *J Clin Gastroenterol* 1993; 16(3): 245–50.

Smith PD, Mai UE. Immunopathophysiology of gastrointestinal disease in HIV infection. *Gastroenterol Clin North Am* 1992; 21(2): 331–45.

Hepatobiliary problems

Bach N, Theise ND, Schaffner F. Hepatic histopathology in the acquired immunodeficiency syndrome. *Semin Liver Dis* 1992; **12**(2): 205–12.

Bonacini M. Hepatobiliary complications in patients with human immunodeficiency virus infection. *Am J Med* 1992; **92**(4): 404–11.

Cappell MS. Hepatobiliary manifestations of the acquired immune deficiency syndrome. *Am J Gastroenterol* 1991; **86**(1): 1–15

.Lafon ME, Kirn A. Human immunodeficiency virus infection of the liver. *Semin Liver Dis* 1992; **12**(2): 197–204.

Herndier BG, Friedman SL. Neoplasms of the gastrointestinal tract and hepatobiliary system in acquired immunodeficiency syndrome. *Semin Liver Dis* 1992; **12**(2): 128–41.

18
GASTROINTESTINAL PROBLEMS IN INFANCY AND CHILDHOOD

Lawrence Weaver and Edward Eastham

GENERAL PRINCIPLES

Paediatric gastroenterology is not simply scaled-down adult gastroenterology. The digestive system undergoes considerable development during early life, and disorders of maturation occur. Diet changes throughout childhood, from milk in the suckling period, through supplementary foods during weaning, to a solid diet in late infancy, with the introduction of a growing variety of foods to adulthood. Not only do the nutritional requirements of the child change with increasing age, but also the gastrointestinal problems, and the symptoms and signs that accompany them. Children with gastrointestinal problems should therefore be considered within the context of their growth, development and diet.

The newborn infant

The newborn infant has a small repertoire of symptoms and signs, many of which derive from the gastrointestinal tract. Contentment and discomfort appear closely related to the state of the gut, which plays a dominant role in the consciousness of the neonate. It may be used to express distress, in the form of vomiting or 'colic.' The heightened awareness, with apparent pleasure or pain, that the newborn experiences from such simple physiological processes as feeding and defaecation, may be manifest by smiles, grimaces and contortions of the face and body. These must be distinguished from symptoms and signs of pathology such as the vomiting of bile or blood, diarrhoea, rectal bleeding and tense abdominal distension.

The toddler

The toddler may vocalise his symptoms, and point to his umbilicus. Abdominal pain, which affects up to 10% of children at some time, more often than not has no identifiable organic basis. Nevertheless it is a symptom that should be taken seriously, and may indicate, if not physical disease, disturbance elsewhere in the child's world.

The gastrointestinal tract can become the focus of many of the child's ills, and a source of concern to the parents. Change in diet may be associated with change in bowel habit. In infancy this may cause alarm, particularly if undigested food is visible in the stool. When the child becomes aware of his parent's interest in this area, his bowel habit may become the subject of differences between them, and retention of faeces, leading to constipation and encopresis, can follow.

The older child

In the older child, weight loss or poor growth are important symptoms of gastrointestinal disease. It is mandatory to obtain, and plot, on age-related centile charts, a child's weight and height at each consultation. If possible, weights and heights before the onset of symptoms should be included.

Children may be vague, shy or inarticulate about their symptoms, particularly if socially embarrassing, and they are sometimes loath to discuss them in the presence of their parents. However, it is important to ask the child to give the history of his illness, in his own words. Direct questions are often best combined with the examination. When recording a history of diarrhoea or constipation it is essential to obtain accurate information of the frequency, size and consistency of the stools passed, and whether or not they contain blood, bits of food or are greasy. Normal bowel habit in childhood is close to that in adulthood: modal frequency of defecation is once daily, and 90% of children fall within the range of three times daily and three times a week.

Although it is sometimes argued that rectal examination has adverse psychological effects, it is important that it is performed when indicated. The child should lie curled up on his side, holding his mother's hand, in a warm, private room. With full explanation the procedure need not be traumatic and often reveals valuable information not obtainable by general physical examination or investigations. The perianal region should be carefully inspected before a well-lubricated finger is gently introduced. Stool on the finger can be tested for blood or pus cells.

The adolescent

The adolescent complains of many of the same symptoms and signs as the adult. However, adolescence is a relatively disease-free period of life and the majority of patients of this age group have chronic conditions, such as coeliac disease, inflammatory bowel disease or cystic fibrosis.

There is no definite age when care should cease to be provided in the paediatric clinic. Many children with cystic fibrosis, for instance, prefer to remain with the doctor who has cared for them all their lives, while children with coeliac disease, who attend simply for a yearly review, may wish to be transferred to an adult clinic when they feel uncomfortable in a waiting room full of toddlers. Transfer of care is optimally done at a joint consultation between paediatric and adult gastroenterologist, when issues unrecorded in the notes can be discussed.

Investigation and diagnosis

Investigation and diagnosis rely as much as possible on non-invasive methods and for all but simple problems, should be undertaken in a clinic dedicated to the care of children. A paediatric dietitian is an essential member of the team caring for children with gastrointestinal problems and there needs to be close collaboration between the paediatrician and paediatric surgeons, radiologists, child psychiatrists, immunologists, nutritional support services, adult gastroenterologists and hepatologists.

The common problems of gastrointestinal and liver disease are discussed in this chapter, followed by an approach to differential diagnosis. The natural history and management of each is outlined. Those exclusive to the child are covered in greater depth than those that affect the adolescent and adult, details of which are given in other chapters.

ABDOMINAL PAIN: REACHING A DIAGNOSIS

Abdominal pain is a common childhood complaint, more often than not transitory and of no identifiable physical cause. Functional abdominal pain (and sometimes other gastrointestinal symptoms such as vomiting and constipation) may be an expression (somatisation) of anxieties, stresses and other difficulties in the child's life. However, pain should always be taken seriously since it is essential to identify the acute abdomen as quickly as possible.

Is it functional or organic?

Recurrent abdominal pain (more than three episodes in three months) occurs in 10–15% of school-age children of both sexes with a peak incidence at nine years of age. It is more frequent in those with a family history of abdominal pain, peptic ulcer, appendicectomy, headache and psychiatric disease. The character and severity of the pain is of little diagnostic significance, but nocturnal pain that wakes the child, and pain that is peripheral rather than umbilical, are more likely to be of organic origin. The child may be of an anxious disposition, with enuresis, sleep disorder or eating difficulties. In around 5% of children, recurrent abdominal pain is a symptom of depressive illness.

▶ **Causes of acute abdominal pain in childhood**

- Appendicitis
- Mesenteric adenitis
- Pyelonephritis
- Henoch–Schönlein disease
- Pneumonia
- Intestinal obstruction
- Gastroenteritis
- Diabetic ketoacidosis
- Renal colic
- Sickle cell crisis
- Abdominal trauma
- Pancreatitis

Investigations that should be performed, but are usually normal, are urinalysis, full blood count, erythrocyte sedimentation rate and plain abdominal radiography. The latter may show signs of faecal retention. Abdominal ultrasound, intravenous urogram or di-mercapto succinic acid scan, liver function tests, serum amylase, endoscopy and barium studies should be reserved for those children who have other symptoms and signs pointing to organic or chronic disease, have growth failure or anaemia, or are suspected of having a surgical cause such as intussusception or volvulus (see below). Rare causes of chronic or recurrent abdominal pain include lead poisoning, porphyria and diseases of the urogenital system.

Is it infant colic?

Infant colic affects about 10% of babies during early infancy. Episodes begin typically in the evening and take the form of inconsolable crying with drawing up of the legs. Colic occurs equally frequently in breast- and formula-fed infants; nevertheless infants who reach a paediatrician often have had more than one change of feed. Colic can be distinguished from hunger by demonstrating satisfactory weight gain. Occult infection (urinary tract infection and otitis media) must be ruled out.

Is it an acute abdomen?

Only about 10% of children with acute abdominal pain require abdominal surgery. However the child with guarding, rebound tenderness, pain that has localised in the right

▶ **Recurrent abdominal pain**

- Affects 10–15% of school-age children
- Nocturnal or peripheral rather than central abdominal pain suggests organic cause
- Check urine for infection
- Do not 'overinvestigate' (FBC, ESR/CRP usually sufficient)
- Over 75% get better with reassurance and explanation

iliac fossa, tenderness per rectum, or abdominal pain associated with gastrointestinal bleeding, should be assessed, as an emergency, in hospital.

Diagnosis may be difficult, and the common causes are not the same as those in the adult (see Chapter 2). Full physical examination, including hernial orifices and rectum, with attention to the urinary tract and respiratory system, will distinguish gastrointestinal disease from other causes. Investigations should include chest X-ray, erect and supine abdominal X-ray, urinalysis, full blood count, urea and electrolytes, and blood culture if the child is pyrexial. Observation in hospital allows the natural history of the disease to unfold. Those conditions in which vomiting is a prominent feature (including causes of intestinal obstruction), or those accompanied by diarrhoea and/or gastrointestinal bleeding are discussed below.

Is it appendicitis?

Appendicitis is the commonest cause of the acute abdomen in childhood. In infants, classical signs are often not present and the diagnosis may be missed. The child with appendicitis presents with abdominal pain that moves to the right iliac fossa where it becomes localised, with rebound tenderness, which may be elicited per rectum. Low-grade fever, leucocytosis, anorexia, vomiting and a change in bowel habit are often present. The symptoms and signs may evolve over several hours, and a mass may become palpable.

Is it mesenteric adenitis?

Mesenteric adenitis may mimic appendicitis, but is frequently associated with signs of acute viral infection: pyrexia, pharyngitis, and lymphocytosis. Adenovirus is a cause. Pain may be intermittent and poorly localised. Observation in hospital should ensure that laparotomy is avoided, but, if performed, it may reveal swollen mesenteric lymph nodes.

Is it Henoch–Schönlein disease?

Henoch–Schönlein disease may present as acute abdominal pain preceding the appearance of the characteristic purpuric rash. It may follow beta-haemolytic streptococcal or viral infection. Haematuria and arthropathy are clues to the diagnosis, which becomes stronger if stools contain blood or melaena occurs. Rarely, painful orchitis may occur.

Is there peptic ulcer disease?

Peptic ulcer disease is rare in childhood. It should be considered in children and adolescents with persistent epigastric pain, especially if associated with haematemesis, or a history of smoking and alcohol consumption. Nocturnal pain and a family history of peptic ulcer are often present. Diagnosis is by upper gastrointestinal endoscopy when gastritis or a gastric or duodenal ulcer may be visualised. Antral biopsies should be taken to identify *Helicobacter pylori*, which is present in around 50% of patients. Gastric ulcers may occur after corticosteroid treatment, in acute stress (e.g. burns) and with salicylates and other anti-inflammatory agents.

Is it pancreatitis?

Pancreatitis is usually idiopathic in childhood, but mumps, cystic fibrosis and trauma (both accidental and non-accidental) as well as other infections, pancreatic duct anomalies and obstruction, and some drugs (frusemide, sodium valproate) are well-recognised causes.

The child presents with acute upper abdominal pain, that is often constant and sometimes associated with vomiting. Diagnosis is confirmed by elevated plasma amylase (and lipase). Abdominal ultrasound may reveal a swollen pancreas and in 10% of paediatric patients, acute pancreatitis is associated with the passage of gallstones.

In recurrent pancreatitis, hyperlipidaemia (particularly hypertriglyceridaemia with chylomicrons), hyperparathyroidism and anatomical abnormalities (such as congenital fusion of biliary and pancreatic ducts) should be sought, but hereditary pancreatitis, the mechanism for which is not yet understood, is the commonest cause of chronic pancreatitis in childhood.

Is there food intolerance?

Food intolerance is more often perceived than real in childhood. Lactose intolerance (see page 257), milk protein intolerance (see pages 256, 264) and coeliac disease (see page 266) affect infants and children, but it is doubtful that abdominal pain alone (without vomiting, diarrhoea and atopic symptoms) is often caused by components of the diet. Certain food additives and preservatives (sometimes present in medicines) can cause symptoms. Infants with milk protein intolerance usually have diarrhoea with or without blood as well as pain (see page 250).

Is there inflammatory bowel disease?

Crohn's disease may present as abdominal pain alone. This is usually associated with localised disease possibly with an abdominal mass, but may very rarely present as an acute perforation with peritonitis. Diagnosis is as for adult disease. Serum C-reactive protein is elevated in over 90% of patients with active disease, so a normal result means that the diagnosis can be excluded with reasonable certainty.

MANAGEMENT OF CONDITIONS CAUSING ABDOMINAL PAIN

Appendicitis

Treatment is appendicectomy. Antibiotics are not usually necessary, but preoperative rectal metronidazole is sometimes given to prevent wound infection. Appendicitis is covered more fully in Chapter 2.

Mesenteric adenitis

Management is conservative, with intravenous fluids, nil by mouth and simple analgesia. Prognosis is excellent.

Infant colic

Although there is no certain evidence that symptoms derive from the gastrointestinal tract, antispasmodics are prescribed, such as dicyclomine hydrochloride, 5mg, 20 minutes before a feed.

Recurrent (functional) abdominal pain

Management should emphasise reassurance, in particular allaying unspoken fears ("he has not got leukaemia or cancer"). Drugs are ineffective. Informal psychotherapy is helpful, and children with depressive illness should be treated by a child psychiatrist. About 75% of children with recurrent abdominal pain get better, but some 'little belly achers' grow up to be 'big belly achers' (see Chapter 1).

Milk protein intolerance

Most thriving infants lose their symptoms by the age of six months, and parental support and reassurance are the mainstay of management.

Anaemia, secondary to gastrointestinal blood loss, should be treated with iron supplements (ferrous sulphate, 60 mg three times daily).

Henoch–Schönlein disease

Treatment is supportive, with intravenous fluids, and blood transfusion if gastrointestinal blood loss is significant. Prednisone, 1–2 mg/kg, is sometimes effective for controlling bleeding and abdominal pain. Antibiotics are not indicated. Intussusception is a well-recognised complication and renal involvement requires monitoring of blood pressure and urinary output. Long-term renal impairment is rare, but relapse of Henoch–Schönlein disease is frequent and 40% of patients may have a second episode.

Peptic ulcer disease

Treatment is as for adults (see Chapter 1): avoid the precipitating cause, H_2 antagonists and anti-*H. pylori* medication, if indicated.

Acute pancreatitis

Treatment is with nasogastric suction, intravenous fluids and pethidine, 1–2 mg/kg, until serum amylase returns to normal (see Chapter 2). Pancreatitis rarely becomes chronic or recurrent in childhood unless there is structural damage to the organ, or an underlying metabolic cause.

VOMITING: REACHING A DIAGNOSIS IN THE NEONATE (0–28 DAYS)

Is there oesophageal reflux?

During the first days of life some degree of regurgitation of feeds may occur due to immaturity of coordination of sucking, swallowing and breathing. Persistent regurgitation (the return of small quantities of feed with no weight loss) is due to gastro-oesophageal reflux. The diagnosis is made from the history. Oesophageal pH monitoring or scintiscan will detect acid reflux and should be performed if there is failure to thrive with significant regurgitation of feeds if other causes of vomiting have been excluded (see table below). Stools may be positive for occult blood if oesophagitis is severe.

Oesophagitis presents with epigastric pain and/or upper gastrointestinal bleeding. It can be caused by caustic ingestion and *Herpes simplex* infection, but is more often asymptomatic, associated with gastro-oesophageal reflux. Diagnosis is by gastrointestinal endoscopy. A hiatus hernia may present with vomiting, failure to thrive and pain or epigastric discomfort from oesophagitis. Aspiration or recurrent pulmonary infection may occur. Diagnosis is made by radiographic contrast studies, which show the hernia, and oesophageal stricture if present (Figs.18.1 and 18.2).

▶ **Causes of vomiting in infancy and childhood**

	Neonate and infant	Child
Obstruction	Intestinal atresias	Appendicitis
	Diaphragmatic hernia	Swallowed foreign body
	Malrotation/volvulus	Bezoar
	Duplication cysts	Achalasia of cardia
	Meconium ileus	As for infants
	Milk plug syndrome	
	Strangulated hernia	
	Intussusception	
	Hirschsprung's disease	
	Pyloric stenosis	
	Gastro-oesophageal reflux	
Infections	Meningitis	As for infants
	Septicaemia	
	Urinary tract infection	
	Otitis media	
	Gastroenteritis	
Metabolic	Galactosaemia	Diabetes mellitus
	Adrenogenital syndrome	Drug overdose
	Reye's syndrome	
	Inborn errors of metabolism	
Food-related	Milk protein intolerance	Coeliac disease
Other	Cerebral injury	Periodic syndrome
		Motion sickness
		Bulimia

Is there a congenital fistula or obstruction?

In the neonate, vomiting with the first feed, particularly when associated with respiratory symptoms, suggests tracheo-oesophageal fistula. This occurs in about 1/2500 births (usually of low birth weight) and is frequently associated with oesophageal atresia and other congenital abnormalities. It may be anticipated by the presence of maternal polyhydramnios, and a drooling baby at birth. Cough, spluttering, cyanosis or apnoea with the first feed should immediately raise the possibility of the diagnosis, and a soft, radio-opaque orogastric tube should be passed. Chest X-ray should be performed, when the obstruction will be seen. If there is air in the gut below the obstruction there is probably a tracheo-oesophageal fistula. There are five types of tracheo-oesophageal fistula (Figs 18.3).

The return of larger volumes of feed suggests obstruction at or distal to the gastric outlet. Congenital causes of obstruction that present soon after birth include duodenal and jejunal atresia, diaphragmatic hernia, duplication cysts and antral web. High intestinal obstruction is often associated with maternal polyhydramnios. Diagnosis is radiological, as described below.

Is there a diaphragmatic hernia?

Diaphragmatic hernia is a neonatal emergency, which presents soon after birth with increasing respiratory distress, a scaphoid abdomen, and signs of intestinal obstruction. It occurs in around 1/2250 births. The apex of the heart is shifted to the right and the chest is dull to percussion. The diagnosis is made by chest radiography, which reveals loops of bowel in the thorax (Fig. 18.1).

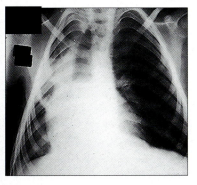

Fig. 18.1 Chest radiograph of a patient with Duchenne muscular dystrophy showing a dilated oesophagus with a fluid level due to severe gastro-oesophageal reflux resulting in stricturing. Aspiration has led to consolidation and collapse of the right lung.

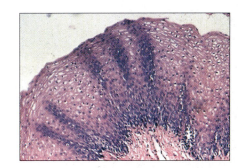

Fig. 18.2 Oesophageal biopsy in reflux oesophagitis showing basal zone thickening and papillary hyperplasia.

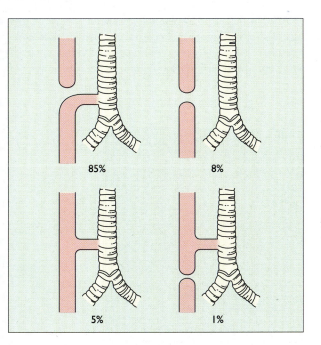

85%   8%

5%   1%

Fig. 18.3 Principal types of tracheo-oesophageal fistula.

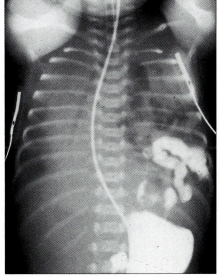

Fig. 18.4 Diaphragmatic hernia. Barium study showing intestine in the left hemithorax.

Is there a duplication cyst?

Enterogenous cysts and duplications can occur throughout the gastrointestinal tract (**Figs 18.5–18.7**). They may be blind-ending, communicate at both ends with the normal gut, are always on the mesenteric border and may be cystic or tubular. They cause symptoms according to where they are sited: those in the thorax produce respiratory distress or upper intestinal obstruction. Those in the small intestine may cause abdominal distension and be palpable, and sometimes give rise to volvulus. When lined with gastric mucosa they may bleed leading to haematemesis or melaena. They can be identified using ultrasound and radiography.

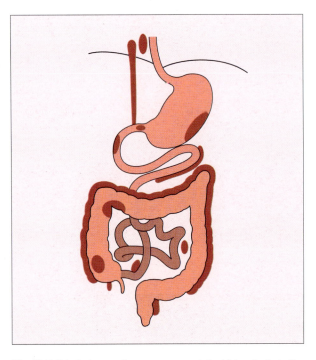

Fig. 18.5 Principal types of enterogenous cysts in children (indicated by the darker shaded areas).

Is there small intestinal atresia?

Small intestinal atresias occur in the duodenum or jejunum at a rate of 1/5000–6000 live births. The former may be associated with annular pancreas, and in 30% of patients with Down's syndrome. The latter may be associated with meconium peritonitis. Both duodenal and jejunal atresia present with vomiting and signs of high intestinal obstruction soon after birth, and the mother may have had polyhydramnios. Vomit will be bile-stained if the obstruction is below the ampulla of Vater, and passage of meconium may be delayed.

Diagnosis is made with erect abdominal radiography, which shows a characteristic 'double-bubble' (**Fig. 18.8**). The stomach and gut before the obstruction may be distended, with fluid levels, and there may be no air in the lower gastrointestinal tract. Speckled calcification suggests meconium peritonitis from an intrauterine perforation.

Is there malrotation?

Malrotation may not be apparent unless volvulus occurs, resulting in vomiting, usually bile-stained, and signs of upper intestinal obstruction. The condition follows failure of rotation of the midgut during its return to the abdominal cavity in embryological life: Ladd's bands cross the duodenum causing partial obstruction and allow the small intestine to twist around a narrow pedicle of mesentery in which the superior mesenteric vessels run (**Fig. 18.9**). Symptoms and signs may be intermittent, but when volvulus is prolonged, the blood supply to the midgut is compromised and gastrointestinal ischaemia occurs with bowel necrosis. This may be accompanied by pain and lower gastrointestinal bleeding.

Abdominal radiographs may show an abnormal gas pattern, but barium meal is necessary to demonstrate non-rotation of the duodenum, sometimes with signs of partial obstruction, and incomplete rotation of the large bowel.

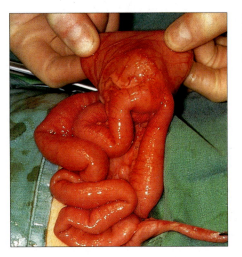

Fig. 18.6 Duplication of ileum: findings at operation.

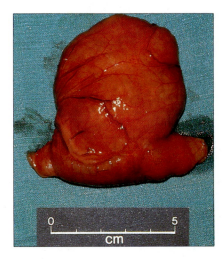

Fig. 18.7 Large mesenteric cyst after excision.

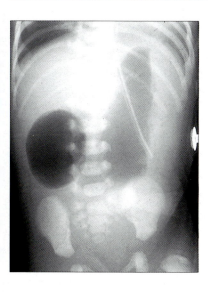

Fig. 18.8 Plain abdominal radiograph showing the 'double bubble' of duodenal atresia.

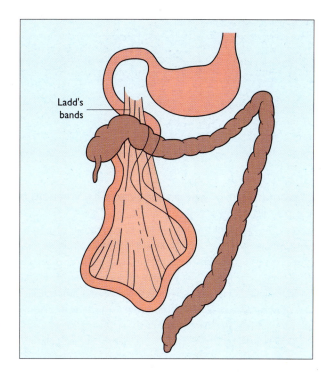

Fig. 18.9 Diagram of the commonest type of malrotation showing Ladd's bands causing duodenal obstruction, and the caecum in the right upper quadrant of the abdomen.

Vomiting later in the neonatal period suggests either a lower intestinal cause or partial obstruction: necrotising entero-colitis, milk plug syndrome, meconium ileus (see cystic fibrosis) and Hirschsprung's disease should be considered. Inguinal hernia is easily detected by examination.

VOMITING: REACHING A DIAGNOSIS IN INFANCY AND CHILDHOOD

In later infancy and childhood, intussusception, malrotation with volvulus, and swallowed foreign bodies are important causes of obstruction. Periodic syndrome (cyclical vomiting) occurs in the anxious child. Vomiting is a symptom of acute gastroenteritis, and of Reye's syndrome. Bilious vomiting suggests obstruction distal to the ampulla of Vater (the descending part of the duodenum). Blood-stained vomiting is discussed below. Vomiting may also be a sign of:

- Infection: otitis media, meningitis, peritonitis, pyelonephritis, hepatitis, malaria.
- Disease of the central nervous system: intracranial haemorrhage, hydrocephalus and other space-occupying lesions.
- Metabolic disorders: diabetes mellitus, galactosaemia, congenital adrenal hyperplasia, thyrotoxicosis.
- Drug overdose.
- Heart disease: cardiac failure.

Is there pyloric stenosis?

Persistent vomiting in early infancy raises the possibility of hypertrophic pyloric stenosis. Pyloric stenosis typically occurs at about six weeks of age in first-born boys; the male to female ratio is 4 to 1. Vomiting follows a feed (when fresh milk enters a stomach that has not emptied), and becomes projectile. The infant becomes dehydrated with a hypo-chloraemic alkalosis. Peristalsis is visible and a pyloric 'tumour' is palpable. These signs may be elicited with a test feed, and confirmed by abdominal ultrasound.

Is there periodic syndrome or cyclical vomiting?

Periodic syndrome or cyclical vomiting occurs in 'highly-strung' children, often in response to stress. There may be central abdominal pain, and vomiting is repeated until bile-stained. It may be severe enough to cause dehydration and metabolic disturbance with alkalosis and ketonuria. The abdomen is soft to palpation. Further investigation is required to rule out physical causes (see below).

▶ **Surgical causes of vomiting in early life**

- Oesophageal atresia with and without tracheo-oesophageal fistula
- Duodenal and jejunal atresia
- Diaphragmatic hernia
- Abdominal wall defects
- Enterogenous cysts and duplications
- Malrotation and volvulus
- Anal stenosis and anorectal abnormalities

▶ **Acute diarrhoea and vomiting**

- Diarrhoea and vomiting in infancy and childhood is usually due to viral gastroenteritis
- Fluid replacement with oral rehydration solution is the mainstay of management
- Breast feeding should be continued, but formula feeding should cease until recovery
- Antibiotics and antimotility agents are contraindicated

Management of conditions causing vomiting

Gastro-oesophageal reflux

Gastro-oesophageal reflux is the regurgitation of gastric contents, which may lead to vomiting, pulmonary aspiration, reactive apnoea, oesophagitis and failure to thrive. Foul-smelling clothes particularly upset mothers. It is due to incompetence of the lower oesophageal sphincter, and possibly to delayed gastric emptying. Common in normal infants, it usually resolves spontaneously by one year of age. Children with mental and physical handicap are prone to gastro-oesophageal reflux and may become malnourished.

Management should include nursing the infant at 30°, head up, and thickening of feeds with Carobel (Cow and Gate) or Nestargel (Nestlé). Metoclopramide or cisapride may be useful in the symptomatic infant with failure to thrive, and antacids and H_2 antagonists when oesophagitis is present. Gaviscon (alginic acid, aluminium hydroxide, magnesium trisilicate and sodium bicarbonate mixture) after feeds may protect the lower oesophagus from the effects of reflux. The older child may benefit from sitting upright after feeds, and sleeping with the head of the cot or bed raised.

Gastro-oesophageal reflux has a good prognosis. Physiological maturation of the lower oesophageal sphincter occurs during the first year, though a few infants who develop severe oesophagitis may eventually require fundoplication. In severely retarded children gastrostomy may be necessary to maintain adequate nutrition.

Pyloric stenosis

Fluid and acid–base balance should be restored before a Ramstedt pyloromyotomy is performed. Early recommencement of oral feeding is recommended, and prognosis is excellent.

Periodic syndrome or cyclical vomiting

Rehydration should be undertaken in hospital. Sedation with promethazine, 15–25 mg, may be required. Psychotherapy can be helpful if episodic vomiting becomes repeated.

Tracheo-oesophageal fistula

The immediate aim of management is to prevent pulmonary aspiration, with continuous suction to the oesophageal pouch if necessary, before transfer to a neonatal surgical unit. Primary oesophageal anastomosis and closure of the fistula is achieved in 75% of patients. The remainder need reconstructive surgery, and may require a feeding gastrostomy before transposition of a colonic segment.

Small intestinal atresia

Management is surgical after aspiration of the stomach and correction of fluid and electrolyte imbalance. Survival is high, but intestinal atresias are frequently associated with other abnormalities of the gastrointestinal tract, and elsewhere, such as vertebral anomalies and ventriculoseptal defects. The management of short gut syndrome, a consequence of resection of the atresia, is outlined below.

Diaphragmatic hernia

Urgent tracheal intubation, with positive pressure ventilation, and decompression of the gastrointestinal tract by continuous suction, should be followed by prompt transfer to a neonatal surgical unit. Prognosis is largely determined by the degree of pulmonary hypoplasia.

Enterogenous cysts and duplications

Treatment is surgical and will depend on the site of the cyst. They should be excised if symptomatic.

Malrotation

Surgical division of Ladd's bands and placement of the large bowel on the left, and the small bowel on the right side of the abdominal cavity should be undertaken if there are intermittent symptoms of obstruction. Volvulus is a surgical emergency, and massive infarction of the bowel may follow operative delay.

Abdominal wall defects

Abdominal wall defects are immediately apparent at birth, or may be detected prenatally by ultrasound or alphafetoprotein screening. They are rare (about 1/10,000 live births) and are frequently associated with chromosomal and other abnormalities. When the small intestine fails to return to the abdominal cavity during early embryological life, a small hernia into the cord may result (omphalocele), or there may be a muscular defect of the abdominal wall at the umbilicus, with herniation of viscera (liver, bladder) as well as gastrointestinal tract (exomphalos) (**Fig. 18.10**). Gastroschisis is the term given to a defect in the abdominal wall to the right of the umbilicus, through which the midgut herniates.

The immediate management of all abdominal wall defects is to cover them with warm, sterile, saline-soaked gauze. Primary closure should then be attempted, though a two-stage procedure, employing a silastic pouch is necessary for large defects.

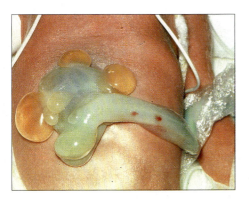

Fig. 18.10
Exomphalos.

UPPER GASTROINTESTINAL BLEEDING

Reaching a diagnosis

Blood-stained vomit (fresh blood or 'coffee grounds') suggests upper gastrointestinal bleeding, the most common sites being the gastro-oesophageal junction (due to oesophagitis, gastro-oesophageal varices), or the stomach (due to gastritis, swallowed foreign body, milk protein intolerance, haemorrhagic disease). Other causes of haematemesis include peptic ulcer, enterogenous duplications and cysts, and haemangiomas.

A history of salicylate ingestion should be sought. The nasopharyngeal region should be inspected for causes of epistaxis. The neonate may ingest maternal blood during passage through the birth canal, or from a cracked nipple during breast feeding. Upper abdominal pain points towards a gastric cause (gastritis, peptic ulcer disease), while a long history of vomiting makes an oesophageal mucosal tear likely. History, symptoms and signs of hepatic disease (spider naevi, hepatosplenomegaly, jaundice, distended abdominal veins, ascites, oedema), if present, suggest oesophageal varices. Bleeding from other sites (e.g. haematuria, bruising) suggest coagulopathy.

▶ **Causes of haematemesis in childhood**

- Epistaxis
- Foreign body
- Oesophageal varices
- Oesophagitis
- Gastritis and gastric ulcer
- Duodenal ulcer
- Salicylates, corticosteroids and anti-inflammatory drugs
- Coagulopathies
- Mucosal tears (Mallory–Weiss)
- Duplications
- Vascular malformations

General principles of management

Most hamatemeses stop spontaneously, but bleeding gastro-oesophageal varices may require sclerotherapy or placement of a Sengstaken tube (see below). Haemoglobin, haematocrit, platelets and coagulation factors should be measured, and a nasogastric tube passed (to confirm bleeding and to wash out the stomach). Abdominal radiograph may show evidence of perforation, mass, obstruction or enterocolitis.

The management of continuing gastrointestinal bleeding is replacement of lost blood. Indications for transfusion depend on age, clinical condition and cause, and a rule of thumb for the older child is to transfuse in any of the following circumstances:

- If haemoglobin is less than 10 g/dl.
- If systolic blood pressure is less than 100 mm Hg.
- If pulse rate is higher than 100/minute.

▶ **Gastrointestinal haemorrhage**

- Bleeding from the gastrointestinal tract is always abnormal and should be investigated
- Fibroscopic endoscopy and contrast studies are used to detect site and/or cause of bleeding
- Significant acute gastrointestinal blood loss should be replaced with whole blood

Fibreoptic endoscopy of the upper gastrointestinal tract may identify the site of bleeding when undertaken acutely, but rarely alters management unless varices are suspected. Drugs that may cause mucosal bleeding should be stopped and an H_2 antagonist given.

Conditions causing upper intestinal bleeding
Gastritis

Gastritis in childhood is often part of the syndrome of gastroenteritis, usually of viral origin. It may also be caused by salicylates and other drugs, including corticosteroids and anti-inflammatory agents. There is increasing evidence that antritis, caused by *H. pylori* infection, occurs in children, but this is not a cause of bleeding.

Haematemesis secondary to gastritis usually subsides with proper treatment of gastroenteritis or removal of the precipitating cause. Blood transfusion may be necessary if blood loss is excessive.

Gastro-oesophageal varices

The commonest site of varices is at the gastro-oesophageal junction, as a result of increased portal venous pressure secondary to hepatic disease. They may be identified by barium swallow, or directly by upper endoscopy.

The management of bleeding varices is a specialised procedure best undertaken by an expert team. Lost blood should be replaced by transfusion. H_2 blockers should be given to reduce gastric acidity and intravenous somatostatin can be very effective, but a Sengstaken tube should be passed if bleeding persists. Sclerotherapy may be attempted to control an acute haemorrhage, but is more usually used to obliterate varices.

DIARRHOEA: REACHING A DIAGNOSIS

Neonatal diarrhoea

Is there necrotising enterocolitis?

Acute diarrhoea in early life is a serious sign. In the neonate vomiting accompanied by loose bloody stools and abdominal distension indicates necrotising enterocolitis (NEC) until proved otherwise (see pages 260–261).

Is there a congenital enteropathy?

Persistent diarrhoea in the newborn points towards a congenital enteropathy of the small or large intestine. Congenital chloride diarrhoea, congenital microvillus atrophy and mucosal enzyme deficiencies (primary lactase deficiency, enterokinase deficiency) are rare, but well-described causes.

Congenital enteropathies present as diarrhoea, which begins soon after birth and is persistent or protracted. The investigation and management of the infant with intractable diarrhoea requires the support of a specialist centre: in most instances intestinal mucosal biopsy is indicated.

Congenital microvillus atrophy is a disorder of the cytoskeleton of the apical region of the enterocyte with atrophy and involution of the microvilli of the small and large bowel. It presents within a few days of birth with intractable secretory diarrhoea, is diagnosed by electron microscopy of a mucosal biopsy, is treated with total parenteral nutrition and has a very poor prognosis. It is probably inherited by autosomal recessive mode, and is one of a family of congenital familial enteropathies. Among the heterogeneous syndrome of intractable diarrhoea of infancy there is a group with autoantibodies to the enterocyte membrane and a group in which the disorder is associated with mastoiditis, but often no specific diagnosis can be made.

Congenital chloridorrhoea is another rare autosomal recessive cause of severe watery diarrhoea in the neonate characterised by very high concentrations of chloride in the stool. There is defective Cl^-/HCO_3^- transport in the ileum and colon. This disorder is present prenatally and is associated with polyhydramnios and premature birth. The newborn has abdominal distension and hypochloraemic acidosis, and requires prompt chloride replacement therapy.

Congenital lactase deficiency presents with profuse watery diarrhoea soon after the introduction of milk feeds. Diagnosis is made by withdrawal of lactose-containing feeds and the demonstration of absent lactase activity on a jejunal mucosal biopsy. It is rare compared with the lactose intolerance, which occurs after weaning in many parts of the world where cows milk is not part of the regular diet.

Is the diarrhoea persistent?

Persistent diarrhoea is defined as the passage of two or more loose, watery stools daily for more than two weeks, with no weight gain. Persistent diarrhoea is commonest in early infancy, in the UK, usually caused by a congenital enteropathy, but in the developing world it begins during the weaning period and is a major cause of malnutrition and growth failure in early childhood. The infant or child is usually malnourished with a weight well below his or her third centile for age. The onset of diarrhoea may be associated with the introduction of a particular item of diet (e.g. cows' milk, gluten).

Weanling diarrhoea

Weanling diarrhoea occurs in a large proportion of the infants of the developing world where it is a major cause of malnutrition and growth faltering. Mortality rates may be as high as 10 million deaths/year, the majority within the first 12 months of life. Diarrhoea frequently begins at weaning, and is associated with gastrointestinal bacterial colonisation, the cessation of breast feeding and the introduction of solid foods.

Until the first introduction of non-milk diet infants usually thrive, are free of diarrhoea and exhibit no evidence of small intestinal damage. Growth failure begins around six months and is associated with a widening 'energy gap' caused by insufficient breast milk intake and inadequate supplementary diet. The latter is frequently watery, of low energy density and protein content, contaminated with pathogenic bacteria and also contains potentially harmful food proteins, which may contribute to the mucosal injury of malnutrition of infancy.

The enteropathy of the diarrhoea–malnutrition complex is the net effect of the interaction of these factors. It is characterised by villus atrophy, crypt hypertrophy and lymphocyte infiltration, and is associated with a loss of functional integrity of the intestinal mucosa, diminished lactase activity, and immunological evidence of persistent gastrointestinal bacterial and protozoal infection. The nutritional advantages of early introduction of weaning foods to fill the energy gap caused by dwindling breast milk intake must be balanced by the risks of introducing infection and causing damage to an immature gut mucosa by the 'foreign' proteins of supplementary foods.

Diarrhoea in the toddler

Toddler diarrhoea is often coincident with increasing ingestion of a solid diet. The stools contain pieces of apparently undigested food (e.g. peas, carrots) and the child's diet is often low in fat and high in carbohydrate. When associated with abdominal pain, and episodes of constipation alternating with diarrhoea, the term irritable bowel syndrome is used. The stool may contain mucus, but not blood, and the clinical picture is of an irritable, hyperactive bowel in a hyperactive child. Children with toddler diarrhoea do not fail to thrive, and the disease usually disturbs the mother more than the child. It is important to rule out infection (particularly giardiasis) and in the presence of poor growth, coeliac disease and cystic fibrosis.

Diarrhoea in childhood and adolescence
Is it gastroenteritis?
Gastroenteritis is usually an acute self-limiting illness in the developed world, caused most commonly by enteroviruses. In the developing world it remains a major cause of morbidity and may lead to chronic diarrhoea, malabsorption and growth failure. Gastroenteritis is commoner in bottle-fed infants than in breast-fed infants, and in conditions of poor sanitation.

Stools should be cultured for bacterial pathogens, examined by electron microscopy for viruses, and under the light microscope for parasites and leucocytes. There are enzyme-linked immunosorbent assay tests for the rapid identification of rotavirus and other enteroviruses in the stool. Other causes of diarrhoea and vomiting should be ruled out (see table below).

▶ Causes of acute diarrhoea and vomiting

- Gastroenteritis
- Coeliac disease
- Milk protein intolerance
- Inflammatory bowel disease
- Appendicitis
- Intussusception
- Hirschsprung's disease
- Diabetic ketoacidosis
- Urinary tract infection
- Congenital adrenal insufficiency
- Haemolytic–uraemic syndrome
- Necrotising enterocolitis

Rotavirus is the commonest pathogen identified in the stool of children with gastroenteritis in the UK, and occurs with a peak incidence in winter, sometimes preceded by a respiratory illness. Other viruses causing gastroenteritis are listed in the adjacent table. Vomiting usually precedes diarrhoea and may be accompanied by fever. Dehydration follows if lost fluid is not replaced. When gastroenteritis is caused by bacteria, the stools may be bloody (dysenteric), indicating the invasive nature of the infecting organism. The course of the disease may then be longer.

▶ Microorganisms isolated during acute diarrhoea

Viruses	Bacteria	Parasites
Rotavirus	Salmonella spp.	Giardia lamblia
Adenovirus	Shigella spp.	Cryptosporidium
Astrovirus	Escherichia coli	Entamoeba histolytica
Small round virus	Campylobacter jejuni	Strongyloides
Calcivirus	Staphylococcus aureus	
Coronavirus	Yersinia enterocolitica	
Norwalk agent	Clostridium difficile	
	Vibrio cholerae	
	Vibrio haemolyticus	
	Aeromonas hydrophila	

IS THERE SECONDARY LACTASE DEFICIENCY?
Secondary lactase deficiency follows acute gastroenteritis and other causes of small intestinal enteropathy (coeliac disease, Crohn's disease, protein energy malnutrition). It is manifest by watery, frothy, diarrhoea related to milk or lactose ingestion. Reducing sugars (lactose, glucose or galactose) are detectable in the liquid stool, and a hydrogen breath test is positive after ingestion of lactose. Lactose intolerance resolves with repair of the injured mucosa, and a lactose-free diet. A lactose-free milk such as Pregestimil (Mead Johnson) or Galactomin (Cow and Gate) should be used for 4–6 weeks, by which time lactose tolerance has usually returned.

IS THERE INFLAMMATORY BOWEL DISEASE?
In chronic diarrhoea in the older child inflammatory bowel disease should be considered and excluded by endoscopy and/or barium examinations as for adult disease (see Chapter 3). Serum C-reactive protein will nearly always be elevated in active Crohn's disease and a normal sigmoidoscopy virtually excludes ulcerative colitis.

IS THERE MALABSORPTION?
Inspection of a stool sample should always be performed as early as possible. Significant fat malabsorption will usually be manifest by an obviously fatty pale stool. Investigation (see page 265) will thereafter follow different lines from that of watery diarrhoea.

MANAGEMENT OF CONDITIONS CAUSING DIARRHOEA

Congenital enteropathies
Nutritional support is the central objective of treatment. Total parenteral nutrition should be used to restore the infant to normal weight and growth. Enteral feeds should not be reintroduced until a clear diagnosis has been made and their composition will depend on the underlying cause.

Weanling diarrhoea

Treatment is preventive: improved sanitation and food hygiene, prompt treatment of acute diarrhoea with oral rehydration therapy (see Gastroenteritis), and vigorous realimentation to reverse growth faltering. It is rarely possible, and probably inadvisable, to provide proprietary formulae or weaning foods to children of the developing world. Appropriate use of traditional weaning foods, with improvement in their energy density, protein content and palatability, may override the enteropathy so that children pass through the criticial weaning period to achieve catch-up growth in later childhood.

Toddler diarrhoea

Sometimes a specific item of diet may be responsible: careful history, withdrawal and challenge with the offending food will identify this. The parents should be reassured that the child will grow out of the disease, usually by school age, and that with normal growth he is making proper use of his food, although bits appear in the stool. Increasing the bulk of the diet (with methylcellulose) may 'regularise' intestinal motility, and sometimes Calogen (Scientific Hospital Supplies), 10 ml three times daily, may apply an 'ileal brake' and reduce stool frequency. Antispasmodics and antimotility agents such as mebeverine, dicyclomine and loperamide are rarely effective.

Gastroenteritis

Rehydration is the mainstay of management. It is essential to assess the degree of dehydration present (see below) and to rehydrate promptly. If the child is more than mildly dehydrated, urea and electrolytes should be measured.

The breast-fed infant should continue with mother's milk. Formula feeds should be discontinued and oral glucose electrolyte solution (150–180 ml/Kg/d) given. Severe dehydration may require intravenous fluids, particularly in the infant who continues to have diarrhoea after cessation of milk feeds. When diarrhoea stops the infant should return to full-strength milk feeds. Antibiotics are not indicated, except for some infants with bacterial (*Salmonella, Shigella* or *Campylobacter*) gastroenteritis and systemic symptoms or

▶ **Causes of persistent diarrhoea in infancy**

Congenital

- Microvillous atrophy
- Congenital chloridorrhoea
- Primary lactase deficiency
- Sucrase-isomaltase deficiency
- Lymphangiectasia
- Adrenogenital syndrome
- Acrodermatitis enteropathica

Dietary

- Coeliac disease
- Milk protein intolerance

Secondary carbohydrate intolerance

- Lactose intolerance
- Monosaccharide intolerance

Infections

- Enteropathogenic E. coli
- *Giardia lamblia*
- Dysenteric infections
- Occult systemic infection
- HIV/AIDS

Surgical

- Hirschsprung's disease
- Intestinal stenosis
- Blind loop syndrome

Pancreatic

- Cystic fibrosis
- Shwachman syndrome

Other

- Necrotising enterocolitis
- Familial protracted diarrhoea
- Immunodeficiency/ AIDS
- Pseudomembranous colitis
- Autoimmune enteropathy

Tumours

- Lymphomas
- Ganglioneuromas
- Histiocytosis X

▶ **Assessment of dehydration in infancy**

	Weight loss	Clinical features
Mild	0–5%	Alert, but thirsty with dry mouth Normal skin elasticity
Moderate	5–10%	Restless with tachycardia Depressed anterior fontanelle Reduced skin elasticity
Severe	> 10%	Worsening of signs above Hypotension and tachycardia Drowsy or comatose

signs. They should be given systemically according to the organism's sensitivity. Antidiarrhoeal agents are contra-indicated. The child should return to full normal diet as soon as possible to avoid growth faltering.

Short bowel syndrome

Short bowel syndrome may follow excision of a significant portion of the small intestine, leading to malabsorption, diarrhoea and growth failure. Loss of bowel may follow pre- or postnatal damage to the gut. Survival without parenteral nutrition is rare when less than 15 cm of small intestine remains after resection. Other factors that determine outcome are:

- Whether the jejunum or ileum was resected (the latter has greater powers of adaptation, the unique ability to absorb vitamin B_{12} and bile acids, and has a longer transit time).
- Whether the ileocaecal valve was preserved.

▶ **Causes of short bowel syndrome**

Prenatal	Postnatal
Vascular accidents	Necrotising enterocolitis
Intestinal atresias	Midgut or segmental volvulus
Abdominal wall defects	Inflammatory bowel disease
Midgut volvulus	Abdominal trauma
Segmental volvulus	Vascular thrombosis

Management

Following intestinal resection there is massive diarrhoea, which requires intravenous fluid and electrolytes. This usually lasts days and is associated with an increased transit rate and gastric hypersecretion. It is followed by a period of gradual intestinal adaptation during which there is growth in the length and diameter of the remaining bowel, and mucosal hypertrophy. Total parenteral nutrition (TPN) is required during this phase. Intestinal adaptation may continue for months, but maximal adaptation is usually achieved by three years of age in the infant who has a neonatal intestinal resection.

Enteral feeds should be introduced cautiously: while they may encourage mucosal growth and function they also stimulate intestinal and pancreatico-biliary secretion, which may contribute to further intestinal fluid loss. An element of pancreatic insufficiency may accompany short bowel syndrome owing to the gastric hypersecretion, rapid transit rate and loss of mucosal enterokinase.

Feeds should be elemental, of high protein and low fat (composed of a protein hydrolysate and medium-chain triglyceride) and lactose-free initially. They should also contain adequate fat and water-soluble vitamins and minerals, particularly calcium, magnesium, iron and zinc. Dietary oxalates should be restricted to reduce the risk of nephrolithiasis.

H_2 antagonists (cimetidine) may help to reduce gastric hypersecretion. Vitamin B_{12} supplements are necessary after terminal ileal resection. Antimotility agents such as loperamide may be effective, but should be used with care. Cholestyramine is indicated if there is evidence of bile acid diarrhoea after ileal resection. Somatostatin analogues have been used for some intractable cases, but require parenteral administration and have many unwanted effects on the endocrine system.

Weaning from TPN to enteral feeding should be done gradually by methodically changing one thing at a time. For example, loperamide should not be stopped and cows' milk formula feeds introduced at the same time; the infant with short bowel syndrome is very susceptible to setbacks in growth and bowel habit. Close attention should be paid to weight gain, stool volume, nutritional status and fluid and electrolyte balance. Properly managed, most infants climb back into the normal weight range by their third year, albeit on the lower centiles. They should be followed through childhood with particular attention to fat assimilation and vitamin B_{12} and fat-soluble vitamin status.

Failure to support infants with short bowel syndrome on enteral nutrition has led to attempts at surgical treatment aimed at slowing intestinal transit time or increasing absorptive surface area by reconstruction of the ileocaecal valve, interposition of colon or antiperistaltic segments, or recirculating loops. Small bowel transplantation offers hope to the infant who remains totally dependent on parenteral nutrition.

RECTAL BLEEDING AND BLOODY DIARRHOEA : REACHING A DIAGNOSIS

Rectal bleeding of any sort (the passage of bright-red or altered blood on the toilet paper, mixed with the stool, or frank bloody diarrhoea) is not normal, and there are many causes:

- In the newborn, particularly the preterm, necrotising enterocolitis must be ruled out, as well as swallowed blood (during birth or from a mother's cracked nipple), gastroenteritis is not a common cause in older onfants.
- Anal fissure is usually associated with difficulty of defecation in the toddler.
- Bright red painless rectal bleeding suggests Meckel's diverticulum.

- When there is pain, the blood is intermingled with mucus and the child has weight loss, Crohn's disease is a likely diagnosis.
- Intussusception and malrotation with volvulus are associated with severe colicky abdominal pain and signs of obstruction.
- Streaking of the stools with blood indicates rectal or anal bleeding. Gastrointestinal bleeding can also be occult, caused by cows' milk protein intolerance, leading to anaemia.
- Blood in the stool may also be a sign of haemorrhagic disease, infarction of the bowel secondary to asphyxia, and other causes of acute intestinal hypoxia.

▶ **Causes of lower intestinal bleeding in childhood**

- Causes of upper gastrointestinal haemorrhage
- Polyps
- Intussusception
- Inflammatory bowel disease
- Anal fissure and haemorrhoids
- Meckel's diverticulum
- Rectal prolapse
- Gastroenteritis
- Henoch–Schönlein disease
- Necrotising enterocolitis
- Antibiotic colitis
- Milk protein intolerance
- Haemolytic–uraemic syndrome
- Coagulopathies
- Salicylates, corticosteroids, anti-inflammatory drugs etc.
- Angiomas, telangiectasia

The darker the blood passed, the higher its probable site of origin: melaena suggests one of the causes of upper gastrointestinal haemorrhage. Haemorrhoids are unusual in childhood.

Is there necrotising enterocolitis?

Necrotising enterocolitis (NEC) is primarily a disease of the preterm infant of very low birth weight and occurs most frequently within the first week of postnatal life. Its incidence ranges from around 0.5–15/1000 livebirths, and in infants of under 1.5 kg it may approach 8%. NEC is a pathological response of the immature intestine to injury by a variety of factors, which have a complex interrelation: damage to the mucosa, the presence of bacteria, and a metabolic substrate (feeds) in the intestine are all necessary for the development of the disease.

Enteral feeds may predispose to NEC by a number of mechanisms and nearly all infants who develop NEC have received oral feeds. Although there is little evidence that NEC is primarily and exclusively an infectious disease, microbial infection is clearly an important aetiological factor. Infants with NEC often have a septicaemia, but no organism is consistently associated with the disease. Blood cultures are often positive and correlate closely with isolates from stool or peritoneal fluid. A damaged gut allows enteric organisms to traverse the mucosa to the circulation.

NEC presents classically with bloody stools, abdominal distension and bile-stained vomiting. Clinical features may be more insidious, with hypothermia, apnoea, signs of infection or disseminated intravascular coagulation (**Figs 18.11–18.16**). Abdominal radiographs show dilated loops of bowel, intaluminal gas and sometimes signs of perforation.

Is there milk protein intolerance?

Milk protein intolerance may follow feeding with cows' milk formula, soya-based formula and even human milk (which

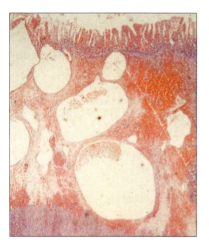

Fig. 18.11 Necrotising enterocolitis: histological section of intestine showing intramural gas.

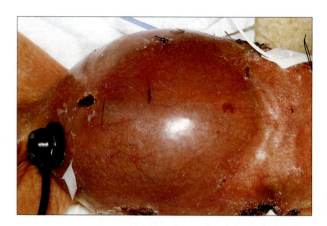

Fig. 18.12 Tense abdominal distension in necrotising enterocolitis.

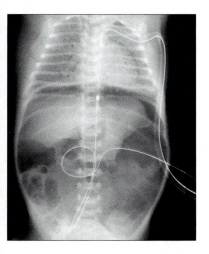

Fig. 18.13 Abdominal radiograph showing intraperitoneal gas following perforation from necrotising enterocolitis.

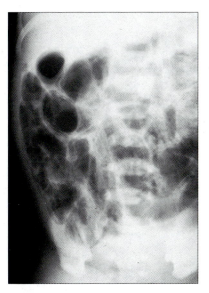

Fig. 18.14 Abdominal radiograph showing intramural gas from necrotising enterocolitis.

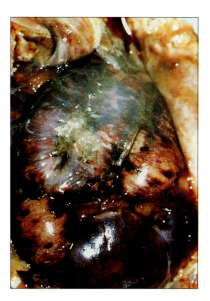

Fig. 18.15 Gangrenous bowel in necrotising enterocolitis.

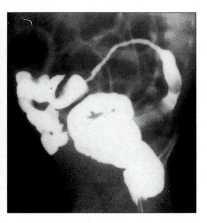

Fig. 18.16 Barium enema appearance of colonic stricture following necrotising enterocolitis.

contains small amounts of cows' milk protein). It is commonest in the first months of life, in infants of atopic parents and has an incidence of around 0.5%. It may affect the stomach or small or large bowel, as well as having non-gastrointestinal effects ranging from acute anaphylaxis to chronic atopic disease (eczema and asthma).

Gastrointestinal manifestations may include occult blood loss with iron-deficiency anaemia, failure to thrive, diarrhoea and vomiting sometimes indistinguishable from gastroenteritis, malabsorption, protein-losing enteropathy, frank gastrointestinal bleeding and colitis.

In the stomach there may be an antritis with eosinophilic infiltration, and in the jejunum a subtotal villus atrophy with crypt hyperplasia and leucocyte infiltration of the lamina propria, reproducible with milk challenge, has been described. Colonic changes include a patchy erythema, loss of vascularity and superficial ulceration with leucocyte infiltration of the lamina propria.

It may sometimes by necessary to do a milk challenge or mucosal biopsy in early infancy to make a diagnosis. Serum IgE may be elevated. It is important to exclude infective causes of enteropathy.

Is there an anal fissure?

Anal fissure is one of the commonest causes of rectal bleeding, precipitated by the passage of hard stools, often in the constipated child. Defecation is painful and the stools are usually flecked with blood, or it may be seen on the toilet paper. The fissure is usually visible posteriorly, but may require proctoscopy to be seen fully. Persistence of the fissure, with local pain, can lead to stool withholding and constipation.

Is there intussusception?

Intussusception presents in infancy and early childhood, with short episodes of colicky abdominal pain. The legs are drawn up and the child may vomit and is very distressed with pallor, but between bouts appears perfectly well. The passage of bloody stools ('red currant jelly') follows, and other signs of intestinal obstruction (vomiting and abdominal distension) are present. A sausage-shaped mass may be palpable and rectal examination will reveal bloody stools.

A polyp, Meckel's diverticulum or duplication cyst may be the leading point of the intussusception, and occasionally swollen intestinal lymph nodes are responsible. Intussusception also occurs in Henoch–Schönlein disease and cystic fibrosis. The commonest site of invagination is terminal ileum into caecum and colon. The diagnosis is confirmed with ultrasound and plain abdominal radiograph, which shows features of obstruction and a soft tissue mass. This

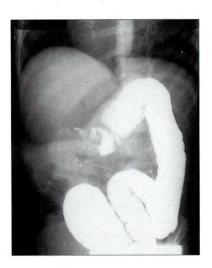

Fig. 18.17 Barium enema showing typical appearances of intussusception. Courtesy of Dr TJ Evans.

should be rapidly followed by contrast examination of the colon (showing the 'coiled spring' sign and site of obstruction, **Fig. 18.17**) and reduction of the intussusception.

Is there a polyp?

Polyps may be single or multiple, are almost always benign and are sometimes familial. All may present with painless gastrointestinal bleeding.

Juvenile polyps of the colon are the commonest: they are single, pedunculated and hamartomatous, frequently within reach of the tip of the finger on rectal examination and may prolapse through the anus. In the child with multiple hamartomatous polyps annual colonoscopy should be done to assess the rate of appearance of new polyps: large or growing polyps should be excised and examined histologically. The risk of malignancy is low, but bleeding, pain on defecation, rectal prolapse and repeated protrusion of polyps from the rectum may necessitate colectomy.

Peutz–Jeghers syndrome describes the association of multiple benign hamartomatous polyps throughout the gastrointestinal tract with perioral pigmentation. There is autosomal dominant inheritance and a slightly, but definitely, increased risk of malignancy.

Familial adenomatous polyposis coli is an autosomal dominant inherited condition. The defective gene has been identified on chromosome 5, but its normal function is not known. Multiple polyps (typically over 100 and often over 1000/colon) are seen on sigmoidoscopy or contrast studies (**Figs 18.18** and **18.19**), and because they are premalignant, management is surgical, with colectomy and ileostomy. Patients with Gardner's syndrome have a more extensive defect in the same gene and have osteomas of the mandible, skull and long bones. In Turcot's syndrome, which is probably part of the same syndrome, polyposis is associated with gliomas and other brain tumours.

The retinal abnormalities may precede the development of colonic polyps and fundoscopy is therefore a useful part of screening for family members. First degree relatives should be screened by flexible sigmoidoscopy at 2–3 year intervals from 13 years of age. Total colectomy should be performed in individuals with the condition at 17–18 years of age. (See also Chapter 6.)

Is there a Meckel's diverticulum?

Meckel's diverticulum is usually not detected unless it contains ectopic gastric mucosa that bleeds. It is the result of persistence of the omphaloenteric duct, a blind pouch 10–150 cm proximal to the ileocaecal valve. Present in 1–3% of the population, bright or dark red, painless rectal bleeding occurs in 60% in childhood and almost always before 40 years of age if gastric mucosa is present. The diverticulum may be very difficult to detect with barium examinations, but a technetium (^{99}Tc) scan will identify the presence of ectopic gastric mucosa (see Chapter 6).

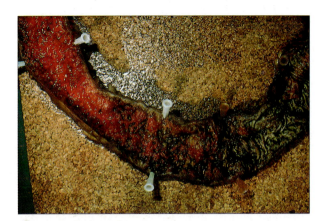

Fig. 18.18 Colon resection specimen in familial polyposis coli showing hundreds of small polyps. Courtesy of Dr TJ Evans.

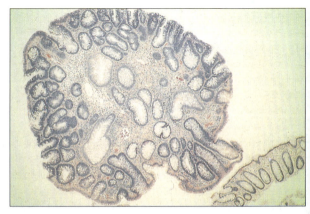

Fig. 18.19 Cross-section of adenomatous colonic polyp. Note the dysplastic cells with darkly-staining nuclei. Courtesy of Dr TJ Evans.

Is it ulcerative colitis?

Ulcerative colitis in childhood usually presents with a change of bowel habit, or with diarrhoea, blood, mucus and sometimes pus. There may be tenesmus, but abdominal pain is uncommon as a presenting symptom (in contrast with Crohn's disease). In infancy, colitis is most often associated with food intolerance. In older children and adolescents there may be a family history of the disease.

The incidence of ulcerative colitis in the UK is about 15–20 new cases/million children/year, or 70–80/million children overall. Growth retardation is a late clinical feature, but extra-intestinal signs, such as fever, erythema nodosum, uveitis and arthritis may occur. Oral and perianal disease is very rare.

The diagnosis is made by radiology and colonoscopy. Double-contrast barium enema shows loss of motility and haustral pattern in the large bowel, with crypt ulcers. The small intestine and terminal ileum are usually normal, but the rectum is almost always involved. At colonoscopy the mucosa looks red with contact bleeding and superficial ulcers. Pseudopolyps may be present. Mucosal biopsies show crypt abscesses, infiltration of the lamina propria with lymphocytes, eosinophils and plasma cells, with goblet cell depletion. Granulomas are rare.

Differential diagnoses include Crohn's disease, amoebiasis and food intolerance (in infants). Stool bacteriology should be carried out. (See also Chapter 3.)

Is it Crohn's disease?

Crohn's disease is commoner than ulcerative colitis in childhood: in the UK there are 90–100 cases/million children. Diagnosis is often delayed because of its insidious onset and non-specific features, which include abdominal pain, weight loss, diarrhoea, lower gastrointestinal bleeding, malaise, fever and delayed puberty. The classical patterns of presentation seen in adulthood (see Chapter 3) are uncommon, although rectal bleeding with oral or perianal ulcers make the diagnosis very likely. Iritis, arthritis, erythema nodosum and clubbing should be sought (**Figs 18.20–18.22**). In the adolescent puberty may be delayed.

Investigations should include full blood count (normocytic, normochromic anaemia occurs) and measurement of erythrocyte sedimentation rate and acute phase proteins in serum such as C-reactive protein (almost always elevated). Lymphocytosis is often present. Serum proteins and liver function tests should be measured: hypoalbuminaemia is often caused by malnutrition and gastrointestinal protein loss.

Diagnosis is made by radiology and colonoscopy. Contrast studies of the upper and lower gastrointestinal tract will reveal the distribution and extent of the disease, while colonoscopy is used to obtain a histological diagnosis. With a paediatric instrument endoscopy can be undertaken in infants and young children, and the terminal ileum can be reached. The diagnostic features of the disease are essentially the same as those in adulthood (see Chapter 3).

Is there amoebiasis?

Amoebiasis is found worldwide and caused by *Entamoeba histolytica*, a protozoan that is ingested, usually in its cystic form, with contaminated food or water. It presents most often with bloody diarrhoea, sometimes mistaken for ulcerative colitis, and may also cause hepatic abscesses. Microscopy of a fresh stool sample examined before it cools reveals motile amoebae containing phagocytosed red blood cells.

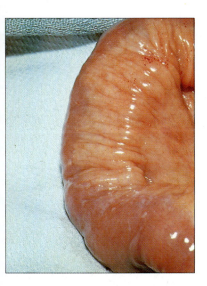

Fig. 18.20 Small intestinal Crohn's disease showing the junction between diseased and adjacent healthy mucosa.

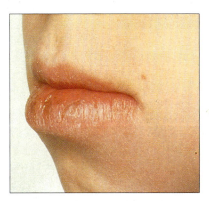

Fig. 18.21 Oral Crohn's disease affecting the lower lip.

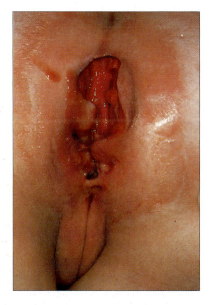

Fig. 18.22 Severe peri-anal Crohn's disease.

Is there a rectal prolapse?

Rectal prolapse alarms and puzzles parents, when they first see the symptomless protrusion of a large pink mass, often after the child has been straining (sometimes squatting) or has had diarrhoea for a while. It is a well-described feature of cystic fibrosis and may be seen in the malnourished child with wasting or weakness of the perirectal tissues.

MANAGEMENT OF CONDITIONS CAUSING RECTAL BLEEDING AND BLOODY DIARRHOEA

Necrotising enterocolitis

The mainstay of treatment of NEC is supportive: rest the gut, control infection, restore metabolic equilibrium and maintain the infant in optimal condition until the bowel heals. Cessation of enteral feeding and removal of umbilical cannulae, correction of anaemia, hypovolaemia and electrolyte imbalance, and vigorous treatment of infection with systemic broad-spectrum antibiotics and metronidazole should be instigated. Parenteral nutrition should be provided and coagulopathy treated. Regular X-rays of the abdomen should be performed to detect perforation or intramural gas. The majority of infants thus managed recover in 7–10 days, after which enteral feeding may be cautiously restarted so long as the abdomen is soft and bowel sounds are audible.

Surgery is indicated in 20–40%, for perforation or for failure to progress. Abdominal paracentesis may sometimes be helpful in the latter. Contrast studies may help to determine the site of obstruction. Postoperative care includes parenteral nutrition until normal peristalsis has returned. Intestinal stricture may occur (**Fig. 18.16**), but overall survival and long-term outcome have greatly improved over the last decade.

Prevention

Guidelines for the prevention of NEC are largely empirical. Early removal of umbilical artery catheters is advised, especially if there is evidence of thrombosis, such as difficulty withdrawing blood, or discoloration of the infant's toes or feet during infusion. Because of the positive relation between fluid intake and incidence of NEC, maintenance of intravenous fluids to a minimum compatible with normal hydration is advised.

In the low birth weight infant enteral feeds should be introduced slowly and a check made by regular gastric aspiration that milk is not pooling in the stomach. Evidence of normal gastrointestinal motility (meconium has been passed, the abdomen is not distended and bowel sounds are audible) should be confirmed. Small, non-nutritional volumes of milk may contribute to the maturation of the gut of the preterm. Human milk should be used in preference to formula. The oral administration of milk or drugs of high osmolarity should be avoided and episodes of hypotension, hypoxia and hypothermia minimised. Prophylactic antibiotics have not been shown consistently to be beneficial.

Intussusception

Hydrostatic reduction should be performed in a centre where surgery is available so that if unsuccessful an operation can be carried out before necrosis of the bowel occurs. Contraindications to non-surgical reduction are signs of peritonitis or perforation, and a history longer than 48 hours. Mortality is less than 1%, and recurrence rate is around 5–10%.

Polyps

Polyp removal may be achieved by sigmoidoscopy or colonoscopy using a diathermy snare. In children with familial polyposis coli, colectomy will inevitably be required, usually at 17–18 years of age (see Chapter 6), but may be required earlier if multiple polyps are found in childhood since the earliest occurrence of carcinoma is at about ten years of age. Six monthly colonoscopy and polypectomy is appropriate if there are less than ten polyps found and all can be removed.

Meckel's diverticulum

Treatment is replacement of lost blood and surgical resection of the diverticulum.

Anal fissure

Local application of lignocaine ointment will ease the pain of passing stools. When the stools have softened, with oral lactulose or some other stool softener (see Constipation) the fissure usually heals spontaneously. Chronic anal fissure may require anal dilatation.

Rectal prolapse

Gentle manipulation of the prolapsed rectum will usually reduce it; sedation may be necessary, and nursing the child with the bottom raised. Stool softeners, such as bran or lactulose, should be used (after ruling out underlying disorders), and if recurrent, submucosal sclerosant injection or insertion of a perianal suture may be necessary.

Milk protein intolerance

Treatment is by withdrawal of the offending milk and substitution with a hypoallergenic protein hydrolysate (Pregestimil).

Ulcerative colitis

When the disease is restricted to the rectum (proctitis), treatment with steroid enemas is often sufficient. Oral sulphasalazine, 30–50 mg/kg/day (up to 2 g) or mesalazine, 400 mg three times daily, should be added if the whole colon is affected, and systemic steroids, prednisone, 1–2 mg/kg/day for 2–4 weeks, when disease is extensive or there are extraintestinal manifestations. Disease progress and response to treatment should be monitored with full blood count, erythrocyte sedimentation rate, white cell count, serum proteins, temperature and weight. Labelled-leucocyte scan and colonoscopy provide more accurate assessment of disease extent and activity, but are not necessary routinely.

Nutritional deficits may result from diarrhoea and/or poor intake. Hypoalbuminaemia and electrolyte imbalance, from intestinal protein and fluid loss, should be corrected, intravenously if necessary. Deficiencies of water and fat-soluble vitamins, minerals and trace metals should be sought and replenished: iron, calcium, zinc, folate and vitamin B_{12} are particularly important.

Surgery is indicated if there is toxic megacolon or perforation (see Chapter 3), or no response to medical treatment. It should be contemplated in chronic steroid-dependent disease when there is growth failure or delayed puberty. Partial colectomy is not indicated and total colectomy results in an ileostomy or ileorectal anastomosis with or without a pouch, but also a permanent cure. Ulcerative proctitis has a good prognosis, with less than 20% of patients eventually requiring surgery.

Crohn's disease

Management should be undertaken in a specialist clinic, preferably jointly with a paediatric surgeon and dietitian. The aim of treatment is to achieve and maintain remission of disease, and to ensure optimum nutrition and growth.

Corticosteroids (prednisone, 1–2 mg/kg, up to to 40 mg/day, for four weeks) will usually control symptoms of disease. Progress should be monitored by measuring erythrocyte sedimentation rate, haemoglobin and serum albumin, and steroids reduced and discontinued as soon as possible. They should not be used long term.

Sulphasalazine, 1–2 g/day, or mesalazine, 400 mg three times daily, are used to maintain remission, and to treat children with colonic disease. Azathioprine, 6-mercaptopurine and cyclosporin are alternative steroid-sparing drugs. Metronidazole, 10 mg/kg/day, may be effective against perianal disease, especially if there are fistulae or abscesses.

Nutrition should be maintained using enteral formulae, unless gastrointestinal bleeding, diarrhoea or extreme malnutrition make parenteral feeding unavoidable. The aim is to provide around 140% of recommended daily requirements, using an elemental diet such as EO28 (Scientific Hospital Supplies). Such formulae are not always regarded as palatable by children and may be flavoured and/or given by nasogastric tube overnight. Children soon tolerate this and can learn to pass their own tube and use a pump at home. With motivation, good organisation and supervision, elemental diets can be effectively used to induce remission of a relapse when disease is largely restricted to the small intestine. They have the advantage of being steroid-sparing and nutrition-providing. During remission the diet should be low residue, high-energy and protein-rich. Formulae such as Polycal (Cow and Gate) and Casilan (Farleys) are often useful.

Indications for surgery are intestinal obstruction, abscess, fistula, severe haemorrhage and toxic megacolon. Disease unresponsive to medical therapy and growth failure unresponsive to nutritional support may require surgical intervention. Resection of a stricture or persistently active section of bowel may improve symptoms and growth.

Amoebiasis
Treatment is with metronidazole, 200–400 mg, according to age, three times daily for five days.

MALABSORPTION AND STEATORRHOEA: REACHING A DIAGNOSIS

Malabsorption results from failure of the mechanisms of digestion and/or absorption of food, leading to loss of essential nutrients in the faeces. The passage of carbohydrate unabsorbed in the small intestine to the colon results in osmotic, watery diarrhoea. Fat malabsorption is manifest as bulky, offensive, greasy, pale stools (steatorrhoea), while protein malabsorption may not be obvious on faecal examination. The principal causes of malabsorption in childhood are disorders of the liver, exocrine pancreas and small intestine.

In making a diagnosis of malabsorption, a full dietary history (with the help of a dietitian) is essential to:

- Obtain a measure of the intake of nutrients.
- Find out whether particular foods (gluten-containing, based on cows' milk) are being eaten by the child.
- Find out the frequency and character of the stools passed.

Inspection of the faeces is essential (**Fig. 18.24**). When malabsorption is marked, failure to thrive, persistent diarrhoea, and signs of specific nutrient deficiencies will be present, including loss of subcutaneous tissue, muscle wasting, abdominal distension, peripheral oedema, bruising, anaemia and short stature. It is vital to plot the child's height and weight on appropriate centile charts.

It is important to distinguish malabsorption from insufficient nutrient intake, and excessive utilisation of nutrients. When malabsorption is suspected pancreatic exocrine, hepatobiliary and gastrointestinal mucosal function should be tested, with the aim of both making a diagnosis and assessing the nutritional and other effects.

▶ **Causes of malabsorption**

- Cystic fibrosis
- Chronic liver disease
- Coeliac disease
- Abetalipoproteinaemia
- Short gut syndrome
- Lymphangiectasia
- Bacterial overgrowth
- Shwachman syndrome
- Inflammatory bowel disease
- Chronic pancreatitis
- Parasite infections (*Giardia lamblia*, Ascariasis, Strongyloidiasis)
- Milk protein intolerance

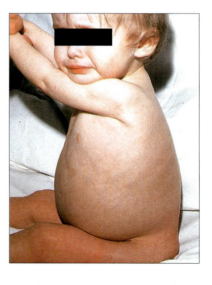

Fig. 18.23 A child with coeliac disease.

Is it coeliac disease?

Coeliac disease (**Fig 18.23**) presents with failure to thrive after the introduction of cereals containing gluten. It may present:

- With signs of malabsorption.
- With frequent, bulky, pale, fatty stools.
- More insidiously, with growth failure, anaemia, abdominal distension or muscle wasting.

Investigations include full blood count, serum iron and folate, proteins, calcium, phosphate and alkaline phosphatase. Circulating anti-gliadin, anti-reticulin and anti-endomyseal antibodies are elevated in untreated coeliac disease with sensitivity and specificity of about 90%. Intestinal permeability tests (lactulose:mannitol or cellobiose:rhamnose urinary excretion ratios) are also elevated, but are less specific, being abnormal in other causes of enteropathy, such as gastroenteritis and cows' milk protein intolerance.

The diagnosis is confirmed by jejunal biopsy, performed either under fluoroscopic control with a Crosby or Watson capsule, or endoscopically. Subtotal or total villous atrophy is seen histologically. Strictly-speaking the diagnosis should be substantiated by a return to normal appearance of the mucosa on withdrawal of gluten from the diet, and a relapse after gluten challenge. However indirect measures such as disappearance of antigliadin antibody and normalisation of intestinal permeability are often used in the place of repeat biopsies.

Is there intestinal lymphangiectasia?

Lymphangiectasia causes protein-losing enteropathy and is detected by jejunal biopsy. The villi are club-shaped, there

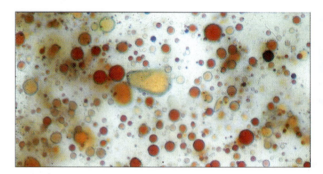

Fig. 18.24 Faecal smear stained with Sudan IV showing fat globules from a patient with malabsorption.

is fat in the enterocytes, and the lymphatics in the lamina propria are dilated. Contrast radiology may show coarse mucosal folds.

Is there abetalipoproteinaemia?

Abetalipoproteinaemia presents with failure to thrive and steatorrhoea, followed later in childhood by ataxia, neuropathy, retinopathy and cirrhosis. Diagnosis is made from low plasma betalipoprotein and cholesterol, and acanthocytes in the peripheral blood (**Fig. 18.25**).

Is there pancreatic insufficiency?

Shwachman syndrome is the next most common cause of exocrine pancreatic insufficiency after cystic fibrosis. Inherited by autosomal recessive mode, it usually presents within the first two years of life. In addition to maldigestion (100%), children have growth retardation (100%), bone marrow hypofunction, with neutropenia, anaemia, thrombocytopenia (80%), recurrent infections (100%) and skeletal abnorm-

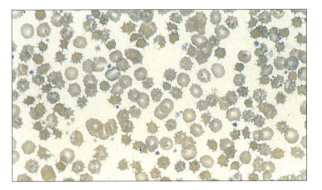

Fig. 18.25 Blood film showing acanthocytes in a child with abetalipoproteinaemia.

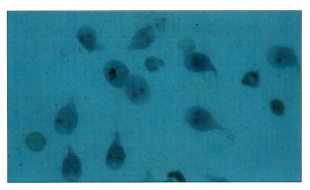

Fig. 18.26 Trophozoites of *Giardia lamblia* in a mucosal smear from a duodenal biopsy (Giemsa stain).

alities (90%). It is distinguished from cystic fibrosis by the sweat test. Blood-immunoreactive trypsin and amylase may be abnormally low, and pancreatic function studies confirm exocrine insufficiency (see Chapter 3). Affected children are below the third centile for height, and skeletal survey may reveal metaphyseal dysplasias, dyschondroplasias and rib abnormalities.

Is there bacterial overgrowth of the small intestine?

Small intestinal bacterial overgrowth usually occurs in a gut with an underlying abnormality, such as a stricture, blind loop or disordered motility. The diagnosis may be made indirectly by a lactulose or glycocholate breath test, or directly by intubation and anaerobic culture of jejunal fluid.

Is there giardiasis?

Giardiasis can mimic coeliac disease. It is caused by *Giardia lamblia*, a protozoan that adheres to the small intestinal mucosa. Infection is acquired by ingestion of cysts present in contaminated food or water. It may be asymptomatic, cause watery diarrhoea or malabsorption. Diagnosis is made by microscopy of the stool (cysts are present in 50%) or duodenal aspirate. It is sometimes detected on the surface of small intestinal mucosal biopsies (**Fig. 18.26**).

MANAGEMENT OF CONDITIONS CAUSING MALABSORPTION AND STEATORRHEA

Coeliac disease

Treatment requires removal of gluten from the diet. A paediatric dietitian should be involved with the management, to ensure that an appropriate full diet containing all essential nutrients is eaten, and to help parents to obtain and prepare gluten-free foods.

A gluten-free diet must be maintained for life (see Chapter 3), and gluten challenge should be avoided during periods of rapid growth, in infancy and adolescence.

Shwachman syndrome

Pancreatic enzyme supplementation should be provided as for cystic fibrosis. Infections should be treated promptly with antibiotics, and steroids (prednisone, 2mg/kg daily) may improve marrow hypofunction. The prognosis is better than that of cystic fibrosis, with a mortality rate of 15–25%.

Small intestinal bacterial overgrowth

Antibiotic treatment, based on the sensitivies of the organisms isolated, should be given, and the underlying abnormality treated. Significant overgrowth usually consists predominantly of anaerobic organisms so if sensitivity is not available, treatment with metronidazole is usually effective.

Protein-losing enteropathy

Protein-losing enteropathy leads to failure to thrive and hypoproteinaemia, with oedema, ascites and pleural effusions. It must be distinguished from hepatic and renal causes

▶ **Causes of protein-losing enteropathy**

Gastrointestinal	Non-gastrointestinal
Ménétrier's disease	Lymphatic obstruction
Lymphangiectasia	Lymphoma
Coeliac disease	Thoracic duct obstruction
Crohn's disease	Constrictive pericarditis
Malrotation/volvulus	Tricuspid valve disease
Lymphosarcoma	Superior vena cava
Giardiasis	
Kwashiorkor	
Ulcerative colitis	
Hirschsprung's disease	

of protein loss, by measurement of stool alpha-1-antitrypsin. The ^{51}Cr-labelled albumin excretion test should be undertaken if this is elevated. Treatment is of the underlying cause, and a high protein diet.

Abetalipoproteinaemia

Treatment is with a low fat diet containing essential fatty acids and fat-soluble vitamins:

• Vitamin A, 15–20,000 IU/day.
• Vitamin K to maintain normal coagulation time.
• Vitamin E, 50–100 mg/kg/day to prevent neurological sequelae.
• Vitamin D (400–800 IU/day) to prevent rickets or osteomalacia.

Intestinal lymphangiectasia

Diet should contain medium-chain triglycerides to reduce lymphatic obstruction.

Giardiasis

Treatment is with metronidazole, 200–400 mg (according to age) three times daily for five days.

Other causes of malabsorption and steatorrhoea, including cystic fibrosis and milk protein intolerance, are discussed elsewhere in this chapter.

CONSTIPATION, SOILING AND ENCOPRESIS: REACHING A DIAGNOSIS

Constipation is the passage of small amounts of hard stool infrequently and with difficulty or discomfort. It may be a trivial and transitory complaint, easily dealt with by the family doctor, or it can be an intractable problem requiring specialist expertise and investigation. It can cause distress to both child and parents, and demands sensible and sensitive management. Physical and psychological factors are blended in its aetiology and an awareness of the contribution of both is essential for successful management.

The bowel habit of infants and children changes markedly between birth and adolescence. During early infancy defecation rate may be higher in the breast-fed than formula-fed, but by four months all infants have a modal frequency of two bowel actions daily. Thereafter this declines so that by the time children begin school it approaches an 'adult' pattern of bowel habit: once daily, with 96% of 3–4-year-old children opening their bowels between three times daily and three times a week; a pattern that persists to old age (**Fig. 18.27**).

Constipation may be a presenting sign of systemic disease, although other diagnostic features are usually obvious when this is the case. It is important to detect any organic cause early. It can be very damaging for a child with a struct-

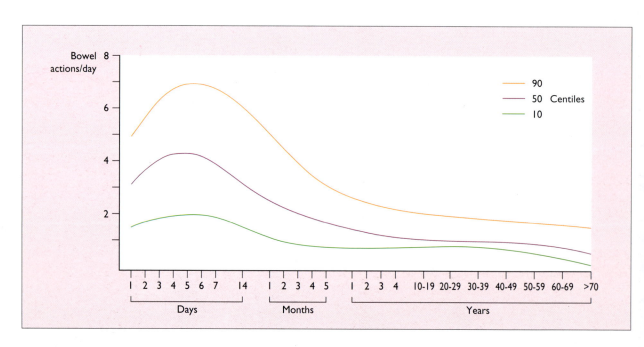

Fig. 18.27 Bowel habit from birth to old age.

► **Organic causes of constipation in childhood**

Neonate	Infant	Child
Anal atresia	Hirschsprung's	Hypothyroidism
Meconium ileus	disease	Short segment
Hirschsprung's	Obstructions	Hirschsprung's
disease	Anal stricture	disease
Obstructions	Hypothyroidism	Hypercalcaemia
Congenital	Hypercalcaemia	Lead poisoning
microcolon	Diabetes insipidus	Diabetes insipidus
Dysmotility	Renal tubular	Renal tubular
syndrome	acidosis	acidosis

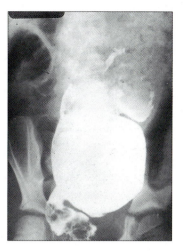
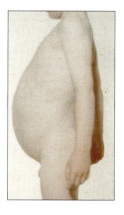

Fig. 18.28 Barium enema in megacolon. Courtesy of Dr TJ Evans.

Fig. 18.29 Child with Hirschsprung's disease, showing distended abdomen typical of late diagnosis. Courtesy of Dr TJ Evans.

ural abnormality of the large bowel to be persuaded by the doctor that he can open his bowels when he cannot, however much he tries. Careful attention to the details of history and physical examination is the key. Although rare, these are all treatable and demand early recognition and prompt treatment.

When constipation is accompanied by abdominal distension and bilious vomiting, a cause of intestinal obstruction should be sought. A tympanic abdomen, local tenderness, a mass, visible peristalsis, hepatosplenomegaly, umbilical protrusion, ascites and inguinal hernias are all signs that assist diagnosis.

Investigation of the constipated child includes rectal examination, plain abdominal X-ray, thyroid function tests, plasma urea and electrolytes, calcium, phosphate and alkaline phosphatase (see table above). Rectal biopsy and manometry should be reserved for children in whom there is strong evidence of a diagnosis of Hirschsprung's disease or other motility disorder.

Is there delayed passage of meconium?

Within 24 hours of birth, 95% of full-term infants have passed meconium, and within 48 hours 99%. Delayed passage of stool beyond this time occurs in more than 90% of infants with Hirschsprung's disease.

In the preterm infant, first passage of meconium may be delayed beyond the second day in 32%. Other causes of delayed passage of meconium are intestinal atresias, ano-rectal abnormalities, meconium ileus (which is almost always a sign of cystic fibrosis, where stools are inspissated and thick, the abdomen is distended and masses may be palpable) and meconium plug.

Is there anal atresia?

Anal atresia or stenosis in the newborn is usually obvious on examination: there is no anus, or the lower bowel is blind-ending. Plain abdominal radiography in an inverted position shows gas outlining the rectal pouch, and a radio-opaque tube may be inserted to define the extent of the atresia. Contrast is necessary to outline a fistula or stenosis. Atresia is often associated with other abnormalities.

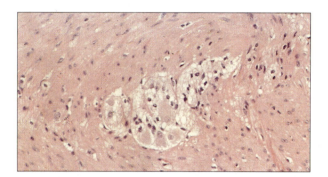

Fig. 18.30 Normal rectal biopsy showing ganglion cells in the muscularis propria.

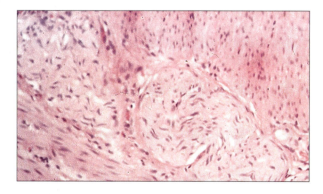

Fig. 18.31 Hirschsprung's disease showing nerve fibres but no ganglion cells.

Is it Hirschsprung's disease?

Hirschsprung's disease occurs in about 1/5000 births and may affect 10% of babies with Down's syndrome. It is due to an embryological defect in migration of neuroblasts, which fail to innervate the distal large bowel, resulting in an absence of ganglion cells in the muscular and submucous plexi (**Figs 18.29–18.31**). A variable length of intestine, extending cranially from the anus, is affected. Most infants present in the neonatal period with delayed passage of meconium (see above), followed by abdominal distension and vomiting.

Decompression of partial obstruction with a rectal thermometer may be followed by continued constipation, or alternatively by frequent stools and enterocolitis, which leads to failure to thrive and perforation. Abdominal radiographs show a gasless distal large intestine, and contrast studies reveal a narrowed aganglionic segment below a dilated large bowel (**Fig 18.28**). Definitive diagnosis is made by histological examination of the rectal mucosa obtained by suction biopsy. The autonomic nerve trunks are thickened, the ganglion cells absent and acetylcholinesterase levels increased (**Figs. 18.30–18.31**). Barium enema shows a funnel or cone of dilated normal bowel above the affected segment. Anal manometry may be necessary to detect short-segment disease.

Is there soiling or encopresis?

Soiling sometimes coexists with constipation and is almost always involuntary. Stool escapes into the underclothes, either because constipation is so gross that 'overflow' occurs, sometimes past impacted faeces, or because there is a neurogenic cause (e.g. spina bifida, myelomeningocoele, paraplegia) with loss of anal sensation and control. The colon distends and loses its tone. The child lacks the reflex urge to defecate and large masses of stool accumulate in the rectum. Liquid stool may seep around the mass and soil the pants, and an incorrect diagnosis of diarrhoea may be made.

Encopresis is the passage of stool in abnormal places, almost always associated with emotional disturbance or mental handicap. Anal sensation and control are normal.

MANAGEMENT OF CONDITIONS CAUSING CONSTIPATION, SOILING AND ENCOPRESIS

Transitory episodes of constipation occur at any age, and prevention relies not only on appropriate diet, but also on adequate intake of fluid. Medication that increases faecal bulk and stimulates the large bowel is not enough alone; the hard dry stool requires hydration to be passed easily. Oral lactulose, 5–30 ml/day for a week or two, is usually sufficient to soften the stool and return bowel habit to normal if the history is short.

The fibre content of the diet should be increased with the help of a dietitian, and intake of high-fibre foods that the child likes best (e.g. beans, raisins) should be maximised. High-fibre breakfast cereals, fresh fruit and vegetables (unpeeled), and wholemeal bread should become a major part of the diet of the whole family.

▶ **Constipation, soiling and encopresis**

- Constipation is usually caused by insufficient dietary fibre
- Simple laxatives are usually required for at least the same length of time as the duration of the constipation
- Enemas and rectal washouts are required only in the most intractable cases
- Management of soiling should follow or accompany treatment of constipation
- Psychotherapy is usually part of the management of encopresis

Chronic functional constipation

Chronic functional constipation often follows an episode of simple constipation. Normal large bowel function is regulated, to a large extent, by the fibre content of diet, and functional constipation often presents first during a dietary transition: at weaning, and in early childhood, when the range and composition of the diet is changing. It may be precipitated by an acute illness, anal fissure, difficulty at home or at school, such as a move, inappropriate toilet training or lack of privacy. The child often does not reach the paediatrician until many months after the onset of constipation, by which time the rectum is distended and contains a mass of hard stool. Owing to discomfort and loss of normal sensation and anorectal propulsive function, the child is unable to either expel or to retain faeces, leading to soiling or overflow incontinence.

It is vital to explain the physiology of the problem to the child and parents; that it is not the child's fault that he is having difficulty passing the stool, or is soiling, and that treatment may last for months or even a year or two. The fibre content of the diet should be increased if possible, but with large doses of laxative this is often unnecessary until the rectum has been emptied and the child is returning to a normal bowel habit.

It is essential to ensure that large doses of stool softener are maintained, and that the family does not 'give up.' Regular follow-up, with positive encouragement of progress is essential. Star charts, with goals and rewards, are helpful. The aim of treatment is to empty the rectum and to keep it empty. This can usually be achieved using a stool softener such as lactulose or docusate sodium (Dioctyl), which should be taken in increasing volumes until the stool is soft and passed easily. Doses of more than 50 ml of lactulose daily may be necessary, for several weeks or months. The dose should not be decreased until it is absolutely clear that the 'backlog' of stool has been expelled and the distended rectum is regaining its tone and assuming a normal calibre.

A rule of thumb is that the duration of treatment with laxatives is as long as the duration of constipation before treatment began. A stimulant laxative, such as senna, may be added to the lactulose when stools are beginning to be passed more regularly. In intractable disease, enemas should be used, but only rarely is evacuation under general anaesthetic necessary.

Soiling

The goal of management is to abolish constipation. Once the rectum is emptied of hard faeces it must be kept empty, with continued laxative treatment, while it reachieves its normal size, tone and function. Long-term outcome is excellent: very few adults soil.

Encopresis

The child may be constipated and require treatment to clear the bowel of hard faeces. Psychological therapy may be behavioural, analytical, or family orientated, with the objective of identifying and rectifying what precipitates the symptom and maintains it, and how the child can learn to defaecate normally.

Anal atresia and stenosis

A defunctioning colostomy is usually necessary, followed by corrective surgery in later infancy. Constipation or faecal incontinence are common complications.

Hirschsprung's disease

Immediate decompression of the gut by daily rectal washouts, or colostomy, is necessary. Definitive treatment involves resection of the aganglionic segment. Neonatal mortality is due largely to delay in making the diagnosis, and from the enterocolitis that may follow.

▶ **Signs and symptoms of liver disease**

- Jaundice
- Pruritus
- Yellow urine
- Poor weight gain
- Grey/pale stools
- Abdominal pain
- Nausea/vomiting
- Haematemesis/malaena
- Anorexia
- Diminished energy
- Abdominal swelling (liver, spleen, ascites)
- Deteriorating school performance

JAUNDICE AND LIVER DISEASE

It is estimated that at least one child dies each week from liver disease in the UK despite a successful liver transplantation programme with around 100 transplants each year and a current survival rate of 80%.

The five main causes of liver damage are:

Obstruction to the flow of bile.
Infection.
Metabolic diseases (usually genetic).
Drugs and poisons.
Poor blood supply.

Symptoms and signs vary greatly, many are nonspecific, and the classic adult signs such as finger clubbing, spider naevi, liver palms, white nails and gynaecomastia are often absent or a relatively terminal event. The commonest presenting features are jaundice, haematemesis and melaena, and the finding (often routinely) of an enlarged liver and/or

▶ **Causes of unconjugated neonatal hyperbilirubinaemia**

- Physiological
- Breast milk jaundice
- Haemolytic disorders
- Increased red cell mass
- Infection
- Hypoxia
- Hypothyroidism
- Dehydration
- Genetic defects in bilirubin metabolism: Gilbert's and Crigler–Najjar syndromes
- Metabolic defects: galactosaemia and fructosaemia
- High intestinal obstruction
- Drugs competing for bilirubin-binding sites

▶ **Investigations of neonatal unconjugated hyperbilirubinaemia**

- Serial determination of total and direct bilirubin concentrations
- Urine microscopy, culture and analyses for reducing substances
- Haemoglobin, reticulocyte count, Coombs' test and blood film
- Blood group of mother and child and search for maternal antibodies and haemolysins
- Blood cultures and bacteriological samples where appropriate.
- Serum thyroid stimulating hormone concentration

spleen. Jaundice becomes clinically apparent in older children when the serum bilirubin exceeds 35 μmol/l, although in the newborn not usually until it is greater than 80 μmol/l.

Unconjugated hyperbilirubinaemia: reaching a diagnosis

Unconjugated hyperbilirubinaemia is usually physiological in the newborn, and is characterised by jaundice without bile in the urine and a raised total serum bilirubin with less than 15% in the direct-reacting form. It is often due to haematological causes and rarely to metabolic or genetic disease. Very high concentrations cause cerebral damage including kernicterus.

Is it physiological?

Physiological jaundice of the newborn is transient, occurring during the first week and after 24 hours after birth. In the full-term infant total bilirubin concentrations usually do not exceed 200 μmol/l between days 2–4, although in the preterm child concentrations of 240 μmol/l are common between days 5–7 and can remain elevated for two weeks. The pathogenesis is complex involving increased bilirubin production, impaired hepatic uptake and excretion, and altered enteric reabsorption.

Is it breast milk jaundice?

Breast milk jaundice has an estimated incidence of 2%, infants remain entirely well and kernicterus has not been described. Bilirubin concentrations may rise to 300 μmol/l or above and jaundice may occasionally be present for 6–8 weeks. The aetiology is unknown, but probably involves a lower calorie intake, steroids (3α, 20β-pregnanediol) in breast milk, and possible inhibition of bilirubin excretion by fatty acid in human milk.

Is it haemolytic?

Jaundice appearing within 24 hours of birth should be considered to be haemolytic until proven otherwise. If the baby is unwell, sepsis, hypoxia and the state of hydration may be important. Hypothyroidism should never be forgotten and in most centres will be detected on neonatal TSH screening using the dried blood spot collected for the Guthrie test. Similarly galactosaemia, although rare, should be ruled out in a baby on lactose-containing feeds by testing the urine for reducing substances.

Is there defective bilirubin conjugation?

Defective activity or complete absence of the enzyme bilirubin glucuronyl transferase is responsible for the Crigler–Najjar syndrome of which there are two types.

- Type I is inherited by the autosomal recessive mode and presents within a few hours of birth with bilirubin concentrations rapidly rising to greater than 340 μmol/l. Usually unresponsive to phototherapy at this stage, and to hepatic enzyme inducers, (e.g. phenobarbitone), repeated exchange transfusions are required although early death with kernicterus can be expected.
- Type II is inherited by the autosomal dominant mode with variable penetrance, and is characterised by less severe hyperbilirubinaemia, which responds to phenobarbitone, levels falling to normal or near normal within 2–4 weeks.

Management

In full-term infants a serum bilirubin concentration higher than 340 μmol/l is associated with a significant risk of kernicterus. Prematurity, acidosis, hypoxia and certain drugs may cause brain damage at lower values. Exchange transfusions, phototherapy and phenobarbitone are the main specific measures for controlling this form of hyperbilirubinaemia. Phototherapy, using lamps that produce radiation in the range of 450–460 nM wavelength, is commonly started when bilirubin concentrations reach around 250 μmol/l in full term infants, and at lower levels in preterm babies. Eye shields prevent the possibility of retinal damage and an increase in fluid intake is necessary to compensate for increased insensible water losses through the skin and sometimes via the gastrointestinal tract due to lactose malabsorption.

When the serum bilirubin concentration exceeds 340 μmol/l in full-term infants, or 250 μmol/l in preterm infants, exchange transfusion(s) with compatible whole blood, replacing twice the calculated blood volume (80 ml/kg), is the most effective method of immediately controlling hyperbilirubinaemia. As a hepatic enzyme-inducing agent, phenobarbitone takes at least 48 hours to become effective and is therefore of no value in the treatment of established dangerous hyperbilirubinaemia.

Conjugated hyperbilirubinaemia: reaching a diagnosis

Characterised by jaundice, with bile in the urine, grey or white stools and a direct-reacting bilirubin of more than 15% of the total, this form of jaundice is always pathological. In a 3–4 week old neonate it is vital to rule out immediately treatable causes, for example:

- Infection (by blood and urine cultures).
- Hypothyroidism (by measuring TSH and T4).
- Choledochal cyst (by ultrasound).
- Galactosaemia (by measuring urine reducing substances).
- Tyrosinaemia (by measuring serum amino acids and urinary succinylacetone levels).

The infant should be transferred to a regional gastroenterology centre for further investigations. The presence or

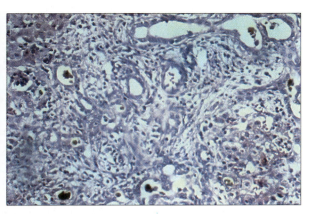

Fig. 18.32 Biliary atresia: portal tract showing bile plugs and proliferation of biliary ductules.

absence of an enlarged liver and/or spleen, and the level of elevation of liver enzymes (alanine aminotransferase, alkaline phosphatase) are not reliable guides to diagnosis, and usually a percutaneous liver biopsy should be performed before the sixth week.

Is there biliary atresia?

In the neonatal period, biliary atresia (**Fig. 18.32**), although rare, must be distinguished from other causes of jaundice to afford the infant the possibility of surgery, which to be effective needs to be carried out before the sixtieth day of life.

Extrahepatic biliary atresia

Extrahepatic biliary atresia is characterised by complete inability to excrete bile associated with obstruction, destruction or absence of the extrahepatic bile ducts anywhere between the duodenum and the first or second order of branches of the right and left hepatic ducts. The incidence is 1/14,000 births and it results from a sclerosing inflammatory lesion initiated in the ductular tissue at around the time of birth or shortly thereafter.

Infants present with conjugated hyperbilirubinaemia at a few weeks of age and if successfully diagnosed and operated upon (Kasai porto-enterostomy) by 60 days, have an 80% chance of surviving with a good quality of life to ten years of age and often longer. Late diagnosis and a non-operative approach inevitably results in death unless liver transplantation is performed. There is an association between this condition and congenital heart disease and situs inversus. Three main types are defined according to the site of the atresia:

- Type I: atresia of the common bile duct with patent proximal ducts.
- Type II: atresia involving the hepatic duct, but with patent proximal ducts.
- Type III: atresia involving the right and left hepatic ducts at the porta hepatis.

▶ **Causes of neonatal conjugated hyperbilirubinaemia**

Idiopathic (approximately 60%)	
Infective	Cytomegalovirus Rubella Herpes simplex Toxoplasma gondii Hepatitis A, B, C Coxsackie Epstein–Barr *Treponema pallidum* Tuberculosis Bacterial septicaemia
Inherited and metabolic disorders	Alpha-1-antitrypsin deficiency Nieman–Pick disease Galactosaemia Fructosaemia Tyrosinaemia Cystic fibrosis Gaucher's disease Wolman's disease Zellweger's syndrome Neonatal iron storage disease Trihydroxycoprostotic acidaemia Chromosomal abnormalities (particularly trisomy 13 and 18)
Bile duct abnormalities	Intrahepatic hypoplasia (Alagille's) Extrahepatic biliary atresia Choledochal cysts
Endocrine abnormalities	Hypopituitarism (septo-optic dysplasia) Hypothyroidism Hypoadrenalism Hypoparathyroidism
Intravenous nutrition	
Vascular abnormalities	
Severe haemolytic disease (inspissated bile syndrome)	
Drugs	

Only types 1 and 2 are amenable to surgery. Diagnosis is made by liver biopsy, interpreted by an experienced histopathologist, and confirmed at laparotomy by operative cholangiogram. Computerised tomography and magnetic resonance imaging have, to date, not been particularly helpful in diagnosis. HIDA scanning is only useful if there is a 'positive' scan (i.e. radioactivity appearing within the bowel indicating a patent bile duct). However, many patients with severe neonatal hepatitis have 'negative' scans and should still be subjected to diagnostic liver biopsy, and if in doubt an operative cholangiogram by day 60.

Is there intrahepatic biliary hypoplasia ?

Intrahepatic biliary hypoplasia is characterised by an absence or reduction in the number of bile ducts in portal tracts within the liver substance. An experienced histopathologist can usually distinguish this easily from biliary atresia where bile duct proliferation is the predominant feature. An adequate biopsy containing at least 20–30 portal tracts must be obtained, and this may require an open wedge resection. Syndromic hypoplasia, also known as **Alagille's syndrome**, is associated with a range of cardiovascular, skeletal, facial, ocular and rarely other system anomalies (**Figs 18.33**). The estimated incidence is 1/100,000 live births, it is probably autosomal dominant with variable expression and reduced penetrance and has sometimes been associated with a short-arm deletion of chromosome 20. Chronic cholestasis dominates the clinical picture although cyanotic heart disease may be the main problem in 10% of patients.

Is there neonatal hepatitis?

The commonest cause of persistent neonatal jaundice is idiopathic neonatal hepatitis. This is more prevalent in the preterm infant and those who have been subjected to hypoxia, infections, multiple drug therapy, abdominal surgery and intravenous nutrition. Other than jaundice and hepatomegaly, splenomegaly may occur in up to 50% of patients, and less commonly, a bleeding diathesis, hypoglycaemia, fluid retention and malabsorption are present. As well as a conjugated hyperbilirubinaemia, serum aspartate and alanine aminotransferases, alkaline phosphatase and gamma-glutamyltranspeptidase are elevated, but are not diagnostic. In more severe disease, prothrombin time may be prolonged and the serum albumin reduced.

Is there alpha-1 antitrypsin deficiency?

Alpha-1 antitrypsin is a potent protease inhibitor existing in at least 34 different allele types, coded for by a single gene on chromosome 14. The different phenotypes are distinguished by isoelectric focussing and labelled alphabetically according to their electrophoretic mobility. About 85% are PiM and the deficiency state is associated with PiZ or Pi nul. Approximately 50% of such infants have abnormal biochemical tests of liver function throughout the first decade and approximately 10% present with symptoms of liver disease. What initiates the liver disease is not clear, but the presence of diastase-resistant PAS-positive 2–20 nm globules around the periportal areas after 12 weeks of age is the characteristic histological feature, associated with clinical features indistinguishable from idiopathic neonatal hepatitis, and if severe, from those of extrahepatic biliary atresia (**Fig. 18.34**). Since this enzyme is an acute phase reactant, serum levels may be

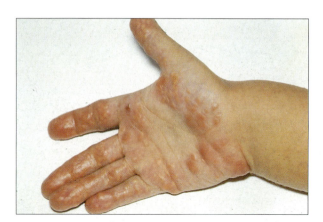

Fig. 18.33 Alagille syndrome showing palmar xanthomata as a consequence of severe cholestasis.

▶ **Extrahepatic features in Alagille's syndrome**

Feature	Frequency
Abnormal facies	75%
Posterior embryotoxon	70%
Skeletal anomalies (vertebral)	50%
Cardiac anomalies classically peripheral pulmonary artery sterosis	95%
Hypogonadism	Variable
Delayed mental development	Variable
Renal dysplasia	Variable
Pancreatic insufficiency	Variable

▶ **Investigations in neonatal conjugated hyperbilirubinaemia**

- Fractionated serum bilirubin (conjugated and unconjugated)
- Liver function tests, including ALT, AST, alkaline phosphatase, albumin, cholesterol and clotting studies
- Stool and urine colour
- Viral and bacterial cultures (see Table 18.17)
- Alpha-1-antitrypsin concentration and phenotype
- TSH and T4
- Urinary amino acids and reducing substances
- Serum amino acids and ferritin
- Sweat test
- Chest X-ray (cardiac lesions, hemivertebra)
- Abdominal ultrasound
- Radionucleotide imaging (e.g. HIDA scan)
- Liver biopsy
- Duodenal intubation
- Bone marrow aspiration
- Laparotomy, operative cholangiogram and definitive surgery

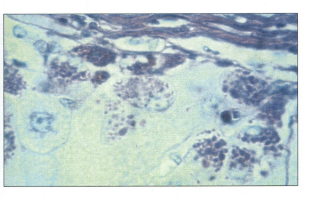

Fig. 18.34 Alpha-1 antitrypsin deficiency: liver biopsy with periodic acid–Schiff (PAS) stain, showing PAS-positive granules of alpha-1 antitrypsin trapped within hepatocytes, particularly in the periportal regions.

elevated in liver disease and thus a 'normal' level may be obtained in neonatal hepatitis, giving a false positive value. It is imperative that Pi typing is performed for all patients with conjugated hyperbilirubinaemia.

Is it Wilson's disease?

Wilson's disease should always be considered as a possible diagnosis in any older child with jaundice or elevated serum transaminase, particularly (but not exclusively) if associated with any evidence of psychiatric or neurological disease. Clinicians should be constantly alert to the possibility of this diagnosis, since early recognition, before the development of cirrhosis and neurological complications, can be effectively treated with pencillamine, trientine or zinc sulphate. Wilson's disease can present:

- Acutely with fulminant hepatic failure and haemolytic anaemia.
- Chronically with varying degrees of liver dysfunction.
- Insidiously with non-hepatic symptoms such as deteriorating school performance, personality changes, recurrent abdominal pain and renal tubular disorders.

Kayser–Fleischer rings are not present in the young before 7–8 years of age. Liver function studies are usually abnormal, but diagnosis is made by lowered serum caeruloplasmin concentration and increased urinary copper excretion after oral penicillamine loading, followed by direct measurement of liver copper concentration.

Management

Whatever its cause, the management of prolonged cholestasis is aimed at improving bile salt delivery to the proximal intestine, maximising absorption of nutrients and correcting deficiencies that may ensue. To improve bile flow, both phenobarbitone and cholestyramine have been used with variable success. The former is an hepatic enzyme-inducer and the latter is effective by binding bile salts in the lumen thereby preventing their reabsorption in the terminal ileum and reducing the 'negative feedback' to the liver. Cholestyramine should be given with food and not at the same time as fat-soluble vitamins. The fat-soluble vitamins A, D, E and K should be supplemented routinely (e.g. ketovite). Depending on prothrombin time, extra vitamin K may be needed as phytomenadione, 1 mg/day. Rickets may develop insidiously or quite acutely and should be treated with monthly intramuscular injection of 40,000 iu cholechocalciferol.

A progressive neuromuscular disorder, usually presenting with loss of the ankle reflexes, has been attributed to vitamin E deficiency after 18 months of age, and is prevented by vitamin E (α-tocopheryl acetate), in oral doses up to 200 mg/kg/day, depending on the vitamin E:lipid ratio.

Because their absorption does not depend on bile salt intraluminal concentration, infant feeds containing medium-chain triglycerides (MCT), (Pregestimil, Pepti-junior or Pregomin) are usually prescribed. For breast-fed infants MCT supplements can be given, and both breast- and bottle-fed infants may require additional calories in the form of glucose polymers.

MANAGEMENT OF CONDITIONS CAUSING JAUNDICE

Neonatal hepatitis

Approximately 80% of infants with idiopathic neonatal hepatitis make a complete recovery between six months and two years of age. Liver biopsy should be performed at six months if liver function tests are still abnormal, as some of these children have histological evidence of chronic active hepatitis, which often responds to oral prednisone.

There is no currently available specific treatment for alpha-1 antitrypsin deficiency and management is that of chronic cholestasis. About 33% of infants will recover, 33% will develop chronic liver disease with cirrhosis, portal hypertension, and hypersplenism, and 33% will deteriorate, and unless offered a liver transplant will usually die before their second birthday. Pi typing of parents and genetic counselling are essential because antenatal diagnosis is possible by chorionic villus sampling. Further children with the condition are likely to follow a similar clinical course as the first child.

Biliary atresia

For children with biliary atresia operated on by 60 days, there is an 80% chance of achieving some biliary drainage, and for 10–15%, a cure requiring no further surgery is achieved. Despite satisfactory biliary drainage however many children continue to develop progressive liver disease and cirrhosis. Biliary atresia is currently the commonest indication for liver transplantation in children.

Inherited disorders of metabolism

Appropriate treatment should be give to those infants with inherited and metabolic disorders such as galactosaemia, tyrosinaemia and cystic fibrosis. Intravenous ceredase (β-glucosidase) has been used for the treatment of non-neuropathic Gaucher's disease, and appears safe and effective in reducing bone pain, splenomegaly and improving the platelet count.

HEPATOMEGALY AND HEPATOSPLENOMEGALY: REACHING A DIAGNOSIS

Hepatomegaly may be due to:

- Hepatitis.
- Cirrhosis.
- Metabolic storage disease.
- Fatty infiltration (hyperalimentation, poorly controlled diabetes mellitus, or acutely, in Reye's syndrome).
- An increase in intrahepatic vascular or lymphatic fluid (congestive heart failure, Budd–Chiari syndrome, lymphangiomata).
- Primary or secondary tumour.
- Rarely, Riedel's lobe (a downward tongue-like, but 'normal' projection from the right lobe, which may cause unnecessary investigation, but may have to be distinguished from an abscess, hydatid cyst or haematoma).

Liver tumours may be benign, malignant or metastatic. Primary liver tumours are the third most common solid abdominal neoplasms in childhood (accounting for approximately 15% of abdominal masses). Benign liver tumours make up about 35%. The commonest is haemangioendothelioma, which presents with hepatomegaly, heart failure and cutaneous haemangiomas. Diagnosis is made by ultrasound, computerised axial tomography, magnetic resonance imaging, angiography and where possible, a liver biopsy.

▶ **Storage disease causing hepatomegaly**

- Glycogen storage diseases: twelve types and subtypes are now recognised
- Mucopolysaccharidosis: including Hurler's, Hunter, San Filippo, Maroteaux–Lausy and Sly diseases
- Macrolipidosis: including Type II (I cell disease)
- Oligosaccharidosis: including sialidosis, mannosidosis and fucosidosis
- Lipid storage diseases: including Tay–Sachs, Gaucher's, Wolman, Taugier, Niemann–Pick, and cholesterol ester storage diseases

Ascites

Neonatal ascites may be a presenting feature of metabolic disorders, including sialidosis, gangliosidosis, Gaucher's disease, Wolman's disease, neonatal haemochromatosis and Neimann–Pick type C. The identification of vacuolated lymphocytes in the peripheral blood, storage cells in the bone marrow and increased urinary excretion of oligosaccharides will then lead to the appropriate diagnosis.

Acute ascites can occur in any patient with underlying liver disease, usually precipitated by sudden events such as alimentary bleeding, intra-abdominal surgery, anaesthesia or the development of hepatoma. Any previously-well child presenting with acute ascites should be suspected as having the Budd–Chiari syndrome, intestinal tuberculosis or disseminated intra-abdominal malignancy.

Investigations should include a diagnostic peritoneal tap with measurement of protein content (to distinguish exudate from transudate), a cytological spin for malignant cells, Ziehl–Neelsen stain for acid-fast bacilli and routine bacteriological culture. Hepatic ultrasound may show an enlarged caudate lobe compressing the inferior vena cava in Budd–Chiari syndrome as this lobe has separate venous drainage and hypertrophies. Hepatic venography and, where clotting allows, liver biopsy may be the only way to confirm the diagnosis. Computerised tomography may show peritoneal malignant deposits as may laparoscopy, which also has

▶ **Liver tumours**

Benign

- Haemangioendothelioma
- Cavernous haemangiomia
- Mesenchymal hamartoma
- Focal nodular hyperplasia
- Lymphangioma
- Adenoma
- Teratoma
- Infective cysts

Malignant

- Hepatoblastoma
- Hepatocellular carcinoma
- Embryonal rhabdomyosarcoma
- Angiosarcoma
- Teratocarcinoma
- Cholangiocarcinoma
- Histiocystosis X
- Non-Hodgkin's lymphoma

Secondary

- Leukaemia
- Lymphoma
- Neuroblastoma
- Wilms' tumour

the potential advantage of obtaining tissue. Intra-abdominal tuberculosis can be present with a negative Mantoux test and Ziehl–Neelsen stain, necessitating the institution of antituberculous therapy (having excluded other causes) before the final cultures are reported.

MANAGEMENT OF CONDITIONS CAUSING HEPATOMEGALY

Hepatitis, cirrhosis and heart failure

The management of hepatitis (either viral, drug-induced, radiation-induced), cirrhosis, congestive heart failure, Budd–Chiari syndrome and abscesses is essentially the same as in adults and is dealt with in Chapters 13, 14 and 15.

Storage diseases

The various storage diseases, resulting in hepatomegaly, with the exception of Gaucher's disease (see above), are treated symptomatically, with correction of hypoglycaemia, appropriate management of mental retardation, and genetic counselling of parents following a histological or biochemical diagnosis of the defect. Liver transplantation offers an ever-increasing hope of long-term survival for many of these patients.

Reye's syndrome

Reye's syndrome is an acute sporadic encephalopathy with panlobular microvesicular fat accumulation in the liver, characterised by a reversible abnormality of mitochondrial structure in liver, muscle and neural tissue (**Fig. 18.35**).

Typically, Reye's syndrome occurs during the recovery phase of what appears to be an unremarkable viral infection, including chickenpox and influenza A. Profuse and persistent vomiting is often the first sign, although neurological signs can occur quickly, with changes in behaviour, agitated delirium, fits and deepening coma.

Biochemical signs of liver dysfunction include elevated serum ammonia and transaminase levels, prolongation of prothrombin time, and, if severe, hypoglycaemia. If the clotting studies allow, a liver biopsy is diagnostic, and shows fatty microvacuolation of the parenchyma, initially seen on frozen section with Sudan dyes. Electron microscopic examination shows swollen pleomorphic mitochondria, loss of dense bodies, loss of glycogen, and triglyceride accumulation in small droplets and, occasionally, proliferation of the smooth endoplastic reticulum and an increase in peroxisomal numbers.

The reported incidence of Reye's syndrome to the British Paediatric Association surveillance programme has fallen from 40 definite cases in 1981/82 to 15 in 1991/92. The current median age of presentation is 16.5 months. The reduction in incidence is probably largely due to the avoidance of salicylates in children under 12 years of age.

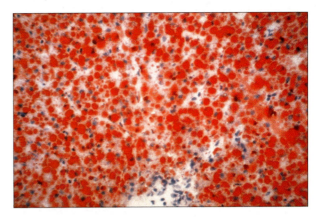

Fig. 18.35 Reye's syndrome showing acute microvesicular fat accumulation (stained red) in a frozen section from a liver biopsy.

Management of Reye's syndrome should take place in the intensive care unit of a regional gastroenterology centre. Therapy is aimed at preventing, minimising and correcting the metabolic abnormalities and controlling increased intracranial pressure. Despite such efforts, 40% of patients still die, and 10–60% of survivors have significant neuro/-logical defects. Treatment usually consists of 10% intravenous glucose given via a central venous line, replacement of clotting factors with fresh frozen plasma, intracranial pressure monitoring and control of cerebral oedema with mannitol, barbiturate sedation and hyperventilation. Oral neomycin, lactulose or enemas, to decrease ammonia production, are frequently used, but there is no evidence that they influence outcome. Similarly, H_2 antagonists are also often prescribed to prevent acute ulcer formation and gastrointestinal bleeding, but there are no controlled trials to justify their use. They have, in fact, been reported rarely to cause an encephalopathy.

Reye's-like syndrome

Reye's-like syndrome can be caused by certain liver enzyme deficiencies and some inborn errors of organic acidaemias (ornithine transcarbamylase, carbamyl phosphatase synthetase, carnitine, β-oxidation defects) and familial erythrophagocytic reticulosis. Where there is a history of an unexplained previous sibling death, or when a child presents with a recurrent Reye's-like syndrome, it is imperative to obtain urine during the acute illness for organic acids and to consider liver biopsy to measure the specifically identified enzymes once recovery has occurred.

Liver tumours

Treatment depends on diagnosis, but may include surgical excision, chemotherapy and even liver transplantation. Haemangioendotheliomas have been treated with varying degrees of success with oral steroids, but a recent intervention study using interferon-α shows promising results.

▶ **Disorders for which liver transplantation may be considered**

Parenchymal end-stage disease

- Biliary atresia
- Alpha-1 antitrypsin deficiency
- Idiopathic hepatitis
- Chronic active hepatitis
- Sclerosing cholangitis
- Budd–Chiari syndrome

Metabolic disorders

- Tyrosinaemia Type I
- Crigler–Najjar Types I and II
- Protoporphyria
- Some glycogen storage diseases
- Some urea cycle defects
- Homozygous Type II hyperlipoproteinaemia
- Haemophilia

Acute hepatic failure

- Acute hepatitis (viral)
- Acute hepatitis (drug)
- Wilson's disease
- Budd–Chiari syndrome

Malignancy

Even where confined to the liver has a poor outcome, with a two-year survival of 25–30%

SPLENOMEGALY AND PORTAL HYPERTENSION

Splenomegaly secondary to liver disease is usually the result of portal hypertension or concurrent infiltration with an abnormal metabolite. The treatment of portal hypertension, varices and hypersplenism is essentially as for adults and is dealt with in Chapter 6. Splenectomy for hypersplenism is rarely indicated in children and should be avoided where possible, particularly if liver transplantation may be considered in the future. Bleeding oesophageal varices respond well to both sclerotherapy and intravenous somatostatin.

ASCITES

Ascites may develop insidiously, usually as a result of portal hypertension secondary to liver disease. Treatment is as for adults, with sodium restriction, diuretics, albumin infusions, and in refractory disease, paracentesis, with or without reinfusions using automated ultrafiltration and, rarely, peritoneal–venous shunts (LeVeen shunt).

FAILURE TO THRIVE

Reaching a diagnosis

Failure to thrive describes the infant or child who does not gain weight or height at the expected rate for his or her age. It is defined by reference to growth charts, on which serial measurements of weight and height have been recorded. When a child's weight remains below the third centile, or crosses centiles downwards a diagnosis of failure to thrive is made.

Full assessment includes a family history of growth in weight and height, pregnancy and feeding, developmental progress, symptoms of gastrointestinal disease, or metabolic disturbance, and a social report from a health visitor or social worker. Physical examination should concentrate on ruling out organic causes and detecting dysmorphic features and signs of abuse, deprivation or neglect. A full dietary assessment should be made by a paediatric dietitian.

Failure to thrive may be due to insufficient intake, excessive requirements or excessive losses of nutrients. The former is the most important and common cause. It is important to distinguish proportional (symmetric) from disproportionate (asymmetric) growth retardation: the former suggests a chronic, often intrauterine cause, while the latter (poor weight gain with preservation of length and head growth) suggests a peri- or postnatal cause.

In the toddler, it is important to rule out coeliac disease and cystic fibrosis (see below). In the older child inflammatory bowel disease, chronic infection, including giardiasis, renal disease (urinary tract infection, renal tubular acidosis, chronic renal failure), immunodeficiency and chronic hepatic disease are other causes.

Full laboratory investigation of unexplained failure to thrive includes full blood count, red cell folate, white cell count, plasma urea and electrolytes, creatinine, calcium, phosphate, alkaline phosphatase, immunoglobulins, liver function tests, stool microscopy, urinary microscopy and culture and chromatography, chromosomal studies, jejunal biopsy, sweat test and skeletal survey. All these tests should be carried out in the child in whom dietary intake is adequate and non-organic causes have been ruled out.

▶ **Failure to thrive**

- Caused by insufficent intake, increased metabolic requirements or excessive nutrient losses
- Principal organic causes to rule out in early childhood are cystic fibrosis and coeliac disease
- Non-organic causes may require coordinated care by paediatrician, dietician, health visitor and/or social worker

▶ **Causes of failure to thrive in early life**

Deficient intake	Increased metabolic demands
Maternal	**Infant**
Poor lactation	Congenital lung disease
Incorrectly prepared feeds	Congenital heart disease
Unusual milk or other feeds	Congenital liver disease
Inadequate care	Congenital infection
	Anaemia
	Inborn errors of metabolism
	Thyroid disease (hyper and hypo)
	Cystic fibrosis
Infant	**Excessive nutrient losses**
Prematurity	Gastro-oesophageal reflux
Small for gestational age	Pyloric stenosis
Oropalatal abnormalities	Necrotising enterocolitis
Neuromuscular disorders	Gastroenteritis
Intracranial disease	Protein-energy malnutrition
Genetic disorders	Milk-protein intolerance
(chromosomal, dysmorphic,	Persistent diarrhoea
skeletal)	Lactose intolerance
	Short bowel syndrome

Is it cystic fibrosis?

Cystic fibrosis affects about 1/2500 live births in the UK. It is due to autosomal recessive inheritance of defects in a gene on chromosome 7, which encodes a membrane transporter protein involved in chloride transport. The gene defect is carried by about 1 in 20 in Caucasian populations. The diagnosis is usually first made soon after birth by immuno-reactive trypsin screening, or in early childhood when respiratory infection, failure to thrive or signs of exocrine pancreatic insufficiency appear. However 15–20% of babies with the condition present in the neonatal period with meconium ileus.

Diagnosis is by the sweat test, using pilocarpine ionto-phoresis. Because it is not always possible to obtain suffic-ient sweat for an accurate test during the neonatal period, particularly in the preterm infant, the sweat test should not usually be done before four weeks. Sweat sodium of 80–120 mmol/l is diagnostic. About 75% of those with cystic fibrosis have the delta F508 genotype. Genotyping can also be used to screen for unaffected heterozygote carriers.

The pancreas is affected prenatally, but infants do not usually have steatorrhoea until there is more than 90% loss of pancreatic exocrine function. Duodenal intubation with stimulation of exocrine pancreatic function results in decreased volume of secretions, with depressed bicarbonate and en-zyme concentrations. Intestinal obstruction and perforation, poor growth, respiratory infections, prolonged jaundice, rectal prolapse and failure to thrive in early life demand a sweat test if no other cause is found. Older children develop signs of chronic pulmonary infection, with clubbing.

MANAGEMENT OF CONDITIONS CAUSING FAILURE TO THRIVE

General principles of management

Nutritional requirements are based on the infant's size, gestation and clinical condition. Reference to appropriate centile charts for weight, length and head circumference, and comparison of the infant's growth centiles with those of his parents, are essential in making calculations of nutritional needs. These should be based on the baby's expected weight for age in order to provide adequate protein and calories for catch-up growth.

Careful observation of the infant's feeding behaviour, and of the mother's abilities to feed (test weighing the infant if breast-fed, and supervision of formula preparation if bottle-fed) should be undertaken. This may require hospital admission, but separation of mother and baby should be avoided unless essential to determine accurate nutritional intake. If there are increased metabolic needs (e.g. in congenital heart and lung disease), tube feeding may sometimes be indicated. Severe emotional deprivation may delay catch-up growth. Failure of adequate dietary intake to promote weight gain suggests underlying disease, such as renal failure or chronic infection (e.g. tuberculosis).

Cystic fibrosis

Management is aimed at optimising nutrition and prevent-ing pulmonary infection. Infants with cystic fibrosis have increased nutritional requirements not only because of the effects of the disease (respiratory infections, steatorrhoea), but also because there may be a basic defect in energy metabolism. There are positive advantages in breast feeding, which should be encouraged as long as an adequate daily intake is ensured. A standard cows' milk based formula supplemented with additional carbohydrate, and micro-nutrients is an alternative. A semi-elemental protein hydrolysate (e.g. Pregestimil) may be useful in the infant who has had meconium ileus or who has growth failure with malabsorption and steatorrhoea. A calorie intake of at least 130% of RDA (150 kcal/kg/d), in which medium-chain triglycerides replace other fats in the diet, should be given. Pancreatic enzyme supplements should be given with each meal, the dose 'titrated' against the degree of steatorrhoea. Fat-soluble vitamins should be provided. Physiotherapy of the chest should be instituted from diagnosis. Prophylactic flucloxacillin reduces the incidence of pulmonary infection.

Early recognition of cystic fibrosis and improved management have ensured that a growing number of affected infants survive to adulthood. With the identification of the defective gene reliable antenatal diagnosis and genetic counselling have become available. It is the responsiblity of the paediatrician who makes the diagnosis of cystic fibrosis in a neonate to ensure that genetic counselling is provided to the parents before their next pregnancy.

Meconium ileus and distal intestinal obstruction syndrome

Meconium ileus and distal intestinal obstruction syndrome (DIOS) are caused by impacted viscid meconium or undigested material in the distal small intestine. Meconium ileus is the presenting feature of 10–15% of infants with cystic fibrosis: there is failure to pass meconium, abdominal distension, bile-stained vomiting and occasionally intestinal perforation. Plain abdominal radiography reveals signs of obstruction (fluid levels) with granular bowel contents. Calcification suggests meconium peritonitis. Diagnosis may be confirmed with gastrograffin enema, which may also relieve the obstruction. If not, surgery is indicated.

In the older child with DIOS, with features of partial or complete obstruction and visible or palpable loops of bowel, acetylcysteine, 10–20 g in 100 ml of water, given as 10 ml three times daily orally, or as an enema using 50 ml of solution with 50 ml water, should be given. Surgery is indicated if medical treatment fails.

Protein energy malnutrition

Protein energy malnutrition is a major cause of failure to thrive in the developing world where it accounts for around 50% of all deaths under five years of age. It is caused by a diet inadequate in energy and protein, often associated with weanling diarrhoea, and exacerbated by recurrent or chronic systemic infection. Micronutrient deficiencies frequently accompany calorie and protein deficit. It may be divided broadly into kwashiorkor and marasmus.

Kwashiorkor

In kwashiorkor, oedema is a dominant sign. It is accompanied by skin pigmentation, hyperkeratosis and desquamation, with sparse discoloured hair. Hidden by the oedema are muscle wasting and weight loss (**Fig. 18.36**). The child is often apathetic and developmentally retarded. Kwashiorkor follows weaning onto a diet inadequate in protein, and may be precipitated or potentiated by measles, gastroenteritis and malaria. There is biochemical evidence of hypoalbuminaemia, hypoglycaemia, hypokalaemia and immunodeficiency.

▶ **Special diets for infants with cystic fibrosis**

- Human milk

- Adapted cows' milk formula (e.g. Gold Cap (SMA), Premium (Cow and Gate)

- High-energy milks (e.g. Formula above with added glucose polymer: Polycal (Cow and Gate), Caloreen (Roussel) or Maxijul (SHS)

- 'Cystic milk' (high-protein, high-energy), prepared from:
  - 8.4 g adapted cows' milk formula, as above
  - 7.2 g glucose polymer, as above
  - 5.6 g dried skimmed milk (e.g. Marvel (Cadbury's))
  - 120 ml boiled water

- Energy density and macronutrient composition/100 ml feed:
  - 7.5 kcal
  - 2.5g protein
  - 2.0 g fat (g)
  - 12.0g carbohydrate

- Semi-elemental (e.g. Pregestimil (Bristol–Myers))

- Protein hydrolysates (Prejomin (Milupa)

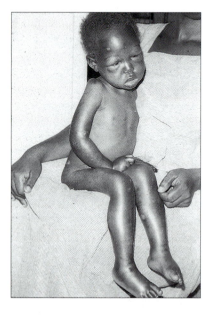

Fig. 18.36 A child with kwashiorkor. Courtesy of Dr RG Whitehouse.

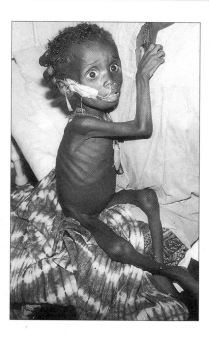

Fig. 18.37 A child with marasmus. Courtesy of Dr RG Whitehouse.

Marasmus

In marasmus the dominant sign is wasting, with loss of subcutaneous fat (diminished skin-fold thickness), a scaphoid abdomen, and muscle wasting. The child is less than 60% weight for height (**Fig. 18.37**). Gastrointestinal function is often depressed, with a persistent enteropathy. Treatment aims to provide adequate energy and protein to restore normal nutritional status, and then to ensure normal growth.

FURTHER READING

Abdominal pain

Apley J. 1975. *The Child with Abdominal Pains*. Oxford, Blackwell Scientific Publications.

Barr RG. 1991. Colic and gas. In: *Pediatric Gastrointestinal Disease*. Walker WA, Durie PR, Hamilton JR, Walker-Smith JA, Watkins JB (eds). Toronto, Decker.

David TJ. 1993. *Food and Food Additive Intolerance in Childhood*. Oxford: Blackwell Scientific Publications.

Eastham EJ. 1991. Peptic ulcer. In: *Pediatric Gastrointestinal Disease*. Walker WA, Durie PR, Hamilton JR, Walker-Smith JA, Watkins JB (eds). Toronto, Decker.

Murphy MS. Management of recurrent abdominal pain. *Arch Dis Child* 1993; **69**: 409–15.

Oesophageal reflux

Davis CF, Young DG. 1992. Congenital defects and surgical problems. In: *Textbook of Neonatology*. Roberton NRC (ed), pp 655–86. London, Churchill Livingstone.

Winter HS, Madara JL, Stafford RJ, Quinlan JE, Goldman H. Intraepithelial eosinophils. A new diagnostic criterion for reflux esophagitis. *Gastroenterology* 1982; **83**: 818–23.

Wright VM. 1991. Congenital anomalies of the esophagus, stomach and duodenum. In: *Pediatric Gastrointestinal Disease*. Walker WA, Durie PR, Hamilton JR, Walker-Smith JA, Watkins JB (eds), pp 366–70, 423–6. Toronto, Decker.

Malabsorption and diarrhoea

Feldman B, Peters J, Belohradsky BH. Shwachman's syndrome. *Pediatr Rev Commun* 1992; **6**: 195–209.

Goodchild MC, Dodge JA. 1989. *Cystic Fibrosis: Manual of Diagnosis and Management.* London, Bailliere Tindall.

Kosloske AM, Musumeche CA. Necrotising enterocolitis of the neonate. *Clin Perinatol* 1989; **6**: 97–111.

Lucas A, Cole TJ. Breast milk and neonatal necrotising enterocolitis. *Lancet* 1990; **336**: 1519–23.

Phillips AD, Schmitz J. Familial microvillous atrophy: a clinico-pathological survey of 23 cases. *J Pediatr Gastroenterol Nutr* 1992; **14**: 380–96.

Schwartz MZ, Maeda K. Short bowel syndrome in infants and children. *Pediatr Clin North Am* 1985; **32**: 1265–79.

Seidman E, LeLeiko N, Ament M et al. Nutritional issues in pediatric inflammatory bowel disease. *J Pediatr Gastroenterol Nutr* 1991; **12**: 424–38.

Sullivan PB. Cows' milk induced intestinal bleeding in infancy. *Arch Dis Child* 1993; **68**: 240–5.

Sullivan PB, Marsh MN, Mirakian R, Hill SM, Milla PJ, Neale G. Chronic diarrhea and malnutrition—histology of the small intestinal lesion. *J Pediatr Gastroenterol Nutr* 1991; **12**: 195–203.

Vanderhoof JA et al. Short bowel syndrome. *J Pediatr Gastroenterol Nutr* 1992; **14**: 359–70.

Walker-Smith JA. Clinical and diagnostic features of Crohn's disease and ulcerative colitis in childhood. *Balliere's Clin Gastroenterol* 1994; **8**: 65–81.

Constipation

Clayden G, Agnarsson U. 1991. *Constipation in Childhood*. Oxford, Oxford University Press.

Weaver LT, Steiner H. The bowel habits of young children. *Arch Dis Child* 1984; **59**: 649–52.

Jaundice

Alagille D, Odievre M, Gautier M, Dommergues J P. Hepatic ductular hypoplasia associated with characteristic facies, vertebral malformations, retarded physical, mental and sexual development and cardiac murmur. *J. Pediatr* 1975; **86**: 63–71.

Glasgow J F T. Clinical features and prognosis in Reye's syndrome. Arch Dis *Child* 1984; **59**: 230–5.

Hall R J, Karrer F M. Biliary atresia: perspective on transplantation. Pediatr Surg *Int* 1990; **5**: 94–9.

Mowat A P, Psacharopoulas HT, Williams R. Extrahepatic biliary atresia versus neonatal hepatitis. A review of 137 prospectively investigated infants. *Arch Dis Child* 1976; **51**: 763–70.

Valaes T N, Harvey-Wilkes K. Pharmacological approaches to the prevention and treatment of neonatal hyperbilirubinaemia. *Clin Perinat* 1990, **17**: 245–273.

Failure to thrive and malnutrition

Frank DA, Zeisel SH. Failure to thrive. *Ped Clin North Am* 1988; **35**: 1181–206.

Waterlow JV. *Protein Energy Malnutrition*. 1992, London, Edward Arnold.

19
STOMAS

COUNSELLING

In the UK there are approximately 50,000 patients with permanent colostomies and 15,000 with ileostomies. Excellent patient-support groups are available (see below), and it is important for the patient to realise from the beginning that:

- He/she is not alone.
- Help is always available.
- A virtually normal life-style should be possible.

It is particularly important that the patient is given adequate explanation and reassurance pre-operatively. This should include an unrushed visit from a stoma care nurse who should also be able to provide the patient with some of the excellent explanatory booklets that are available. It should usually be possible to arrange a visit from a volunteer stoma patient (or 'ostomate') who can give first hand experience and reassurance.

Useful addresses

- British Colostomy Association, 38/39 Eccleston Square, London SW1V 1PB.
- Ileostomy Association of Great Britain and Ireland, Amblehurst House, Black Scotch Lane, Mansfield, Nottinghamshire, NG18 4PF.

SITE OF THE STOMA

The stoma should be sited over the centre of the rectus muscle, and usually below the umbilicus for a permanent stoma. The precise site should be decided pre-operatively

▶ **Pre-operative preparation for stoma patients should include:**

- Counselling from a stoma care nurse
- Visit from a stoma patient volunteer (if possible)
- Literature on stoma care
- Careful siting of the stoma using a water-filled stoma bag

with the patient wearing a stoma appliance containing 200 ml water and tested in the sitting and standing positions. The intestine should pass through the rectus in a straight line to the stoma.

Continent pouch

Parks' ileo-anal pouch

It is increasingly common for an ileo-anal pouch (Fig. 19.1) to be constructed in young patients requiring colectomy for ulcerative colitis or polyposis to remove the need for a stoma.

A reservoir is constructed by doubling back the distal 50 cm of ileum and joining the limbs of the 'J' together. There are various ways of forming the pouch, which some surgeons construct as an 'S' or 'W' shape either hand-sutured or stapled. The simpler pouch structures generally work at least as well as those that are more complicated. The pouch is then anastomosed to the lower 1–2 cm of rectal mucosa at

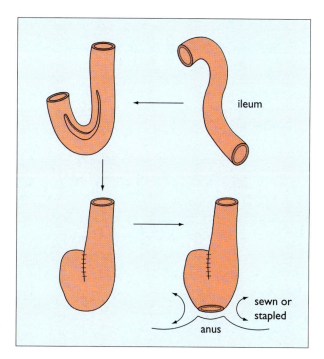

Fig. 19.1 Construction of a J-shaped ileo-anal pouch.

the top of the anal sphincter. This leaves a small risk of malignancy in the rectal mucosa, which therefore necesitates long-term annual surveillance, but this is simply achieved.

The results are generally very good. Average stool frequency is about four bowel actions during the day and one at night. About 65% of patients are completely continent, while about 5–10% of patients have troublesome problems requiring more than a pad. Postoperative complications are quite common however, local leakage and sepsis requiring reoperation in up to 40% of patients.

Pouch construction is contraindicated in Crohn's disease because of a very high rate of pouch inflammation. Milder inflammation (pouchitis) occurs in up to 50% of patients with ulcerative colitis following pouch construction, but not in patients with polyposis. The pouchitis usually responds well to either sulphasalazine or metronidazole.

▶ **Parks ileo-anal pouch**

- Excellent results in about 65%
- Most patients need to get up once at night
- Contraindicated in Crohn's disease
- Pouchitis affects up to 50% of patients with ulcerative colitis
- Pouchitis is usually mild and responds to sulphasalazine or metronidazole

Kock pouch

A continent ileostomy, described by Kock (**Fig. 19.2**), is sometimes performed either to avoid the inconvenience of continual wearing of an appliance or in the occasional patient with severe contact dermatitis. The stoma is sited in the lower abdomen. A reservoir is constructed out of a 'U' loop of ileum and a valve fashioned by retrograde intussusception of the ileum into the pouch. The patient then empties the pouch using a soft catheter. The operation is relatively difficult and suture-line leakage can be a problem. If the pouch has to be taken down then about 45 cm of ileum will have been 'wasted.' Continence rates of 70–95% are reported.

MANAGEMENT OF STOMA-RELATED PROBLEMS

Fluid and electrolyte problems

The average ileostomy patient with a conventional Brooke spout ileostomy has a three-fold increase in faecal volume, to about 500 ml/per day. Faecal sodium loss usually increases four-fold to about 40 mmol/day, but potassium loss actually diminishes slightly if the ileostomy is working normally. The kidneys compensate by excreting a low volume of low sodium, but otherwise concentrated urine.

Patients will have greater fluid and electrolyte losses if they have:

- Persisting small bowel disease (e.g. Crohn's disease).
- An extensive small bowel resection.
- Intercurrent gastroenteritis.
  Gastroenteritis may result in rapid and very serious loss of fluid, sodium and potassium.

Fig. 19.2 Construction of Kock continent ileostomy.

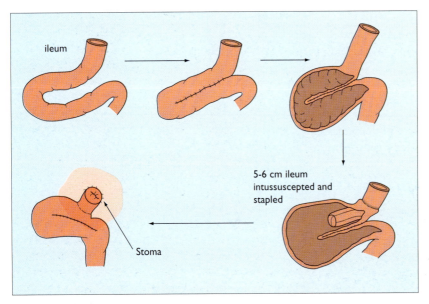

ileum

5-6 cm ileum intussuscepted and stapled

Stoma

In patients with a chronically high ileostomy output loperamide (up to 16 mg/day) is often useful and is preferable to codeine. The fluid and electrolyte intake should be deliberately increased if faecal volume is persistently higher than 1 litre/day. Absorption is much better if carbohydrate is included in the fluid/electrolyte mixture.

The World Health Organization recommend a solution for fluid and electrolyte replacement comprising:

- Water, 1 litre.
- Glucose, 20 g (four heaped 5 ml spoons).
- Trisodium citrate dihydrate, 2.9g (just less than one level spoon).
- Sodium chloride, 3.5 g (just less than one level spoon).
- Potassium chloride 1.5 g (half a spoonful).

If all these constituents are not available then one teaspoonful of salt (120 mmmol) and four teaspoonfuls of sugar in one litre of water should be taken as a daily supplement.

All patients with an ileostomy should be encouraged to increase their fluid intake because of the increased risk of urinary calculi that results from the chronically concentrated urine. In occasional patients with a persistent high output it may be necessary to consider maintenance somatostatin therapy (e.g. octreotide, three times daily subcutaneously). This form of therapy is very expensive however and also increases fat malabsorption. In patients with persistent high output it is important to exclude partial stoma obstruction as a cause.

Trace element and vitamin deficiencies

Calcium and magnesium losses are increased, but do not usually cause clinical problems. Vitamin B_{12} deficiency is usually only a problem if appreciable terminal ileum has been resected (i.e. 20–30 cm) or if there is terminal ileal disease. Bile salt deficiency may occur and is responsible for an increased rate of gallstone formation, but bile salt supplements cause unacceptable diarrhoea so are not appropriate.

▶ **Fluid loss from an ileostomy stoma**

- Averages about 500 ml/day
- Loss > 1 litre/day requires replacement therapy
- Replacement therapy should be with a salt/sugar/water mixture (e.g. as recommended by the World Health Organization, see text)
- Loperamide, up to 16 mg daily, may be useful
- Persistent high output may be due to obstruction

Odour

The offensive odour of faeces results mainly from the production of short-chain fatty acids such as butyrate by bacterial fermentation of unabsorbed carbohydrate (fibre). Reduction in dietary fibre may therefore be helpful. Modern stoma appliances have good leak-proofing and the addition of activated charcoal, which is often incorporated in the appliance, should help avoid odour. Ileostomies usually give little problem with odour.

Obstruction

Obstruction at the stoma may present with either pain or increased fluid losses and should always be considered in the patient with persistently high ileostomy losses.

Causes include:

- Poor construction of the stoma.
- Adhesions.
- Local sepsis.
- Obstruction by dietary fibre (e.g. fruit pith).

Digital examination, barium examination of the stoma and endoscopy via the stoma may all be required to establish the diagnosis. Obstruction by dietary fibre may be relieved in hospital by irrigation using a soft catheter. Other problems are likely to require surgical revision of the stoma.

Herniation

Significant herniation is rare around ileostomies, but may affect up to 25% of colostomies. It is then a potential cause of obstruction and usually makes appliance fitting difficult. Surgical repair usually requires the use of a prosthetic patch.

Bleeding

A small amount of bleeding is to be expected during cleaning of the stoma. Postoperative bleeding may require ligation of a mesenteric or submucosal vessel. Persistent chronic bleeding from a colostomy should raise the possibility of metachronous carcinoma.

Malignancy

Carcinoma in an ileostomy is extremely rare. Carcinoma in or close to a colostomy is fairly common and arises either as a result of recurrence of the initial tumour or development of a metachronous tumour. Change in colostomy habit or persistent bleeding therefore need investigation.

Ischaemia

Ischaemia is usually an immediate postoperative problem, which becomes apparent in the first 48 hours. Some duskiness is common, but progressive darkening is worrying. The stoma should be carefully inspected and if the discoloration extends through the abdominal wall then laparotomy and stoma revision is required.

Late ischaemia may occasionally occur due to intermittent prolapse. Distal ischaemia with sloughing of the spout can result from overtight appliance flanges.

Effluent dermatitis

Effluent dermatitis affects the area immediately around the stoma that is in contact with faeces. Barrier creams containing zinc may be useful. Candida infection should be considered particularly in patients who have recently received broad-spectrum antibiotics. A local fungicide such as clotrimazole should then be used.

Contact dermatitis

Allergy to the adhesive or appliance material results in dermatitis corresponding to the shape of the adhesive material. Patch testing should be perforned until a suitable appliance material and adhesive is identified. Rarely it may prove impossible to identify a suitable adhesive and when it is occasionally severe it may be necessary to convert to a continent (e.g. Kock) ileostomy.

Psychological and sexual problems

The extent of psychological problems will be affected by many factors including the patient's age, marital status and previous health.

- In a young married patient who has had a poor quality of life because of troublesome colitis, colectomy and ileostomy often brings a huge sense of freedom and relief and remarkably few marital or social problems.
- For the older patient who has suddenly been through the combined traumas of cancer diagnosis and colostomy, adjustment may be much more difficult and depression is common.

Continual after-care and support from the stoma-care nurse and general practitioner will help to reduce this.

In a young unmarried patient there will almost always be anxiety that the stoma will be offputting to a potential spouse. Some help may be obtained from introduction to other young patient volunteers who have been in a similar situation.

Sexual problems occur in up to 30% of patients, but are less common in younger patients and in those who had satisfactory previous sexual function. Impotence caused by surgical damage to the pelvic autonomic nerves during colectomy is fortunately now very rare, affecting less than 1% of patients.

Life expectancy for ileostomates is normal.

Stomal obstruction during pregnancy is a problem and a careful watch should be kept on stomal function. Vaginal delivery is possible for about 65% of patients.

FURTHER READING

The operations

Becker JM. Ileal pouch-anal anastomosis: current status and controversies. *Surgery* 1993; **113**: 599–602.

Keighley MRB, Grobler S, Bain L. An audit of restorative proctocolectomy. *Gut* 1993; **34**: 680–4.

Kock NG, Myrvold HE, Nilsson LO, Philipson BM. Continent ileostomy. An account of 314 patients. *Acta Chir Scand* 1981; **147**: 67–72.

Parks AG, Nicholls RJ, Belliveau P. Proctocolectomy with ileal reservoir and anal anastomosis. *Br J Surg* 1980; **67**: 533–8.

Sagar PM, Taylor BA. Pelvic Ileal reservoirs: the options. *Br J Surg* 1994; **81**: 325–32.

Pathophysiology

Bingham S, Cummings JH, McNeil NI. Diet and health of people with an ileostomy. *Br J Nutr* 1982; **47**: 399–406.

Nightingale JMD, Lennard-Jones JE, Walker ER, Farthing MJG. Oral/salt supplements to compensate for jejunostomy losses: comparison of sodium chloride capsules, glucose electrolyte solution, and glucose polymer electrolyte solution. *Gut* 1992; **33**: 759–61.

Psychological aspects and counselling

Doughty D. Role of the enterostomal therapy nurse in ostomy patient rehabilitation. *Cancer* 1992; **70** (5 Suppl.): 1390–92.

Jeter KF. Perioperative teaching and counselling. *Cancer* 1992; **70** (5 Suppl.): 1346–69.

Rubin GP, Devlin HB. The quality of life with a stoma. *Br J Hosp Med* 1987; **39**: 300–6.

Young CH, Shipes E. Sexual implications of stoma surgery. *Clin Gastroenterol* 1982; **11**: 383–96.

20
ENTERAL AND PARENTERAL FEEDING

ENTERAL FEEDING

Indications

- **Malnutrition** should be the major indication, but is surprisingly hard to define:
- **Weight loss** of more than 10% is worrying, but depending on the circumstances, may not necessarily correlate with prognosis.
- **Skin-fold thickness** may be unreliable in patients with oedema.
- Serum **albumin** falls rapidly in patients with sepsis or inflammation as part of the acute phase response so does not always mirror nutritional state (although a serum albumin higher than 35 g/l is reassuring).
- **Muscle wasting** or **weakness** are more important indications, but often poorly quantified.

In practice **the most important indications** for enteral feeding are often either:

- A history of **inadequate dietary intake** (e.g. in a patient with alcoholic hepatitis).
- A history of **swallowing difficulty**, which will inevitably lead to malnutrition if enteral support is not provided.

In **Crohn's disease** enteral feeding is increasingly used in adequately nourished patients for its ability to induce remission in patients with active small bowel disease (see Chapter 3).

▶ **Common indications for enteral feeding**

- Malnutrition
- Inflammatory bowel disease
- Hepatic failure
- Renal failure
- Swallowing difficulties (e.g. tumour, cerebrovascular accident , motor neurone disease)
- Surgery or trauma

Type of feed
Nitrogen source

Amino acid- or peptide-based ('elemental') feeds tend to be used much more than necessary on the theoretical assumptions that they will be better absorbed and less allergenic. There is little objective justification for this. They are more hyperosmolar, less palatable and much more expensive than whole-protein feeds and are very rarely indicated. Clinical comparisons have generally shown no significant improvement in nitrogen absorption from elemental feeds compared with whole-protein ('polymeric') feeds. Even after total pancreatectomy, where there are sound theoretical reasons for using an elemental feed, a study has failed to show significant benefit over polymeric feeds.

In Crohn's disease the early studies used elemental feeds on the assumption that it was important to avoid potentially allergenic whole protein. Good results have now been shown in Crohn's disease using whole-protein feeds, but there have been some important discrepancies, with some whole-protein feeds producing poor results in terms of induction of remission. Since many of these patients are well nourished on starting treatment yet still respond well it is a reasonable assumption that in most cases enteral feeding is beneficial in Crohn's disease mainly because of the 'bowel rest,' (i.e. rest from fat or fibre) that it entails rather than because of its nutritional effect. Evidence is growing that the discrepancy between different polymeric enteral feeds may be because of their differing fat contents (see below).**A whole-protein feed should therefore usually be tried before resorting to an elemental feed.**

In **liver failure**, specialised feeds with a low content of aromatic amino acids (phenylalanine, tyrosine and tryptophan and low in methionine) and rich in branched-chain amino acids have been used in attempt to reverse the imbalance of plasma amino acids that is associated with encephalopathy. Evidence that these feeds produce a better outcome is unclear at present.

Most enteral feeds are available as 'standard' and 'high-nitrogen' feeds. Patients who are hypercatabolic as a result of burns or sepsis usually require the high-nitrogen feed, which contains up to 10 g nitrogen/litre and a non-protein

Polymeric (whole-protein) feeds are:

- As effective
- Less hyperosmolar
- More palatable
- Cheaper

▶ Enteral feeds in Crohn's disease

For patients with Crohn's disease or short bowel the enteral feed should have a very low content of long-chain triglycerides

calorie to nitrogen ratio of about 100 kcal/g nitrogen compared to the standard feed, which contains up to 7 g nitrogen/litre and a calorie/nitrogen ratio of about 130 kcal/g.

Calorie source

Most enteral feeds use glucose polymers as the main carbohydrate source and this generally proves satisfactory. In most feeds the fat content (a mixture of long-chain and medium-chain triglycerides) constitutes about 30% of the calorie content. This may cause problems in patients with a short intestine or with intestinal disease such as Crohn's disease. In these patients there is increasing evidence that feeds may be more successful if they contain a much lower fat content (e.g. 1% of calories) or if most of this fat is in the form of medium-chain triglycerides.

Vitamins and trace elements

Most commercial enteral feeds are nutritionally complete and contain adequate trace element and vitamin contents for several weeks' feeding.

Supplement or whole feed?

For patients with a short intestine or small bowel Crohn's disease one of the main aims of enteral feeding is usually to 'rest' the small intestine; in particular to avoid feeding with long-chain fat and, in patients with stricturing disease, to avoid fruit and vegetable fibre. In these patients the polymeric feed should be given as the only feed, but there can usually be free access to clear fluids and occasional tea or coffee providing that the milk intake is low.

When malnutrition is the main indication and there is no reason to suspect any intestinal abnormality then there is no reason why the enteral feed should not be used as a supplement to normal food providing that a careful measure is kept of dietary intake.

By which route?

Oral

Oral feeding should always be used if possible. The whole-protein feeds are much easier to make palatable than the amino acid-based feeds. Some of them are supplied ready flavoured, but they can also be flavoured with easily available flavourings such as 'Nesquick.' The feeds then have a similar taste and consistency to melted ice cream. They are probably easier to take if cooled in the refrigerator. Savoury tastes are difficult to achieve so the feeds are undeniably boring, but should not be unpleasant. In our experience about 75% of adult patients can manage these feeds orally.

Fine-bore tube feeding

Fine-bore tube feeding may be necessary either because the patient cannot tolerate the feed by mouth or because of swallowing difficulties due to mechanical or neurological problems. It is most important that a fine-bore tube is used as very severe oesophagitis causing stricturing can result from the use of standard nasogastric tubes for more than a few days.

Various designs of tubes are available. The presence of a weighted tip seems generally to give little advantage and the most commonly used tubes are wire-stiffened during insertion. They should be lubricated with a smear of lignocaine gel and passed slowly with the patient upright and taking intermittent sips of water. The position should be checked by chest X-ray, partly to ensure that the tube has passed into the stomach, but also to ensure that it has not looped back on itself. The wire should not be reinserted once it has been removed because of the risk of perforation.

In patients with gastroparesis (e.g. due to diabetes), it may be necessary to site the tube endoscopically to allow placement of the tip into the duodenum.

▶ For successful oral enteral feeding:

- Use a whole-protein feed
- Flavour with milk shake or 'Nesquick' flavouring
- Keep cooled in a refrigerator
- Make up fresh each day (unless ready prepared)
- Don't put the patient off by making disparaging remarks about the feed

Bolus feeding is associated with a greater risk of diarrhoea or aspiration and the feed should generally be given by continuous infusion using a peristaltic pump. Most of the feed can generally be given at night to allow the patient to disconnect during the day for free mobility.

About 2–2.5 litres of feed are usually given every 24 hours. Nasogastric aspiration should be performed every 2–3 hours for the first 24 hours, and feeding stopped if more than 100 ml of feed is aspirated. There is no advantage in starting with half-strength feeds. Absence of bowel sounds is not necessarily a contraindication to enteral feeding providing there is no marked abdominal or gastric distension.

DIARRHOEA

Diarrhoea occurs in up to 30% of patients. It is most commonly associated with broad-spectrum antibiotic therapy and is not an indication for half-strength feeding. Stool samples should be screened for pathogens including *Clostridium difficile* and loperamide may be useful. It should rarely be necessary to stop the enteral feeding.

Gastrostomy feeding

Percutaneous endoscopic gastrostomy is used increasingly in patients with swallowing problems, usually due to neurological disorders. A variety of techniques are described. The most widely used technique involves passing an endoscope into the stomach, which is then transilluminated through the anterior abdominal wall (**Fig 20.1**). A needle is then inserted through the abdominal wall at the point of transillumination and a wire passed through the needle into the stomach. The wire is then grasped by an endoscopic snare and pulled out through the mouth and used to guide the gastrostomy tube, which is pulled back down over the wire. The tube is kept in position by a soft plastic distendable plug, which can be deflated externally to allow removal of the tube at a later date without repeat endoscopy.

Complications are uncommon, but prophylactic antibiotics should be used because of the risk of local sepsis or leakage. As soon as the tube is satisfactorily sited feeding can begin.

INTRAVENOUS FEEDING

Indications

Patients should not be fed intravenously via a central line if:

- They are capable of being fed enterally.
- They are unlikely to require intravenous feeding for more than one week.

This is because of the considerable risks associated with central venous feeding.

▶ **Diarrhoea in enteral feeding:**

- Is usually related to antibiotic therapy
- Is not an indication for half-strength feeds
- Is less likely with continuous than bolus feeding

Composition of intravenous feed

For central line feeding there is increasing use of standardised feeding regimens given in three-litre bags, which are changed once daily. A typical feed contains 14 g nitrogen and 2100 kcal, of which 60% are given as carbohydrate and 40% as fat (usually an emulsion containing 50% long-chain and 50% medium-chain triglycerides). Trace elements and vitamins are included. Electrolytes are adjusted according to the requirements of the patient. Heparin, 1000 U/l is usually included. Insulin may also be included, although many units prefer to give it, as necessary, via a separate infusion so that it may be adjusted more flexibly.

By which route?

Central venous catheter placement

A central venous line is needed for prolonged intravenous feeding. The line should be placed via the subclavian or internal jugular vein with its tip in the superior vena cava (and not advanced into the right atrium).

The line should be placed by someone skilled at central venous puncture using scrupulous sterile technique and with the patient tipped head down to remove the risk of air embolism. The line is usually 'tunnelled' subcutaneously so that the point of entry through the skin is distant from the point of entry into the subclavian vein.

INITIAL COMPLICATIONS OF LINE INSERTION

Initial complications of line insertion include:

- Pneumothorax.
- Haemothorax due to puncture of the subclavian artery.
- Cardiac tamponade due to myocardial puncture.
- Chylothorax due to puncture of the thoracic duct (when catheters are inserted from the left side).
- Infusion of intravenous feed into the pleural cavity.

AVOIDANCE OF LINE SEPSIS

This is the most important aspect of intravenous feeding. Line sepsis can be rapidly fatal as a result of shock, adult respiratory distress syndrome and renal failure. At best the occurrence of line sepsis requires resiting of the catheter with its attendant risks and the fever and acute phase response that it generates usually delays the patient's re-

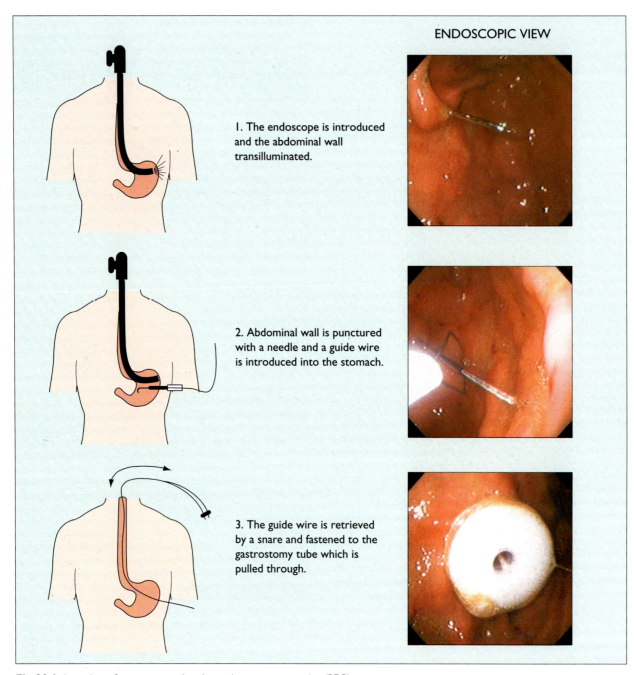

ENDOSCOPIC VIEW

1. The endoscope is introduced and the abdominal wall transilluminated.

2. Abdominal wall is punctured with a needle and a guide wire is introduced into the stomach.

3. The guide wire is retrieved by a snare and fastened to the gastrostomy tube which is pulled through.

Fig 20.1 Insertion of percutaneous/ endoscopic gastrostomy tube (PEG)..

covery by about a week. Sloppy care commonly results in line sepsis rates of up to 33%, whereas well-organised nutrition teams are able to achieve sepsis rates of less than 3%.

Most people are sufficiently aware of the need for sterility when the line is inserted, but seem unaware that infection is most commonly introduced when connections in the line are casually handled to allow use of the line for administration of intravenous drugs or for drawing off blood samples for tests. It cannot be overemphasised that the line should be used for feeding only. An alternative, which is increasingly common is the use of multilumen catheters with one lumen used strictly for feeding and the other lumens available for monitoring and administration of drugs and other fluids. This carries a theoretical risk of infection, but seems to be a reasonable compromise.

A dedicated nutrition team that includes specially-trained nursing staff and takes overall control of intravenous feeding has been shown to be the only practical way of achieving adherence to good practice guidelines and attaining a low sepsis rate.

▶ **Intravenous feeding: indications and contraindications**

> **Contraindications for central line intravenous feeding**
>
> - Patient suitable for enteral feeding
> - Unlikely to require intravenous feeding for more than one week
>
> **Indications for intravenous feeding**
>
> - Abdominal surgery
> - Intra-abdominal sepsis
> - Intestinal failure (ileus, obstruction, resection, fistula)

▶ **Measures to avoid line sepsis**

> - Scrupulous sterile technique for line insertion
> - Insertion site then covered with adhesive dressing, which is left unchanged unless damp.
> - Subcutaneous tunnelling of line (relatively unimportant)
> - Tight quality control over sterility of feeds
> - Good sterile technique for bag changing
> - Handling of catheter junctions always with sterile gloves
> - Chlorhexidine spray and cover junctions after handling
> - Use the line only for feeding

Peripheral line feeding

There has been increasing use of peripheral line feeding since it became realised that most patients do not require more than 2000 kcal/day unless markedly catabolic. This reduces the need for high-strength glucose solutions, which are particularly prone to causing thrombophlebitis. Lipid solutions seem to have some protective effect and peripheral line feeding using a 2000 kcal mixture that includes lipid can generally be infused through a peripheral vein catheter for 2–5 days before phlebitis develops. This means that this is probably the route of first choice when intravenous feeding is only likely to be needed for 10–14 days. Topical glyceryl trinitrate has been reported to reduce the rate of thrombophlebitis.

Monitoring

Blood glucose should be checked four times daily. Electrolytes, phosphate, blood gases and weight should be monitored daily, and liver function tests twice weekly.

Complications unrelated to central line

The commonest metabolic complications are hyper- and hypoglycaemia, hypophosphataemia and hypercalcaemia. With close monitoring and appropriate adjustment of therapy they do not usually cause major problems. Much greater problems used to be encountered when high strength glucose/ high insulin regimens were used.

Jaundice

Jaundice is the most significant non-line-related complication of intravenous feeding. It is usually due to intrahepatic cholestasis, which is in turn often multifactorial. It is not convincingly associated with any particular type of feed. Its incidence has been reported to be reduced by metronidazole and it is likely that sepsis-associated cholestasis is often involved. If sepsis can be excluded, drug jaundice should be considered and any possibly hepatotoxic drugs stopped if possible. Biliary sludge is thought commonly to contribute to the cholestasis and improvement has been reported with ursodeoxycholate therapy. If the jaundice persists intravenous feeding may have to be stopped, but an alternative is to move to intermittent (e.g. nocturnal feeding).

Feeding at home

The successful management of long-term home **parenteral nutrition** is highly specialised and should be managed by a nutrition unit with a particular interest. The patient or a close relative will need to be fully educated about the management of the line and avoidance of sepsis. Feeding can usually be confined mainly to the night to allow freedom during the day. There is increasing use of implantable ports, which are a cosmetic improvement, but will not necessarily diminish the risks of sepsis unless scrupulous care is maintained. Most patients tend to look after their lines extremely well and commonly go for very long periods without the need for line change.

Home enteral feeding can often be done without lines or pumps if the patient is able to take a whole-protein feed by mouth. If nocturnal fine-bore tube feeding is necessary then considerably more support and instruction is required. Advice should be given about avoidance of aspiration, in particular raising the head of the bed (by at least 20 cm) and regular visits by an experienced nutrition nurse should be arranged.

▶ **In jaundice associated with parenteral feeding suspect:**

> - Sepsis
> - Drugs
> - Biliary sludge

FURTHER READING

DiLorenzo J et al. Percutaneous endoscopic gastrostomy. What are the benefits, what are the risks? *Postgrad Med* 1992; **91**: 277–81.

Fernandez-Banares F et al. Enteral nutrition as primary therapy in Crohn's disease. *Gut* 1994; **35**(1 Suppl.): S55–9.

Gauderer MW. Gastrostomy techniques and devices. *Surg Clin North America* 1992; **72**: 1285–98.

Payne-James JJ, Silk DBA. Enteral and parenteral nutrition. In *Diseases of the Gut and Pancreas*, 2nd ed 1994. Eds Misiewicz, Pounder, Venables. pp. 1105–1135. Oxford, Blackwell.

Raouf A et al. Enteral feeding as sole therapy for Crohn's disease: A controlled trial of whole protein versus amino acid based feed and a case study of dietary challenge. *Gut* 1991; **32**: 702–7.

INDEX

NB The diagnosis, natural history and management of each condition are highlighted in italics

abdominal 218
ascites 213
gastrointestinal 73, 89–90
jaundice 193
Turcot's syndrome 262

U
Ulcerative colitis
ankylosing spondylitis 77
arthritis 77
bile duct carcinoma 77, 205
cancer screening 80–81, 134
in children 263, 264–265
colonic cancer 78, 80–81, 133–134
diagnosis 65–67
diarrhoea 76
diet 80
dilatation 78
dysplasia 80–81
episcleritis 77
extra-intestinal manifestations 77–78
fibromuscular strictures 81
natural history and management 76–81
pregnancy 80
proctitis 76
pseudopolyps 81, 134
pyoderma gangrenosum 77
rectal histology 66–67
rectal mucosa 65
sclerosing cholangitis 77
surgery 80
Ulcerative jejuno-ileitis 92
Ultrasound
gallbladder 6–8, 34
jaundice 185–186
pancreas 8, 35, 74
pelvic 41
transvaginal 41
Urea 237
Urine, acute retention 32
Ursodeoxycholic acid 27, 203, 205
Uveitis 81

V
Vagotomy 17
postoperative problems 49–50, 153–157
see also Gastric surgery
Varices
colon 128
oesophageal *see* Oesophageal varices
small bowel 128
Vasculitis 223
Vasopressin 126
Veno-occlusive disease 124

Venous hum 214
Venous thrombosis, mesenteric 40, 123–124
Verner–Morrison syndrome 70
Vipomas 70, 97
Vitamin B$_{12}$
deficiency 74–75, 96
supplements 92, 156
Vitamin deficiencies
primary biliary cirrhosis 202
stomas 285
Volvulus
abdominal pain 10
diagnosis 10
large bowel obstruction 55
natural history and management 56
Vomiting 143–146
bulimia 148–149
in children 250–254
diagnosis 143–146
natural history and management 146
Von Willebrand's disease 132

W
Waterbrash 17, 19, 159
Watson–Alagille syndrome 206
Weight loss 147–150
diagnosis and management 147–148
after gastric surgery 156
malignancy 147
metabolic disease 148
parenteral feeding 287
Weil's disease (leptospirosis) 183, 193
Wernicke's encephalopathy 199
Whipple's disease 72, 92
Whipple's procedure 208, 209
Whipworm 89
Wilson's disease
acute liver failure 227
in children 275
diagnosis 183
natural history and management 196–197
Wind 151–152

Y
Yellow fever 193
Yersinia enteritis 63, 87–88

Z
Zinc deficiency 72–73
Zollinger–Ellison syndrome
diagnosis 4, 153–154
diarrhoea 70
after gastric surgery 153–154
natural history and management 17–19